MW01626157

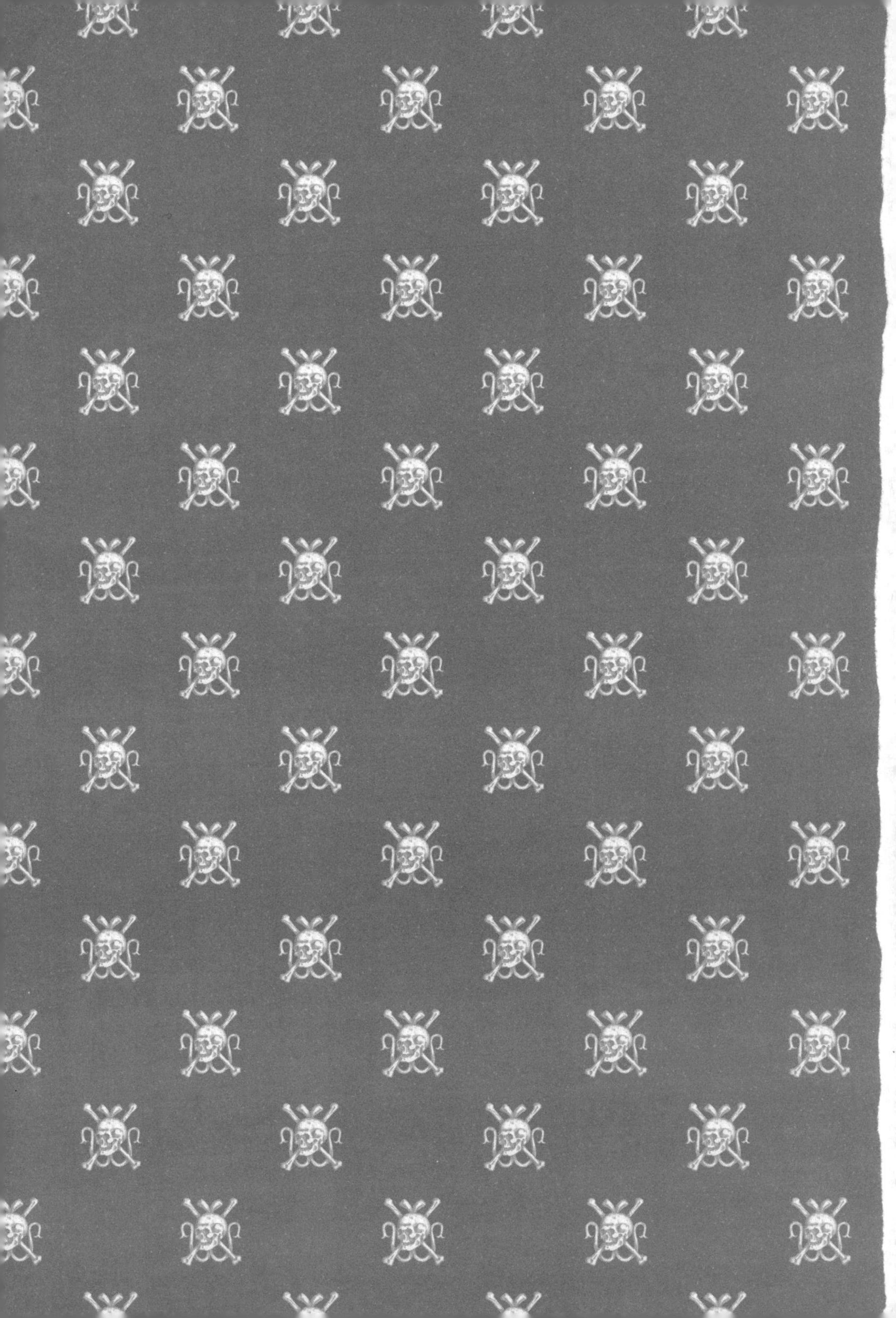

The MORBID ANATOMY *ANTHOLOGY*

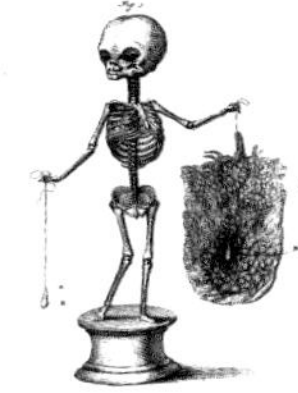

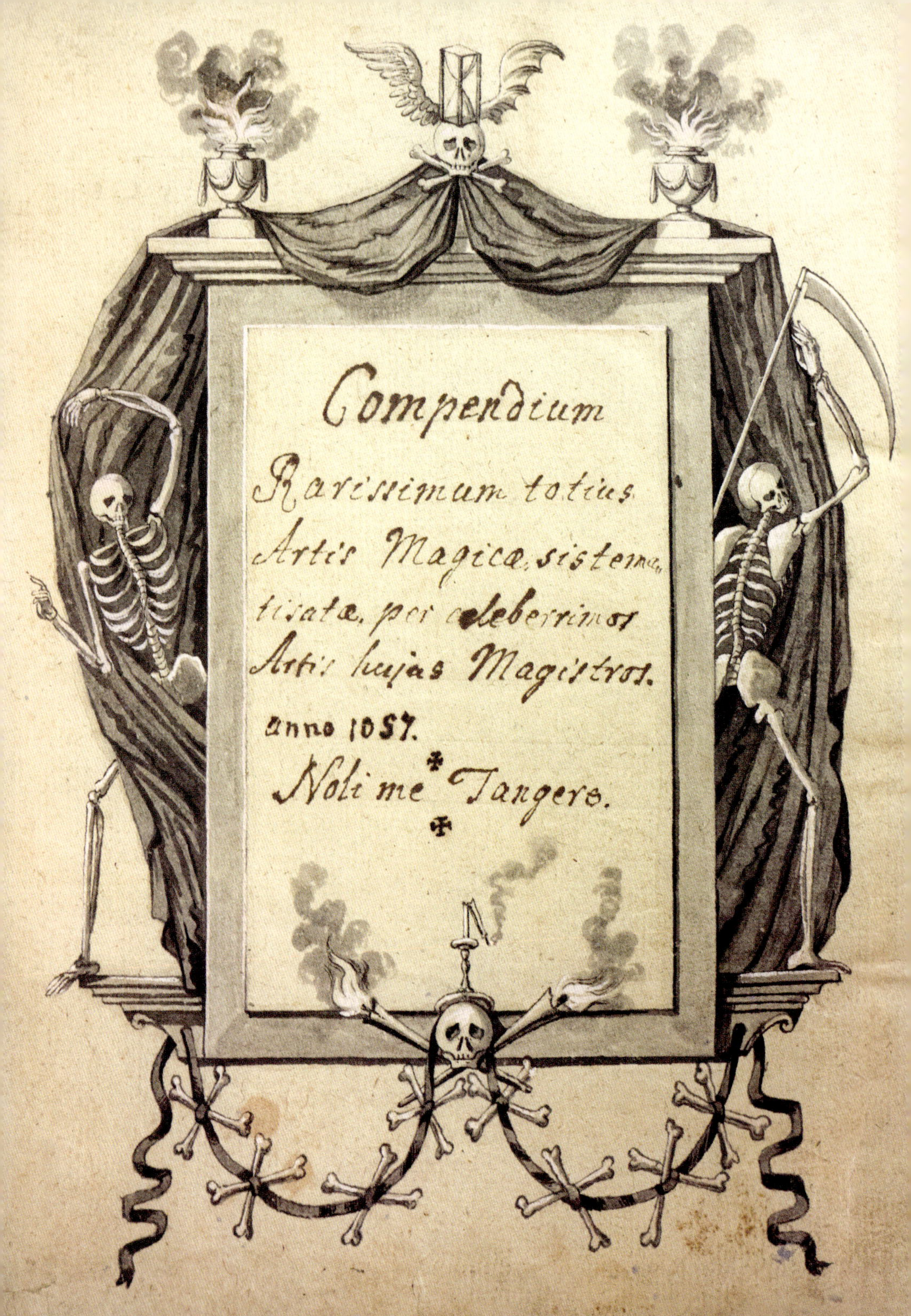
Compendium
Rarissimum totius
Artis Magicæ sistema-
tisatæ per celeberrimos
Artis hujus Magistros.
anno 1057.
Noli me Tangere.

The MORBID ANATOMY *ANTHOLOGY*

edited by
JOANNA EBENSTEIN
and COLIN DICKEY

The Morbid Anatomy Anthology
Edited by Joanna Ebenstein and Colin Dickey

Morbid Anatomy Press
Brooklyn, New York
www.morbidanatomymuseum.org

ISBN: 978-0-9893943-0-7

Second Edition, printed 2015.

Art direction, design and production by Joanna Ebenstein, Morbid Anatomy.

Cover image: Plate from Beach, W.; *An Improved System of Midwifery: Adapted to the Reformed Practice of Medicine: Illustrated by Numerous Plates, to Which Is Annexed, a Compendium of the Treatment of Female and Infantile Diseases, with Remarks on Physiological and Moral Elevation*. New York: Scribner, 1851; Courtesy of The National Library of Medicine.

Endpaper image: From a tomb at Pisa's Camposanto Monumentale, kindly redrawn by GF Newland.

Image on following spread: Hand-painted plate from *Compendium rarissimum totius Artis Magicae sistematisatae per celeberrimos Artis hujus Magistros...* c.1775; Courtesy of the Wellcome Library, London.

Printed in China

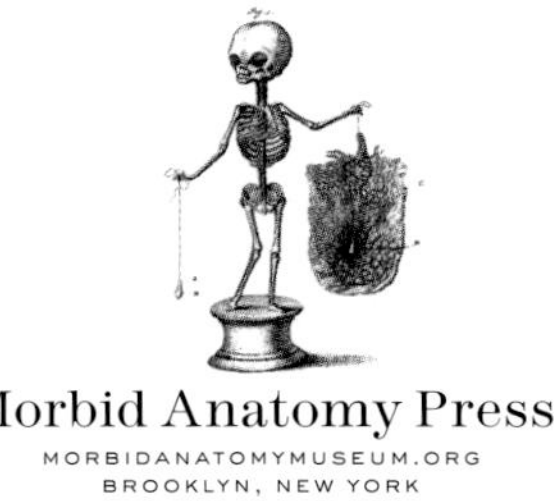

Morbid Anatomy Press
MORBIDANATOMYMUSEUM.ORG
BROOKLYN, NEW YORK

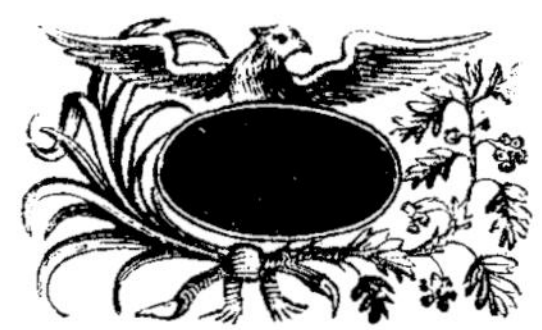

TABLE OF

CONTENTS

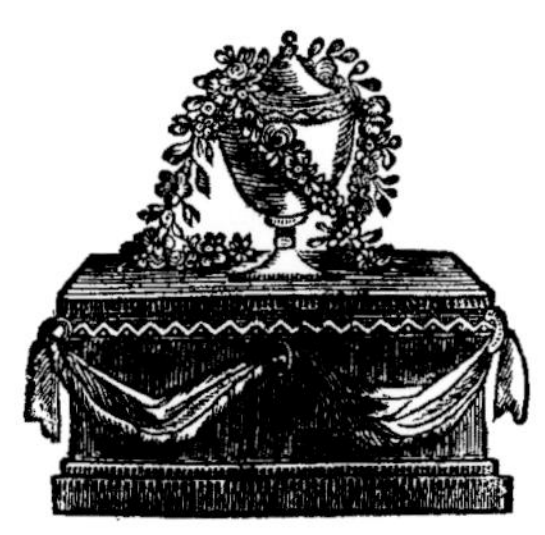

[PART II]

[PART III]

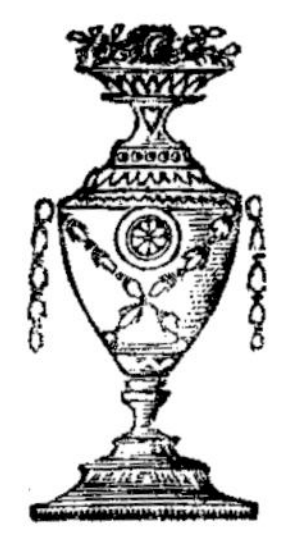

The

MORBID ANATOMY *ANTHOLOGY*

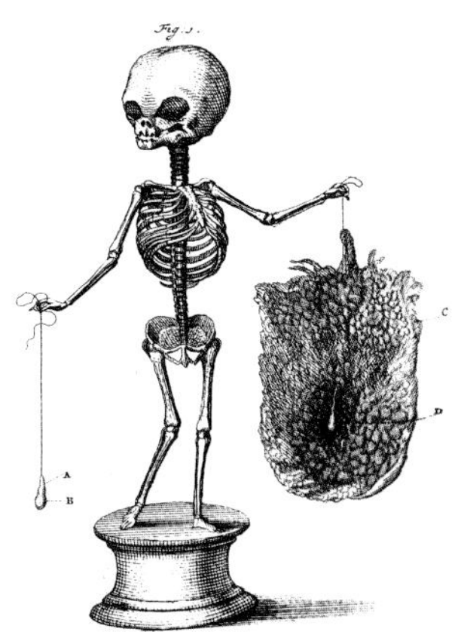

FOREWORD

JOANNA EBENSTEIN

I FOUNDED MORBID ANATOMY IN 2007 AS A BLOG, A SATELLITE project of an exhibition I was working on: "Anatomical Theatre: The Body, Disease and Death in Medical Museums of The Western World", shown at the Alabama Museum of the Health Sciences. To collect material for this exhibition, I embarked on a one-month "pilgrimage" in search of photographic material for this survey of the uncanny artifacts housed in the great medical museums of Europe and the United States. I traveled from country to country with only a backpack and my camera. My goal with the exhibition was to bring the art and history of medical museums to a wider audience, and to reframe their artifacts as artistic and cultural objects, rather than simply antiquated science.

I found myself fascinated by the ways in which context could create meaning; the ways the human body could become, in different situations (or sometimes all at once!) an exhortation to contemplate the transience of life, an object of desire, a word in a curatorial essay. I was drawn by the strange alchemy that transformed an object in a museum into a specimen, and by the ways in which all forms of human knowledge production—and none more than science—could be seen as autobiographical, revealing the very human need to find stories and meaning. I was especially interested by the way that science so often sublimates very human

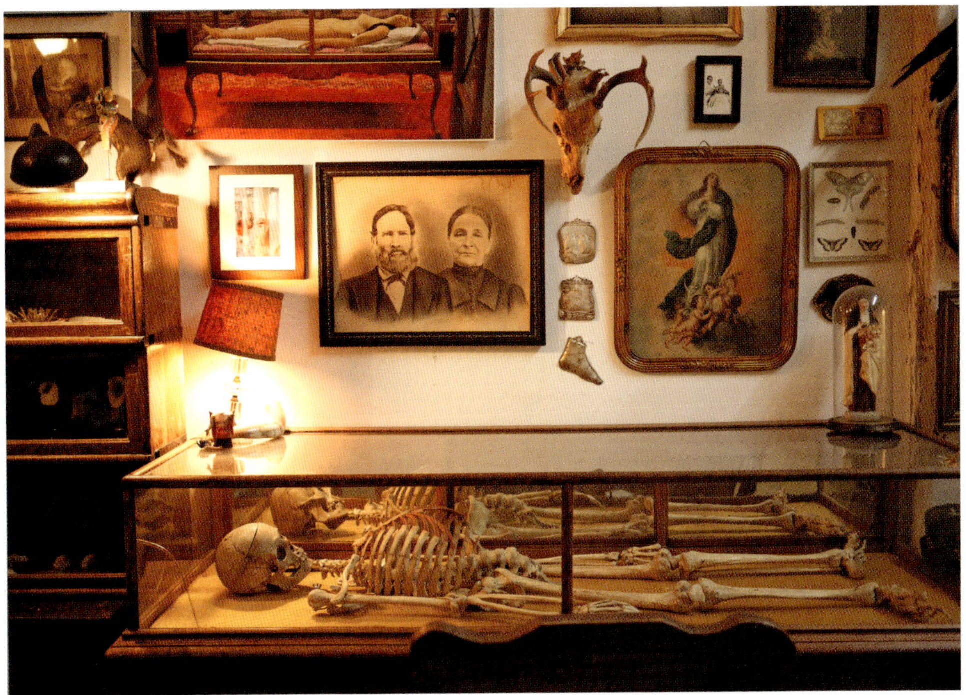

The Morbid Anatomy Library in Brooklyn, New York. Photo by the author.

drives such as the desire to collect, the impulse to order, and sexual curiosity.

When I returned from this trip, I was overwhelmed by the volume of material I had collected. Thousands of photos, scores of links to online exhibitions and museum collections, piles of books and articles from the very kind and patient curators who encouraged my interest with Xeroxed articles and book suggestions. When I closed my eyes at night, I saw rows of babies in jars.

The Morbid Anatomy blog was born from an impetus to organize this material for use in my own work. It never occurred to me that it would be of interest to anyone else. I simply created the blog that I would want to read. The name was drawn from the medical world, "Morbid Anatomy" being the term for the study of diseased organs or tissues. To me, the phrase also operated as a kind of medical double entendre, with which to problematize ideas of what constituted the morbid. Why, I wanted to ask, was it deemed morbid to be interested in death? Death, after all, is the greatest mystery of human life, and everyone who ever has lived has died or will die, and so will I. How could being concerned with such an important thing be seen as morbid?

With a background in intellectual and art history, I had long been intrigued by the ways in which an interest in death had been expressed in other times and cultures. Memento mori, the incorruptible saints in Catholic churches, post-mortem photography, Santa Muerte, anthropomorphic taxidermy, phantasmagoria, ossuaries, mummies on display, the fetal skeleton tableaux of Frederik Ruysch, the Anatomical Venuses of Clemente Susini... Clearly death has not always been deemed an inappropriate subject for art and contemplation. How had death become strange to us? How could looking at the past teach us something about the cultural relativity of our own views? Was I morbid, or was it, in fact, morbid to ignore death, to refuse to grapple with its meaning and implications?

On my blog Morbid Anatomy, I have excavated the history and material culture of death on a near daily basis since its inception in 2007. To my surprise, this decidedly niche material attracted a readership right from the start. Over the past six years, interest in this material has grown and broadened in ways that I simply would not have believed when I began this project. Morbid Anatomy—which was really my own self-indulgent project in which I allowed myself publicly to obsess over my lifelong fascinations—has grown not only in readership but also in scope.

The greater Morbid Anatomy project has now expanded considerably beyond the blog to include the Morbid Anatomy

Library, my own research library and collection of curiosities open to the public; the forthcoming Morbid Anatomy Museum, also in Brooklyn, New York; the Morbid Anatomy Press, publisher of the book you hold now in your hands; and "Morbid Anatomy Presents", a series of lectures and workshops held around the world. Since our first lecture in 2009, the series has drawn representatives from my favorite museums, such as Mütter Museum, The Vrolik, The Hunterian and The Wellcome Collection; favorite scholars such as Mel Gordon (author of *Voluptuous Panic: The Erotic World of Weimar Berlin*), Stephen T. Asma (author of *Stuffed Animals and Pickled Heads: The Culture and Evolution of Natural History Museums*) and Mark Dery (author of *The Pyrotechnic Insanitarium*) and artists who teach the arcane skills I had always wanted to learn, such as anthropomorphic taxidermy (Susan Jeiven), Victorian hair work (Karen Bachmann), and wax moulage making (Eleanor Crook, Sigrid Sarda). We also added two scholars-in-residence to work with the holdings of the Morbid Anatomy Library: Evan Michelson of Science Channel's hit television show *Oddities* and researcher Salvador Olguín, both of whom wrote pieces for this volume.

It was through Morbid Anatomy Presents that I met Colin Dickey, the co-editor of this volume. I had heard about his book *Cranioklepty* and invited him to give a lecture at the Morbid Anatomy Library. As fate would have it, on the night of his reading, a nearby venue was hosting their annual taxidermy contest and so, after Colin's (standing room only) lecture, the intrepid among us, including Colin and his wife Nicole, headed over there, where a number of Morbid Anatomy regulars were competing. This evening cemented our friendship, and Colin became one of our most frequent lecturers.

On one of Colin's visits to New York, he mentioned what a shame it was that the great body of work which constituted the Morbid Anatomy Presents series was so ephemeral in nature. Had I never thought of doing a book which would immortalize some of the lectures? Indeed I had—as a book collector and book designer who has spent all my professional life in publishing, how could I not? I simply had no idea how to go about making it happen. Colin presented an intelligent, comprehensive plan. "Great," I said, "let's do it!" And voilà! Here is the book you hold in your hands.

In the following pages, you will find a variety of previously unpublished pieces. When I look at the list of contributors and read the pieces in succession, I am delighted, amazed and truly humbled. One of my principal aims with the greater Morbid Anatomy Project was to make knowledge accessible, to create a space where everyone could share ideas, to exhume histories that are largely unacknowledged in polite society with intelligence, dignity and wit. I hope you will agree that this book stays true to that original spirit.

INTRODUCTION

JOANNA EBENSTEIN & COLIN DICKEY

FOR SEVERAL YEARS NOW, THE MORBID ANATOMY LIBRARY HAS hosted dozens of scholars, museologists, artists, writers and enthusiasts from around the world who have lectured, presented, and conducted workshops on a wide range of subjects at our humble Brooklyn, New York, space. This book started as a means to document that conversation, and bring it to a wider audience beyond Brooklyn.

Many of these pieces in this book had their origins in events at Observatory, including Daniel K. Smith's history of anthropodermic bibliopegy (books bound in human skin), which began as a talk he gave in February 2012. Likewise, Elizabeth L. Bradley's essay on human zoos was originally delivered as part of the Congress for Curious People, a two-day conference organized jointly by the Morbid Anatomy Library and the Coney Island Museum. Other pieces here are original contributions written specifically for this book by longtime visitors, oftentime speakers, and friends of the Morbid Anatomy Library. With essays such as these, as well as Amber Maykut's documentation of Sue Jeivens' anthropomorphic mouse taxidermy workshop held at the library, we hope that this book will continue to broaden the conversation that began in New York over four years ago.

From the start, the Morbid Anatomy Library has been home to a wide range of disciplines, approaches, and methods of inquiry.

In the same spirit, this book brings together writers and artists from a variety of disciplines and approaches. We have made no attempt with this book to be exhaustive or all-inclusive, and while it represents some of the absolute best examples of what Morbid Anatomy is known for, it can be no more than a cross-section of an ongoing and diverse conversation.

The makeup of the volume which follows expresses this mix. All of the thinkers in the following pages—from professional writers to autodidacts—pull the threads of the past to weave new stories about the present, finding a way to bring to light the things that have fallen through the cracks of good taste or the temper of the time. As we read these pieces, we were intrigued by the ways in which traditional methods of scholarship can be used in personal ways, making outsider scholars out of all of us. We were also interested in the unexpected themes that crop up again and again: themes such as exhumed histories; nostalgia (time travel); the crisis of knowing; the liminal; the attraction but impossibility of expressing the inexpressible or unseeable; the *n*.

In his piece on Giulio Camillo's utterly unknowable Renaissance memory theater, Mel Gordon exemplifies this spirit of inquiry when he writes, "true knowledge is always hidden, veiled in corporal disguise, a shifting constellation of arresting ciphers." Add to this Amy Herzog's insight that we long "to recognize the self through an encounter with the unknown," and Salvador Olguín's attempt to put into words the elusive paradox of lady death in Mexico: "she's as dark as night, but also as clear as the light of disillusionment." These and the other essays in this volume express a relentless curiosity, and something of the elusive essence of the powerful longings that drive the writers in the pages that follow—if not all writers—to know (and express) the unknowable, be it history or invisible knowledge; to use the tools at our disposal; to plumb the depths of human psychology; to evoke (if not directly express) the unknowable; and to capture the tantalizingly impossible but siren-like draw of the longing to crawl into an always unknowable past with words, pictures, scholarship, projection, art and imagination.

In these pages you'll find a loose overlapping constellation of inquiries. The anatomist Frederik Ruysch, known for his innovative means of preserving tissue and body parts, as well as his macabre tableaux involving children's skeletons, appears in several essays here, including Carl Schoonover's short, poetic take on *dura mater*, and Dániel Margócsy's scholarly framing of Ruysch within the Early Modern context. Early self-made museologists like Walter Potter and Pierre Spitzner reappear throughout as well, and essays by Kate Forde, Amy Herzog, and Pat Morris all question in various ways what it means to collect and display.

Both Caitlin Doughty and Stephen T. Asma approach the politics of Medieval reproduction, albeit in radically different ways, while Chiara Ambrosio and Paul Koudounaris explore the nexus between religion and death in, respectively, Southern Peru and Naples, Italy. Meanwhile, Zoe Beloff's and Elizabeth L. Bradley's essays offer two very different ways in which the living human can be put on display for various ends.

In addition to the way the topics of these pieces often resonate with one another in unexpected ways, this book also offers a wide range of differing but complementary methodologies. Alongside essays that adopt a more traditional scholarly mode are first person meditations and reflections on the body and death—everything from art collector Richard Harris discussing the pieces in his collection, to Ross MacFarlane's detailed analysis of one figure in particular, from Evan Michelson's first person account of a trip to the Palermo catacombs, to Simon Chaplin's tracing of the etymology of the word "ottamy" and the strange history hidden therein.

John Troyer's end-of-life planning worksheet, for example, represents one very practical take on how we face death, while Shannon Taggart's photographs of Spiritualist communities pre-sent a completely different approach to our dialogue with the dead. Mark Dery's essay on postmortem photography, in turn, offers yet another, very different, approach to picturing the dead.

Throughout, our goal was to gather together a variety of voices. Ronni Thomas' essay on nineteenth century diableries (3D stereograms of Hell) may, along with Vadim Kosmos' history of death-themed cabarets, offer a lighter side to how we conceptualize death, the decaying body, and the afterlife, but in doing so help to fill in a complicated picture in which reverence must be complemented with laughter, in which grief and joy commingle.

In many ways, David Pescovitz's opening essay represents a frame for the whole book: we envisioned this as a Wonder Cabinet, a Cabinet of Curiosity. As Pescovitz writes, "the world is filled with wonder, and curiosity is something to be cultivated at every opportunity." It is in the spirit of persistent inquiry, and of relentless curiosity, that this book was put together.

PART I

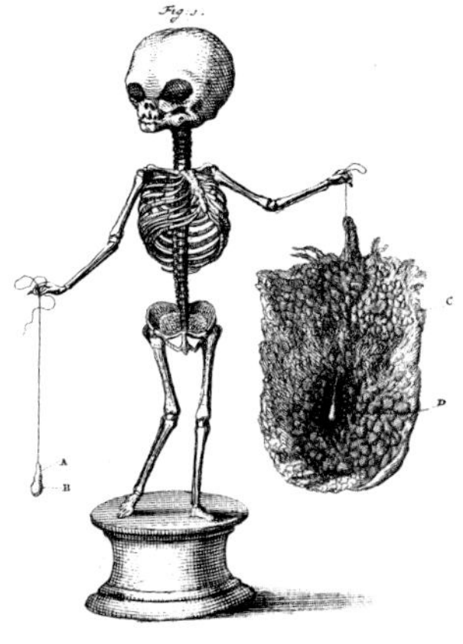

WHAT A WONDERFUL WORLD

DAVID PESCOVITZ

SEVERAL YEARS AGO, I BECAME FASCINATED WITH CABINETS OF curiosity. The Renaissance predecessor to modern day museums, these cabinets, sometimes entire rooms, were filled with a mishmash of objects, both natural and artificial, that embodied the wonder of the world. (The German term for these collections, *wunderkammer*, literally means "chamber of wonders.") Inside, you might find a mummy's hand, a "unicorn's horn," exotic seashells from distant lands, odd insects pinned and cataloged, and possibly even a two-headed lizard in a jar of formaldehyde. As Tradescant the Elder, one of the most notable cabinet keepers in history, requested in a letter to the Secretary of the English Navy in 1625, this was a quest for "Any thing that is strang."

Inspired by this celebration of science, art, and the strang(e), I found an old Chinese tea cabinet at a flea market and began to build my own *wunderkammer*. I quickly filled the shelves with items of the type I thought were "supposed" to be in any *wunderkammer* worth its weight in weirdness—antique medical instruments, a Balinese shadow puppet, a snake stuffed in a perpetual strike. Things became more interesting once the collection process became more organic and I added items that genuinely spoke to my personal sense of the curious: a one-to-one millionth scale model of Frank Lloyd Wright's Fallingwater, fabricated by engineers Ken Goldberg and

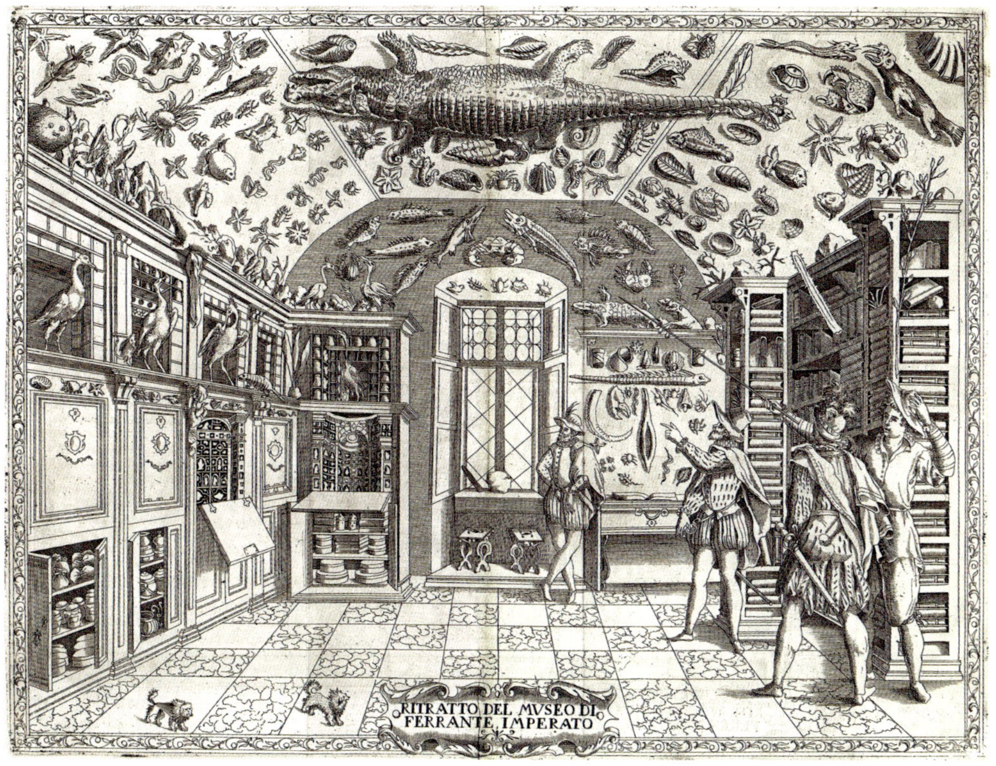

Cabinet of Curiosities, Imperato, Ferrante. Dell'historia naturale. *Napoli: C. Vitale, 1599.*

Karl Böhringer using techniques borrowed from microscale manufacturing; a primitive eye-gouging weapon from Rarotonga; a Houdini automaton's autograph; a resin model of a telerobotic insect outfitted with solar cells for wings.

This small cabinet in the corner of my office serves as a constant reminder for me that the world is filled with wonder, and that curiosity is something to be cultivated at every opportunity. Indeed, we're at our best when we're curious. And the beauty of curiosity is that we're all naturals. Curiosity is how babies learn. In fact, sparking someone's curiosity, at any age, seems to be perfect pedagogy. And, as the professor says in *The Day The Earth Stood Still*, "It isn't faith that makes good science... It's curiosity."

Now, I wouldn't dare suggest that there's a Renaissance revival afoot, but I'm optimistic that the pendulum is swinging at least slightly back toward the heyday of natural history, citizen science, backyard astronomy, and other spirited intellectual pursuits. Several recent museum exhibitions have explored the cabinet of curiosity as an organizational principle, including one dedicated to the appropriately odd juxtaposition of art and cryptozoology. The *wunderkammer* aesthetic has even bubbled up into popular consciousness.

Many blogs, including the one I co-edit, Boing Boing, have been described as virtual cabinets of curiosity—storehouses of unusual links, odd memes, fringe culture, and weird news. Nearly every major city has at least one carefully curated "Olde Curiosity Shoppe" selling strange *objets d'art* and natural oddities packaged as Victorian chic. In fact, I was recently struck by the obviously *wunderkammer*-inspired display of mounted insects and red coral on sale at a mainstream home decor store in the mall. And in the ultimate evidence of a trend, "reality" TV has put its distorted lens on the subject with the show *Oddities*.

Underground or prime time though, I'm heartened by this appreciation of curiosity that, unbridled, is also fueling today's passionate DIY movement. A growing number of ingenious individuals are fashioning robots in their garages, hacking together open-source DNA sequencers, and building backyard weather balloons. On one hand, these makers are dissatisfied with off-the-shelf products. On a deeper level though, they're driven by a daring inquisitiveness about what lies "under the hood" of today's technology, how they can better what they buy (or build it from scratch), and what they can learn along the way. For these makers—in the tradition of crafters, tinkers, scientists, engineers, artisans, and hot rodders who came before—the process is the product.

I'm optimistic that in the coming few years, the DIY movement will reach not only widespread awareness but widespread participation. I'm optimistic that smart companies, instead of criminalizing hackers, will *encourage* these user-innovators and solicit their feedback to design better products. I'm optimistic that science education in the United States can be saved if students are given the opportunity to learn by doing, not just by reading about what someone else has done.

When I watch a screwdriver-wielding maker eagerly voiding another warranty, I see a spark of the same childlike curiosity that fills a baby's eyes as he first explores his world, optimistic that something wonderful lies ahead.

[An earlier version of this essay appeared as a response to the EDGE.org Annual Question of 2007, "What Are you Optimistic About?," and in a book of the same name.]

GIULIO CAMILLO

Renaissance Scholar, Con Man, & Father of the Kabbalistic Theater

MEL GORDON

AMONG THE STRANGE MIX OF VISIONARY AND UTOPIAN PHILosophers, eye-fluttering mystics, technological soothsayers, and primitive science-fantasy writers of the Renaissance, few measure up—in notoriety and stunning brilliance—to the Tuscan scholar and Kabbalistic inventor Giulio Camillo (1480–1544). A contemporary of Leonardo da Vinci and Nostradamus, Camillo was said to have built a "wooden contraption" for the King of France that accurately prefigured cybervision, virtual-reality entertainments, and computer data-processing. In his final treatise, *L'Idea del Theatro*, Camillo claimed that even a short visit to his "Theater-Machine" would endow the spectator with all the ineffable and hidden knowledge of the ages.

How Camillo's theater actually functioned and what its hermeneutic purpose was has been the subject of an enduring debate for nearly five hundred years. Questions concerning the mysterious theater's intricate design and shape, even its physical whereabouts, have haunted Renaissance historians and fellow aestheticians since its rumored disappearance in the late 1540s. So secretive was Camillo's experiment that many in his lifetime doubted its very existence; yet

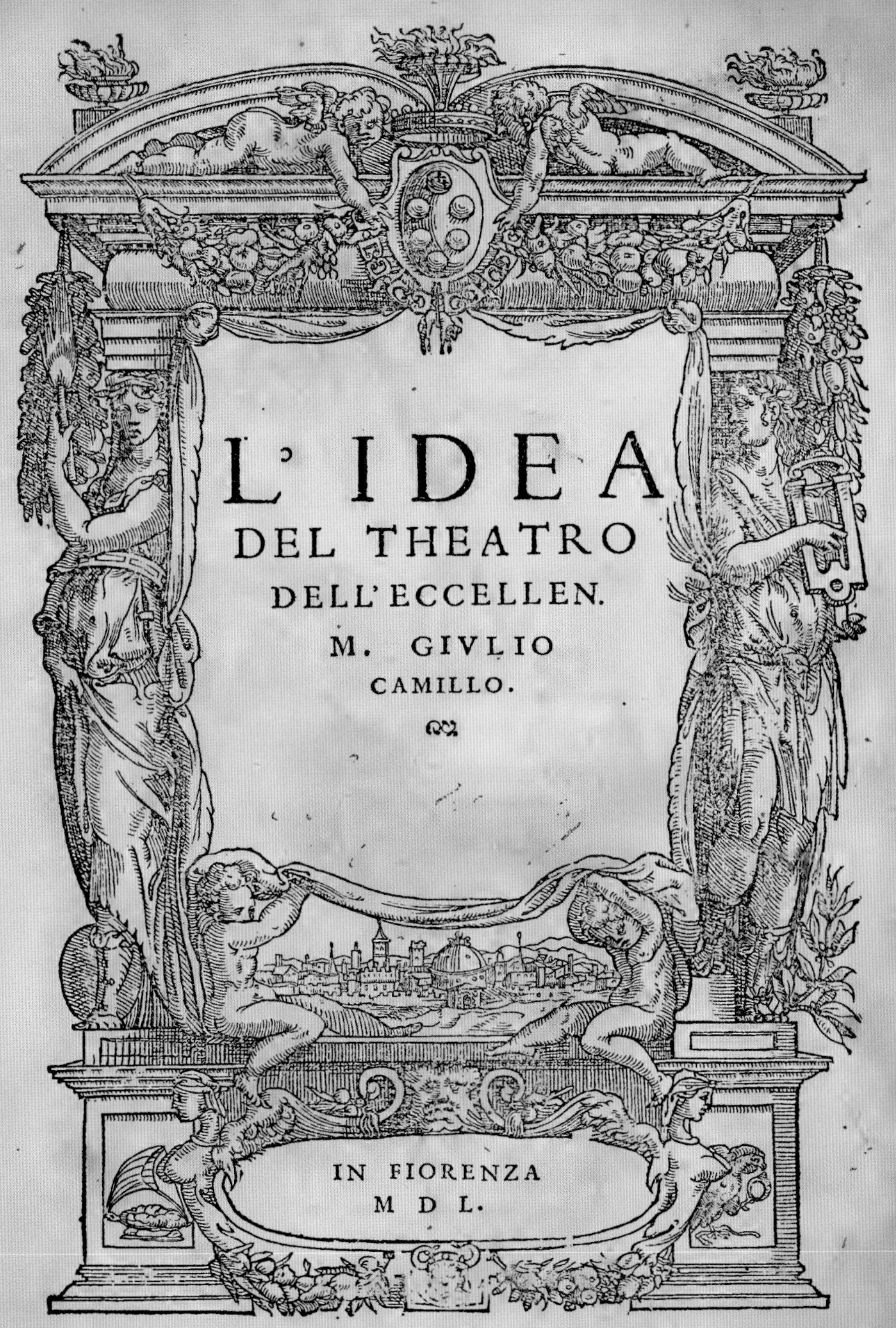
L'IDEA
DEL THEATRO
DELL'ECCELLEN.
M. GIVLIO
CAMILLO.
IN FIORENZA
M D L.

Image previous page: Title page from Camillo, Giulio, and Lodovico Domenichi. L'Idea Del Theatro Dell'Eccelen. M. Givlio Camillo. *Fiorenza: Torrentino, 1550.*

sixteenth-century diary entries and personal letters from French and Italian courtiers confirm its corporeal reality and mental efficacy. One former skeptic enthused that it was more fantastic, more profound than any of the seven wonders of the ancient world.

Within a few months of the master's death in 1544, a bizarre cottage industry devoted to *Camilliana* burst across Western Europe. Bickering teams of Latin scholars and assorted literary detectives traced Camillo's steps and searched private archives for precious clues that might reveal one more detail about the "divine project." Like mad itinerant priests of some lost and fragmenting religion, they issued dozens of tantalizing tracts and articles—each a contradiction of the previous discovery. But after the course of two or three generations, the manic sleuthing for that architectural elixir of sacred knowledge cooled and then expired as speculative sixteenth-century science and art slowly passed into more refined, neo-Aristotelian hands. Certainly by the 1740s, when the first encyclopedic theater chronologies were being assembled in Paris, Camillo's amphitheater and theoretical writings were long forgotten. (And naturally today no comprehensive theater history as much as lists this theatrical cyber-temple of Renaissance Europe.)

International interest in Camillo revived during the 1960s with the publication of Francis Yates' *The Art of Memory.* A highly respected Medieval scholar, Yates declared that *L'Idea del Theatro* might have been the inspiration for the first Elizabethan ring-shaped theaters. According to Yates, Camillo's imagistic enterprise represented a transitional moment between the medieval "art of memory"—an archaic and quasi-scientific technique that trained academicians in the internal formalization and precise recollection of Latin rhetoric for clerical and scholarly oration—and the dissemination of national sentiment in the newly constructed arena of popular British theater. In short, the seeds of the heroic Shakespearean age were sown somewhere in the royal back lots of François I's Paris.

Into the twenty-first century, conjecture and speculation about Camillo continues. In 1997, a three-day conference in Rome, entitled "Giulio Camillo and His Virtual World," offered fifteen presentations and panel discussions. (Currently, the listing "Giulio Camillo" or "memory theater" calls up some seventy spooky websites.) It is as if the Svengali progenitor of cyberspace is still signaling to us from some not-very-distant, pre-electronic past.

What Do We Really Know about Giulio Camillo?

Giulio Camillo was born in 1480 in a village northeast of Venice, nine years before Pico della Mirandola published his Kabbalistic treatise, *Heptaplus*. He studied philosophy and jurisprudence at the University of Padua and, beginning in 1521, held a chair in Dialectics at the University of Bologna. Some scholars believe that Camillo also taught local students at his own private academy in San Vito. Although it is unlikely Camillo married, he had a daughter, Cornelia, who with her husband, Giuseppe Maetano, and former pupils from San Vito, later assisted him in the construction of the first "Ideal Theater."

By 1529, both Camillo and his secretive theater project provided Venice's intellectual circles with rich material for personal invective about his pursuit of young women and other illicit activities. In addition, Camillo's corpulent size and habit of stuttering before unfamiliar audiences made him a model subject for relentless student parody at the university.

Despite all of this, Camillo soon came to the attention of King François I. A devotee of Kabbalistic and occult studies and supreme patron of Renaissance artists, particularly Italian architects, François I heard about Camillo's curious enterprise from Lazare de Baïf, the French Ambassador to Venice. (Besides granting him praise for his military's vacuous conquests, French history traditionally celebrates François' attachment to gold-digging mistresses and haute cuisine as the figure of the First Modern Frenchman.) In the spring of 1530, François formally invited Camillo to Paris. With an entourage of Count Claudio Rangone (soon to be a cardinal) and the pan-European courtier Girolamo Muzio, Camillo surfaced immediately at the French court. To the astonishment of Muzio, Camillo privately demonstrated a mnemonic device for Rangone that assisted the count in rote memorization—through graphic/visual induction—of several complicated Latin and Italian poems.

Camillo's first meeting with the king, according to Muzio, was even more wondrous. And at its conclusion, an intrigued François awarded Camillo six hundred scudi (or five hundred gold ducats)—with the promise of another twelve hundred scudi—for the realization of the magical amphitheater. The enormous down payment was coupled with the unusual proviso that Camillo never divulge or publish any "secrets of his method." Well over six months passed before Camillo returned to Bologna in the winter of 1531. Upon his return, he possessed substantial funding and the indispensable services of Muzio as loyal retainer and official secretary.

Exactly what titillated, excited, or amazed François during Camillo's initial presentation is unclear. Mystified French court sources prattled for decades that Camillo unveiled a table-sized machine that promised to school their linguistically-challenged sovereign in the ancient enigmas of Latin grammar. This would account for Camillo's earlier sessions in mental legerdemain with Rangone that shocked Muzio, as well as the generous and impulsive response of a dyslexic and parsimonious monarch. Most Italian scholars believed Camillo successfully revealed the first physical manqué of the Ideal Theater to the king, or at least spoke about its construction and internal machinations. This theory assumes that Camillo's theater project was already in a final state of completion, or that the famously inept professor suddenly possessed heightened powers of persuasion and effective showmanship. (Neither of these theories is consistent with the twisted history of the project or Camillo's legendary introverted disposition.)

From March to September 1532, Camillo domiciled in Bologna and Venice, where he recuperated from a serious knee injury. It was during this period that the first hard information on the theater project materialized. It came by way of Viglius Zuichemus, an Italian disciple of Erasmus, the radical Humanist theologian, who regularly wrote his teacher about the political scuttlebutt and curious activities in pre-Lenten Venice. Safely hidden away from Inquisition edicts in Swiss exile, Erasmus read Viglius' March 1532 letter with great skepticism. His otherwise rational student enthused over an inventor known as Giulio Camillo, who was said to have created an amphitheater filled with hanging papers, figurines (or human figures) and images arranged within "boxes" through "stupendous labor and divine skill." Even local Humanists ("Ciceronians") claimed that a single exposure to Camillo's theatrical display enveloped the spectator with the superhuman ability "to discourse on any subject no less fluently than Cicero." At first, Viglius passed off these hothouse testimonials as "fables" or Levantine exaggeration, but a passing inquiry with the reputable Humanist philosopher Bapista Egnatio sparked serious and nagging doubts. Bapista had actually inspected Camillo's theater: he told Viglius it was still more marvelous in the viewing than its eager promoters claimed.

In early June 1532, Viglius was ushered into the theater by Camillo himself. Expecting a mere artistic or intellectual novelty, Viglius instead was thoroughly awe-struck by the beauty and profundity of the scenic environment. He wrote to Erasmus that the theater was a "miracle... It depicts in fact everything that the human mind has conceived and what we cannot see with our physical eyes—but is secreted away inside the human soul—except through special signs." According to Viglius, the theater was constructed from wood and filled with so many individual images, three-dimensional ornaments, and scraps of information that Viglius expounded that no single author in a lifetime could amass them all in a literary opus. Yet, lest he seemed too nonplussed or insufficiently critical, Viglius also commented on Camillo's poor command of Latin and stammering delivery in his native Italian. Moreover, a "religious frenzy" sometimes swept over the "Master Architect" as he began to illustrate aspects of the theater's technical apparatus.

Ignoring François' summons for over one year, Camillo eventually returned to Paris in 1534. Like their Venetian counterparts, French intellectuals constantly ridiculed Camillo as a raving charlatan and gossiped about his cerebral pretensions and outsized personality. One story making the rounds was certainly true: During an outing with French aristocrats, various Italian hangers-on, and the Cardinal of Lorraine, a wild lion escaped from the royal compound and charged Camillo's group. While the others scrambled to safety, the obese and nearly immobile Camillo found himself the sole and stationary target of the enraged quadruped. But instead of pouncing on the hapless Tuscan, the lion circled him gamely, lay down at his feet and then began to caress Camillo's hands with its tongue. The solar beast and the solar man bonded.

The theater of Giulio Camillo was built somewhere in Paris between 1534 and 1537. (Gilbert Cousin, another spy for Erasmus, confirmed its Paris existence in a historical memoir written in 1558.) But after an inaugural presentation in 1537, Camillo complained in a letter to the Italian poet Pietro Aretino that François reneged on the project's full funding. Camillo's lament appears to imply that the long-heralded Theater-Machine was only partially constructed and therefore did not fulfill the regal expectations of the warring monarch and his coterie of specialists. Unsaid or unknown to Camillo was the severe financial crisis affecting the greatly over-extended French Empire. François' vast treasury was much depleted. Following in the footsteps of other disappointed Italian artists, like Michaelanglo and Benvenuto Cellini, Camillo returned to his homeland.

True to his word, the ailing and depressed Camillo kept the "secret of his method" for several years. During that difficult period, scholars from all nations naturally impugned the veracity of those who claimed to have witnessed the "miracle." Counter-*Camilliano* was growing.

Finally in October 1543, Muzio arranged a formal audience in Milan with the Marchese del Vasto, one of the nastiest and most Machiavellian characters of his age. (The Spanish-born tyrant was widely known for his extreme greed, cowardly behavior in battle, sadism, and general perfidy, including the assassination of François' envoy to Portugal.) This arch-enemy of France (and rival-collector of itinerant Italian artists) corresponded with Muzio concerning the Ideal Theater, "Genuine or not, I want it." To which the young disciple replied, "You shall have it, Signore!"

The working relationship between Camillo and the marchese is unclear. Some letters, procured by Gian-Giuseppe Liruti, contend that Camillo visited the Milanese dictator several times, starting in 1539, and that the marchese had "more than once seen and examined" the startling Theater-Machine during that period. This would account for the Marchese's increasing enthusiasm over Camillo's otherworldly device, particularly when the reign of the Spanish commander began to show outward signs of weakness and instability.

Between October 1543 and January 1544, Camillo laid open the final "secret of his method" to the marchese. The professor was paid five hundred scudi for seven mornings of lectures, five of which were devoted to the explanation of the amphitheater and two to unknown allied subjects. Irritated by the hostile presence of the Milanese court, Camillo insisted that his instruction be conducted within the marchese's private chambers, where his words and demonstrations were very well-received.

Then realizing that his master had little time left to conclude the exalted project—and that del Vasto's days were numbered as well—Muzio convinced the marchese to request from Camillo a book-length manuscript of the five completed lectures. True to form, Camillo responded in anger, maintaining that he had neither the time, energy, nor desire to undertake such a mammoth endeavor. Anticipating Camillo's heated retort, Muzio skillfully manipulated the maestro into accepting the task by playing on Camillo's authentic gratitude to his strange and sympathetic patron. And finally, to inalterably seal the agreement, Muzio offered to transcribe all of Camillo's angelic words.

The great procrastinator and maker of labyrinths found himself trapped. For seven days in January or early February 1544, Camillo dictated the philosophical underpinnings, precise imagery, and overall arrangement of his clandestine theater. Reclining on adjoining beds from morning to midday, the professor repeated the five lectures, which Muzio reorganized into seven book chapters. (Some Renaissance scholars believed Muzio's transcription was a compendium to the original lectures, not a transcribed copy.)

Although he desperately wanted to return to Venice, Camillo probably never left Milan after his service to the marchese. Local doctors had prescribed fresh-air walks and bloodletting to combat his chronic shortness of breath but Camillo's limbs had become so bloated by then that he could neither stand nor could the attending physician locate a vein for the application of medicinal leeches. Camillo died on May 15, 1544, at the house of an old friend.

The cyber-founder was buried in the Church of Santa Maria delle Grazie. Five years later, Muzio persuaded Lorenzo Torrentino, the official printer to the Duke of Florence, to publish Camillo's grand opus, *L'Idea del Theatro*. It first appeared in April 1550.

Beginning with its first chapter, what is most striking about *L'Idea del Theatro* is Camillo's frequent references to Jewish Kabbalistic sources, such as the *Sefer Yeztira* and the *Zohar*, and how he joins them to Hermetic occult iconography. The many intellectual controversies that chased Camillo and the amphitheater in his lifetime (and after) all fail to address this central aspect of *L'Idea del Theatro*: Camillo's core inspiration from and practical interest in the Kabbalistic canon.

Meaning "received" wisdom, "Kabbalah" refers to an antinomian body of sacred Jewish, mystical teachings from various oral and written traditions. The devotional study of Kabbalah and the practice of ecstatic techniques—such as *gematria* (the transposition of letters and numbers in holy texts) or "ritual crying"—developed among Jewish religious scholars in southern Spain and Palestine during the thirteenth and fourteenth centuries. Following the mass expulsion of Jews from Spain and Portugal in the 1490s, during Camillo's adolescence, Kabbalistic manuscripts were first translated from their original Hebrew and Aramaic and published in Latin and vulgate languages. Overnight, an arcane and esoteric Jewish doctrine imbued contemporary Christian Neoplatonism with more authentic source materials and innovative practices. Explication of Holy Scripture was coupled with the mystical arts of astrology, chiromancy, metoposcopy (forehead reading), meditation on the sounds and sights of Hebrew letters and sacred names, numerology, the creation of artificial lifeforms, spirit evocation, and the drawing of magical symbols.

Camillo's seemingly self-defeating behaviors—his obsessive secrecy, his unwillingness to publicize, and his fanatic introversion—are all reflected in the shrouded world of Kabbalistic teaching and the rare transmission of its arts. Correspondingly, only with extreme reluctance did Camillo allow spectators to enter his amphitheater, despite their uniform ardor. In this sense, Camillo was unlike the run-of-the mill charlatans who appeared with some frequency in the foyers of Renaissance courts; Camillo, at every juncture, avoided the public arena and offers to publish.

Historians generally link those reclusive aspects of Camillo's personality to his uncertainty over the work or to a constitutional neurosis. But the preface of *L'Idea del Theatro* gives another reason: true knowledge is always hidden, veiled in corporal disguise, a shifting constellation of arresting ciphers. For Camillo, the god of the Kabbalah (the Ein-Sof) was even more mysterious, more indirect than the omnipotent creator of the Old and New Testaments. After the world was formed, the Kabbalistic Supreme Being himself retreated from creation and went into hiding. Like the persecuted Jews of Iberia facing Inquisitorial courts and uncertain exile, the god of Kabbalah learned to mask his identity and communicate only to a selected few and then only through the most mysterious of means.

If we accept Camillo as a Christian Kabbalist (as his writings and associations clearly suggest), a nagging question concerning the inchoate amphitheater can be answered: that is, if Camillo's invention is in fact a didactic "Palace of Memory," what does it teach us to remember? In eighty-six densely written pages, *L'Idea del Theatro* articulates something other than an advanced Ciceronian design for the recall of Latin speeches. In fact, Cicero is hardly mentioned at all and Camillo's explanation of "natural and artificial memory" bares little resemblance to Renaissance definitions as set down in the academy. (No wonder classical scholars for centuries had difficulty in comprehending the "marvelous project.") The Ideal Theater that so dazzled its skeptics served a different function than to exercise or enlarge one's oratory skills: its Kabbalistic goal was to stimulate in the spectator the memory of something deeper, more precious, more innately repressed. It was a scenic device to "reverse our exile from Paradise," to return to us a lost knowledge.

According to Jewish folklore and the Gnostic traditions of Kabbalah, each fetus in its mother's womb possesses all the ineffable wisdom of the universe. But at the moment of birth, an invisible angel Gabriel flies through the air and touches the skin between the nose and mouth (hence the ridges there), which causes the infant to cry and give up its divine understanding. For Kabbalists, the single purpose of human life is to reestablish that connection with the godhead, to relearn the absolute knowledge we once possessed before we were violently "kidnapped from Paradise." Giulio Camillo's theater attempted the ultimate in practical Kabbalah—to recapture humanity's lost Eden through the induction of prenatal memory.

The Memory Theater of Giulio Camillo

We know Camillo's "wooden contraption" consisted of

seven ascending platform stages that were divided into seven rows ("The Seven Pillars of Solomon's House of Wisdom"). One-hundred-and-twenty distinct Homeric, Hermetic, and Zoharistic signs and figures were "displayed" within the forty-nine theatrical spaces. The size of the seven-by-seven grid and how the emblems moved (or were changed) inside the framed spaces is unknown and remains one of the subjects of scholarly contention. Also how long the figurines and images remained in place—and therefore, overlapped on the bank of forty-nine chest-shaped "stages"—is indeterminate.

Those who believe Camillo's amphitheater was relatively small, about fifteen feet high and twenty-five to thirty feet wide, an early *Wunderkammer*, assume that images were tucked away in cylinder-shaped containers. Others conclude that the Kabbalistic Machine-Theater must have been quite huge—maybe warehouse sized—and utilized sophisticated roller-like equipment to manipulate the movement of the icons. Since contemporary descriptions support both theories, it seems likely the theater existed in differing versions.

What Happened to Camillo's Theaters?

The search for Camillo's famed amphitheaters began with the publication of *L'Idea del Theatro* in 1550. Interestingly, inquiries by the earliest generation of Camillo scholars in Venice and Paris never seemed very dogged or well directed; for example, none of Camillo's protégés, like Muzio or Camillo's immediate family, were contacted. Most investigative parties quickly concluded that the theaters must have been thoroughly destroyed or existed only in the ever-expanding imaginations of deranged believers.

The first written evidence that some elements of Camillo's Kabbalistic project were extant appeared in 1559 in the form of a small guidebook, entitled *La Villa*, which listed the inventories of various private Milanese art collectors, including those from the outlying villa of Pomponio Cotta. According to Bartolomeo Taegio, Cotta prized among his rarest acquisitions "the lofty and incomparable fabric from the marvelous Theatre of the most excellent Giulio Camillo." (The "pictures" assembled by Cotta from the theater were described in the book as "marvelous" and mural-like, which strongly suggests that Camillo's Italian amphitheater, built in 1532, was considerably larger than a mere *Wunderkammer*.)

In the mid-1600s, Bernard de Montfaucon, a French antiquarian collector, hunted for Camillo's Parisian amphitheater but found no traces of it. One place he failed to explore was François' Château de Madrid, a strange construction in the center of the Bois de Boulogne that served no known purpose. Designed more like a Baroque prison maze than a luxurious country estate, the Château de Madrid was said to be built as a memorial to François' imprisonment in the Spanish capital. Completed around 1530, the outlandishly styled Madrid may have been Camillo's ideal, isolated working space. Its gilded interiors with many sets of embedded panels and elevated landings mimics the casket-like grid of *L'Idea del Theatro*. If Madrid was not in fact Camillo's actual amphitheater by design, then King François I had already anticipated a Kabbalistic division of scenic space and allowed Camillo to set his forty-nine framed wooden stages inside the foyer and main room of the Château.

Both the Milanese emblems and the Château de Madrid (reconstructed after François' original, which was destroyed during the Revolution) remain in place today, waiting to be explored by future historians of Giulio Camillo.

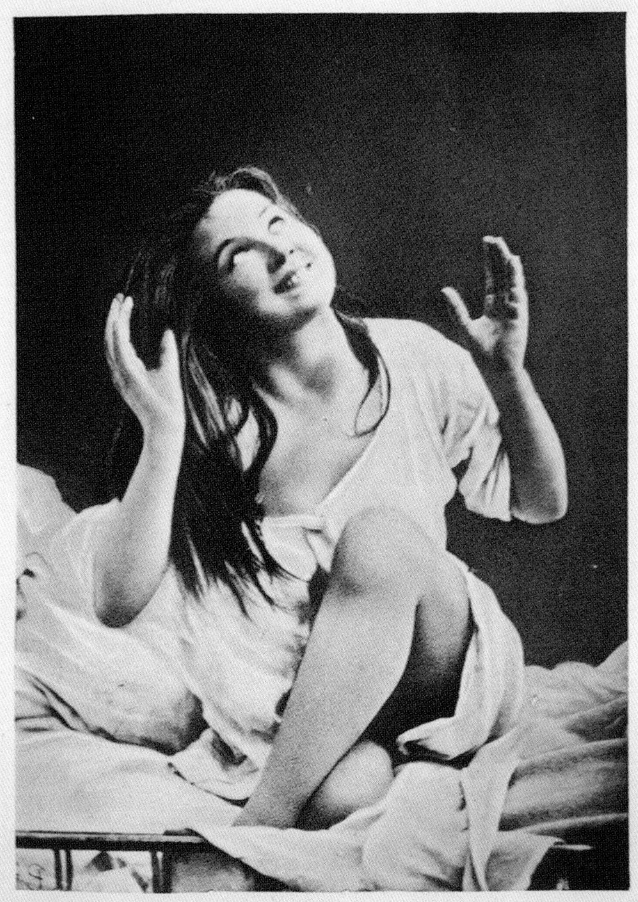

Planche XXIII.

ATTITUDES PASSIONNELLES

EXTASE (1878).

STAGING THE UNCONSCIOUS

ZOE BELOFF

AS A FILMMAKER AND MEDIA ARTIST, I'M FASCINATED BY THE IDEA of graphically recording mental states, finding ways to show the intangible workings of the mind. In what follows, I discuss two of my projects, *Charming Augustine* (2005), a stereoscopic 16mm film, and *The Somnambulists* (2007), a video installation.

Both works focus on mental states once known as hysteria. They are inspired by case histories, photographs and films made by doctors at the turn of the last century. They explore a complex interweaving of ideas from psychology, performance, art and moving image technology.

Why Hysteria?

Hysteria encompassed a vast range of symptoms, from the temporary paralysis of a limb, or uncontrollable movements, to full-scale delirium where the patient conversed with people only they could see. What tied these symptoms together was that they were performed, acted out. One might say that hysteria, like cinema, only existed in the moment of its performance.

But where did unconscious, compulsive acting out end, and acting in the traditional sense begin? What was the relationship between scientific document and spectacle? In *Charming Augustine*, I wanted to evoke this strange area where science meets theater, where women used their bodies to perform their desires in extraordinary and disturbing ways, and explore its connection to the birth of narrative cinema.

Augustine

In the late nineteenth century, the great neurologist Jean-Martin Charcot (1825–1893) presided over the hospital of the Salpêtrière in Paris where he was know as "the Napoleon of the neuroses." Here several thousand woman and some men were treated for mental disorders. In order to understand the elusive nature of hysteria, Charcot believed that it was important to document and codify its symptoms. To do this, he turned the hospital into a veritable factory of image making, employing the latest technology. Though photographing the insane was already a well-established practice, a single photograph could not possibly hope to capture an attack of *la grande hystérie*. The first case to be represented with a sequence of photographs was that of a woman referred to variously as "X," "L" or "Augustine": a young girl who arrived at the Salpêtrière in 1875, aged fifteen and suffering from hysterical paralysis. These were published along with a detailed account of her day-by-day case history in the second volume of *Iconographie photographique de la Salpêtrière* (1876–1880).

Previous Image: "Attudes passionnelles: Ecstacy," Photograph by Régnard, Published in Iconographie photographique de la Salpêtrière, vol II, *1876–1880. Courtesy of Wellcome Library, London.*

The doctors were captivated by her frequent hysterical attacks, which they described as the most perfect examples of *la grande hystérie*. And they photographed her over and over again. Though her gestures look melodramatic to us, one must not forget that Augustine was also deeply disturbed. She had visions and heard voices. Her body would go into spasms where it was completely out of control.

Though sequential images were recorded, they were far from instantaneous snapshots. Because of the long exposure time, they represent not movement caught on the fly, but defined poses, in a way similar to how a storyboard pares a scene down to just the high points. It was here that Augustine's illness pushed photographic technology to its limits and beyond, bringing into existence a new, hybrid way of seeing. It was a proto-cinema of sequential, still images, each representing a key moment of her hysterical attack. I think of it as a bridge between past and future.

Melodrama in Embryo

The doctors considered these photographs hard evidence in the scientific sense. Yet when we look at images of Augustine something else develops. Under cover of the concept that the camera could not lie, or as we say, under cover of darkness, the scientist embraced fiction and the doctors staged illness as drama.

Clearly some of the photographs of Augustine were highly sexualized.[1] And yet to say that she was simply the plaything of the doctors is, I think, too simplistic. Did she not want to be, at least at first, the star of the asylum, to please and provoke? We will never know because we only have her story from the other side, the medical case history. But it seems to me that Augustine was open about her sexuality. She wanted to tell her doctors everything: her adventures, her affairs, her traumatic experiences. But the doctors didn't listen, so she enacted her sexual encounters before their eyes. Here was the problem. The doctors transcribed everything she said, but it never occurred to them that her experiences had anything to do with her mental disturbance. Perhaps her story was too much, too excessive. Instead they preferred to look at her, too study her like a model and to pacify her with drugs. Charcot used to say that, when hypnotized, hysterics made perfect models for artists because they were so expressive.

[1] *The first people to read hysteria as a kind of provocative and highly sexualized performance were André Breton and Louis Aragon, in their essay "Le Cinquantenaire de l'hystérie (1878–1928)," which is illustrated with photographs of Augustine, and even goes so as far as to suggest that the doctors had illicit sex with their female patients.*

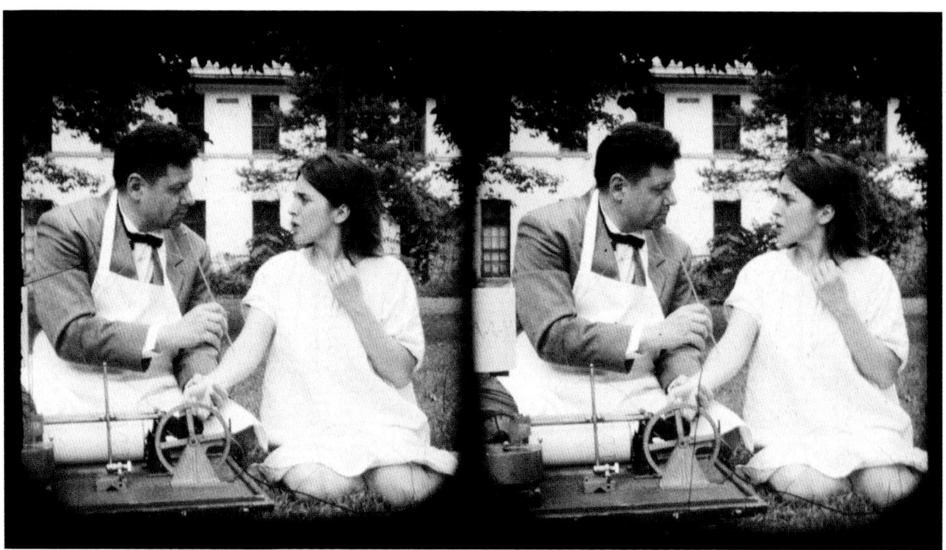

Image above: Zoe Beloff, stereo frames from the film Charming Augustine. *Courtesy of Zoe Beloff.*

I was fascinated by the transcripts of what Augustine said in states of delirium and the accounts of her dreams. Their publication, side by side with the photographs, seemed to me to express a desire on the part of the doctors to make a synchronous sound *avant la lettre*. The technology wasn't quite there. So in some ways I thought of myself as making the film the doctors wished they could make, all these years later.

I think of *Charming Augustine* as an attempt to explore cinema's origins in the relationship between the psychic apparatus and technology. While the roles of Étienne-Jules Marey and Eadweard Muybridge in the birth of cinema are well known, less attention is paid to French photographer Albert Londe who worked with very similar cameras at the Salpêtrière. While Marey attempted to study the mechanics of the body, Londe aimed to reveal the secrets of the patient's minds with his motion studies camera. In my film I wanted to show that while Marey may have invented the mechanics of cinema, it was the doctors and patients at the Salpêtrière who together, perhaps unwittingly, supplied the psychic drive that would come to flower in the works of D.W. Griffith.

Sigmund Freud turned away from the visual in favor of verbal evidence for the existence of the unconscious. He intentionally did not look at his patients, perhaps in part because he wanted to discourage this crazy acting out. He was interested in stories, in the novelistic. But in an early formulation of hysteria, Freud wrote, "hysterics suffer mainly from reminiscences." And it is the way in which the performance of hysteria embodied memory that drew it toward cinema.

In "Screen Images, Film Memory" (1976), Stephen Heath describes how close narrative cinema is to the case history. He explains how film as it was developed commercially reproduced the novelistic which could be simply titled, "family romance." The past in the film and the trouble of the past must be always worked through for narrative resolution.[2]

Freud worked at the Salpêtrière and must have been familiar with Augustine's case history. Of course her story lends itself to melodrama, from her childhood in a convent school where she rebelled against the nuns to her rape by her mother's lover, her breakdown, and her eventual escape from the asylum dressed as a man. I think of Augustine as the first "star" of a cinema about to be born, acting out her own very disturbed "family romance."

In my film I aimed to find a way to represent her inner life in a way that was not possible during her lifetime. Though I took film's intertitles and dialog strictly from the case history, the visual language of the film changes over time. There are three distinct parts. At first I simply present a medical document following the description of the case history. The shots are simple and static, like a series of clinical lantern slides recreating, as closely as possible, the existing photographs of Augustine.

[2] *Steven Heath, "Screen Images, Film Memory,"* Edinburgh'76 Magazine: Psycho-analysis, Cinema, Avant-garde *(1976), 41.*

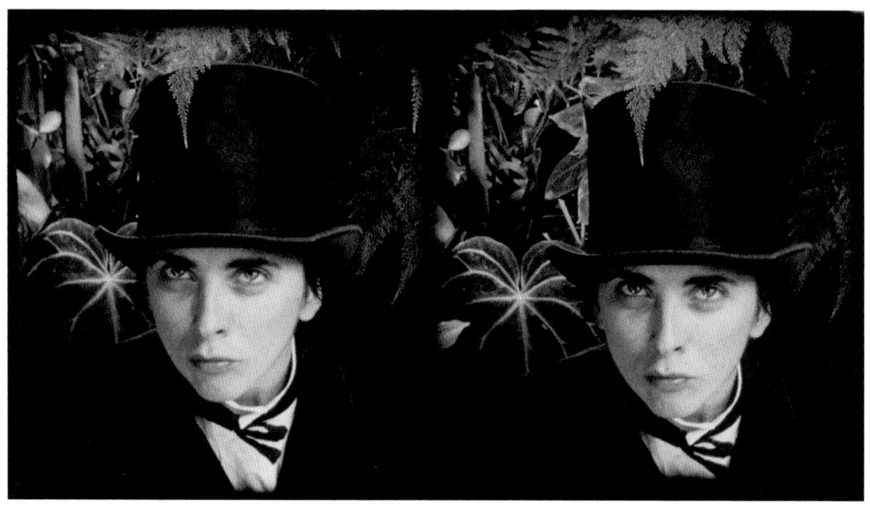

The second part of the film starts once more from the beginning of the story, and this time I attempt to show the world from Augustine's point of view. I accompany the depiction of her delirium with the music of Claude Debussy's *Pelléas et Mélisande* (1902), because I pictured her imagining her life as opera. Maybe in the same way that later, women could imagine themselves as suffering heroines like Jane Wyman in *Magnificent Obsession* (1954). I think the hysterical imagination is extravagant in this way.

In the final part of the film, Augustine becomes "disenchanted," both in the contemporary sense of that word and in its original meaning of being awakened from a magnetic sleep or hypnotic trance. She takes action and finally escapes from the asylum dressed as a man. It is here the language of the film most closely resembles that of a D.W. Griffith two-reeler.[3]

[3] The film that was most inspirational to me both in terms of cinematic language and acting was Griffith's The Painted Lady (1912), in which Blanche Sweet gives an extraordinary performance as a young woman who loses her lover and her mind.

A Film Twenty Years Before Cinema Existed?

A key question for me technically was how to make a film about a time before cinema existed, something that directors

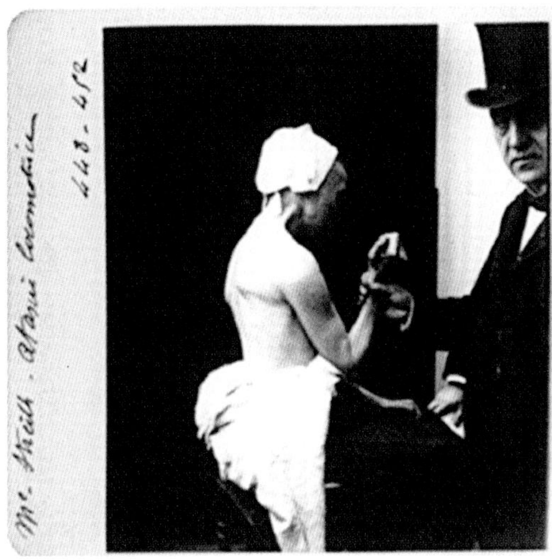

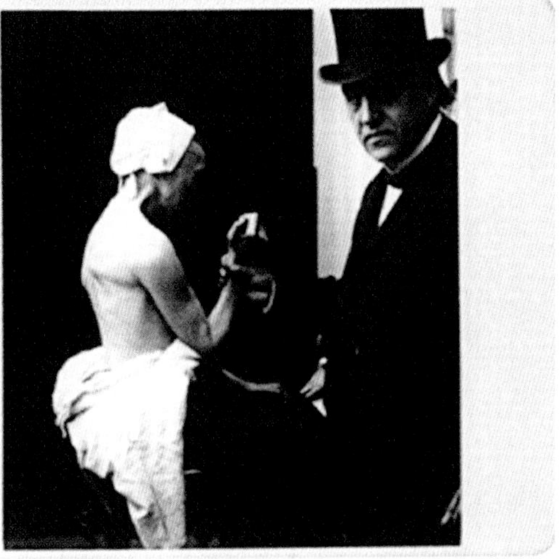

of historical dramas do not usually concern themselves with. I wanted the audience to see cinema afresh, as though it had just been invented. I shot *Charming Augustine* in black-and-white reversal film using a Stereo Bolex 16mm camera. This camera not only produces a 3D image, but one with a vertical aspect ratio. To project it, one needs a silver screen. The wide-angle lenses make it necessary for the projector to be in the same space as the audience. In fact, I think of spectators as being put in a similar situation to scientists a hundred years ago, huddled around their noisy, experimental apparatus.

Though the camera itself is anachronistic, I felt the format suggested a different direction that cinema might have taken had it been invented in the 1880s.[4] I was inspired by the fact that photographers at the Salpêtrière used both stereoscopic cameras and motion studies cameras, and I imagined what it might have been like if they had managed to combine them into a motion picture camera, twenty-five years before the Lumière Brothers invented their cinematograph. One must remember that before the cinematograph, film's aspect ratio had not been

Image left: Zoe Beloff, stereo frames from the film Charming Augustine. *Courtesy of Zoe Beloff.*

Image above: Photographer unknown, *Jean-Martin Charcot et une patiente ataxique,* 1875. *Courtesy of Zoe Beloff.*

[4] *The Stereo Bolex was invented in 1954 so people could shoot their home movies in 3D. It did not catch on with the public.*

set. For example, in the early 1890s Marey experimented with different aspect ratios depending on what he was shooting, a vertical aspect ratio for a rabbit falling, a horizontal one for a horse running.

Ultimately what I wished to convey was fragile, spectral, and hypothetical—a moment in time when the moving image was on the brink of existence in a form not yet standardized.

The Somnambulists

The Somnambulists is an installation comprising five miniature theaters into which moving images are projected. It centers on the idea of "staging the unconscious." Each theater presents a hysterical drama. These include two musicals based on case histories by Pierre Janet (1859–1947) as well as the specters of actual hysterics filmed by doctors a hundred years ago.

The largest theater is made of wood and painted in the style of a Victorian toy theater, 150 centimeters wide and 106 centimeters high. Gallery viewers see what appears to be perfectly formed, three-dimensional, colorfully attired actors about forty centimeters high, performing a musical drama. The effect is closer to that of hallucination than a projection. The illusion is created with high definition 3D video, projected onto a rear screen mounted behind the stage.

The four smaller theaters are approximately forty-five centimeters wide, forty-five centimeters high and fifty-five centimeters deep. They are also made of wood and colorfully painted to resemble small dioramas. In two of them, the viewer peers through an entrance into a courtyard, where a young woman appears to be having a hysterical attack. In another, the viewer looks through a window into what appears to be a mental asylum where they see a disturbed child throwing a fit. The fourth is a Chinese-style theater where a funny Frenchman

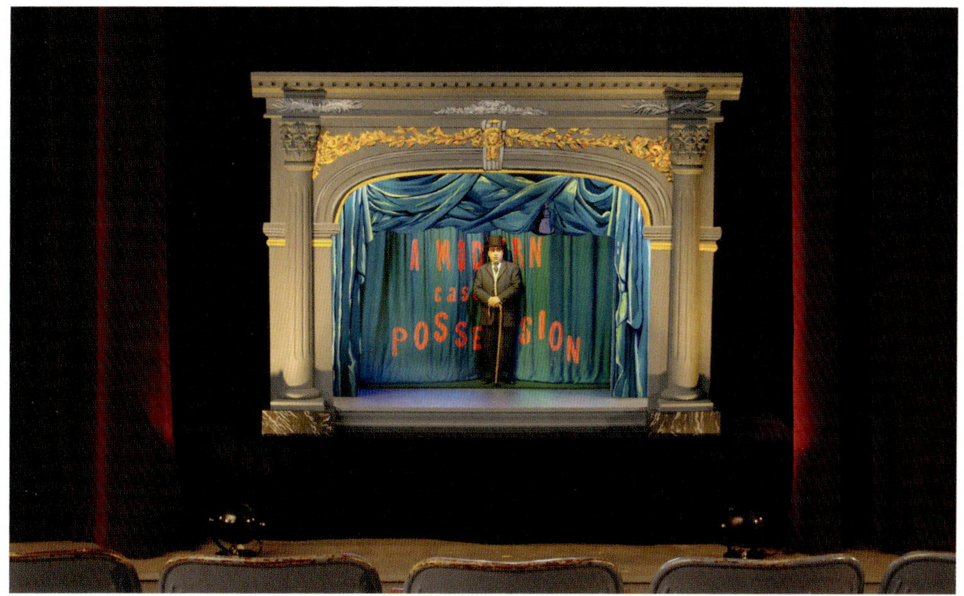

Image above: Zoe Beloff, installation view of The Somnambulists *featuring "Pierre Janet as Master of Ceremonies". Courtesy of Zoe Beloff.*

performs a comic musical number. The figures are black and white and appear to hover in real space rather than being projected on a surface or screen.

The Somnambulists was inspired by several remarkable developments at end of the nineteenth century. While earlier physicians like Charcot believed that hysteria was a neurological disorder, ultimately treatable with drugs, Pierre Janet (who also worked at the Salpêtrière) believed that the symptoms of hysteria were the unconscious acting out or performance of psychological trauma. Along with Freud, he was one of the discoverers of the unconscious and, like Freud, believed that the key to treatment lay in listening to his patients.

With the invention of the cinematograph, doctors began to film their patients. At the same time, hysteria acquired a certain frisson in the popular imagination. Acting crazy became all the rage in the Paris cabarets. For example, the French comic Dranem had a hit song with *Neurasthénic.* There were many other similar songs floating around, like *Nerveuse* or *Tata's Tic.* There were eccentric gommeuses singers in their extravagantly

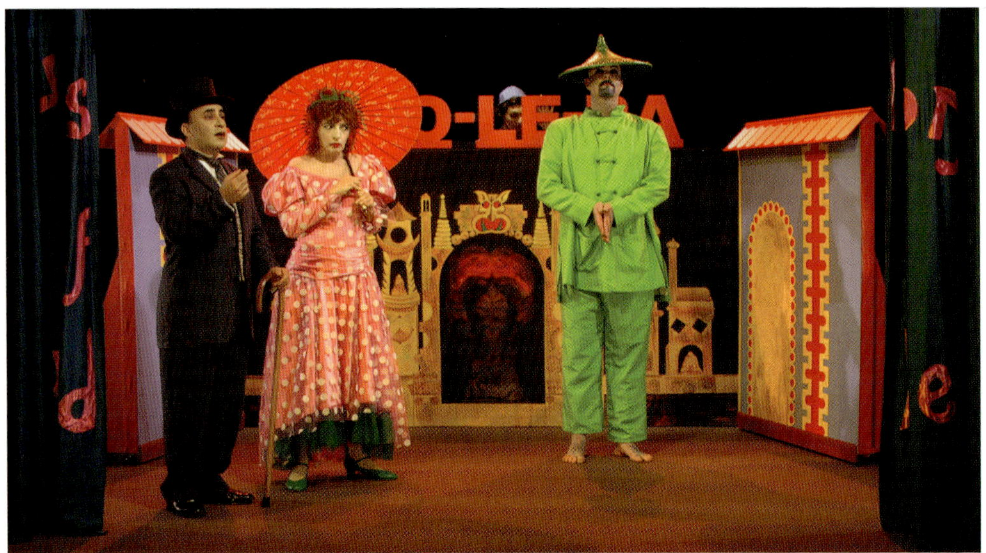

Image above: Zoe Beloff, frame from Historie d'une idée fixe. *Courtesy of Zoe Beloff.*

silly costumes and épileptique singers who threw themselves around on stage and invented nonsense words.[5]

The Doctor as Master of Ceremonies

The centerpiece of the installation is the large theater where two plays based closely on Pierre Janet's case studies, "Histoire d'une idée fixe" (1894) and "Un cas de possession et l'exorcisme moderne" (1898) are presented.[6] I chose to stage them as musicals, not simply because the cabaret was the language of popular culture but more importantly because I wanted to find a way to convey Janet's radical method of treatment.

He realized that his patients' hysterical attacks provided a visual and auditory window into the unconscious workings of their minds. Aware that they could neither hear nor respond to him in the throes of their delirium, Janet discovered that he could communicate by entering into their imaginary world, as a second actor. It was as though he had entered the theater of their minds and, as master of ceremonies, was able to manipulate their fears so that their hallucinations had happy endings. He described it thus: "In order to provoke intelligent signs and conjure up phenomenon in rapport with what the patient still sees, one must enter into her dream."[7]

"Histoire d'une idée fixe," concerns the case of Justine, a woman of forty who would plunge into a delirium where she hallucinated that the specter of "cholera," a naked blue cadaver, was trying to ensnare her. It was at this moment that Janet entered into her private drama. When Justine cried out, "The cholera it's going to take me," he responded, "[Y]es it's taking you by the right leg" and Justine violently recoiled. Using this method he manipulated Justine's hallucinations, transforming the terrifying "cholera" into "Cho-le-Ra," a Chinese general she had been greatly impressed with at the Exposition Universelle in 1898. In fact when Janet finally made the general get up and walk, she burst out laughing.

"Un cas de possession et l'exorcisme moderne" recounts the story of Achille who returned home from a business trip in 1890 only to plunge into a deep depression, finally lapsing into a coma. Just when his wife had given up hope, he leapt from his bed convinced he was possessed by the devil. Only once Janet had hypnotized him did the patient reveal the source of his transformation. During his business trip he had been unfaithful to his wife. Returning home he was overcome by self-loathing, literally believing himself to be consigned to hell. With the aplomb of a stage magician, Doctor Janet conjured up a vision of Achille's wife, who promptly forgave her poor husband.

Theaters of the Mind

One might say that the doctor, the patient and the patient's fears all become performers on a "mental stage." In my play I

[5] *A wealth of information on the relationship between French music hall performance, early cinema and clinical hysteria can be found in Rae Beth Gordon,* Why the French Love Jerry Lewis: From Cabaret to Early Cinema *(Stanford, California: Stanford University Press, 2001).*

[6] *Pierre Janet, "Histoire d'une idée fixe,"* Revue Philosophique XXXVIIII *(1894): 121–168 and Pierre Janet, "Un Cas de possession et l'exorcisme moderne" in* Névroses et idées fixes *(Paris: Felix Alacan, 1898), 375–389.*

[7] *Janet, "Histoire d'une idée fixe," 125.*

wish to show how Janet used his remarkable semiotic technique to manipulate his patients' minds, moving their "mental furniture," which consisted of images, words, sounds and smells, all equivalent and open to substitution. For example, in the case of Justine, Janet changes Justine's hallucination of "the blue cadaver" through manipulation of the word "cholera" into the hallucinated image of a Chinese general "Cho-le-Ra"—whom he dissolves once again into the component letters "C H O," which then recombine in infinitely mutable figures of speech swirling around in Justine's mind.

In his essay, "Histoire d'une idée fixe," Janet makes the point that Justine's case shed light on the question, "what is an idea?" He writes, "We see that the idea of cholera is actually in her, arrived at if one might say to the *n*th degree of perfection; an ensemble, a system of images, imprinted on all of her senses, so that each one is very clear and very complex and becomes realized and objectified in the form of hallucinations and movements."[8] It is this concept of the embodiment of ideas in a visual or aural form and their manipulation on a symbolic level that makes Janet's ideas so interesting to me as an artist.

[8] *Ibid.*, 126.

Charming Augustine had to be a film, precisely because it was about the pre-history of cinema. For *The Somnambulists* I had to find a visual equivalent to the patient's hallucinations where real and virtual figures appeared together. The fact that their fears took the form of absurd characters like blue cadavers or devils, which would not have been out of place in a Victorian pantomime or cabaret, made theater the obvious choice. I tried to create a theater that is real and tangible, only the actors are virtual, 3D projections. I shot each play in one take without cuts or camera movement because I wanted to make it quite clear that it was Doctor Janet, as "master of ceremonies," who was in charge of manipulating his patients' "mental scenery."

Afterlife

The smaller theaters present actual cases of hysteria filmed by doctors. I worked with footage shot by the Romanian neurologist Gheorghe Marinescu, the Belgian neurologist Arthur van Gehuchten, and the American doctor Abram Elting Bennett. To show how madness entered the popular imagination, I included one short 1905 sound film of Dranem, the "Comique Idiot," singing a song.

Rather than simply present the archival footage as I found it, I decided to separate the figures in the films from their backgrounds and project them into small dioramas whose construction was inspired by the patients' original settings. I used an updated version of the Victorian stage illusion "Pepper's Ghost," with beamsplitter glass and small, concealed DVD players, so that these figures seem to exist within the real space of what is actually a painted miniature.

My inspiration for these dioramas stems both from natural history displays and from a scene in the book, *Locus Solus*, written in 1914 by Raymond Roussel. The first decades of the twentieth century saw the construction of the great dioramas, like those at the American Museum of Natural History; these spectacles are considered scientific documentation, though they play very much upon illusionism and fantasy. In them, both space and bodies are manipulated and reconstituted. I find them deeply melancholy. They show us a moment that never existed, frozen in time for all eternity. I always feel like I'm looking into the afterlife.

And in a sense I am. The dioramas were made with the knowledge that these animals and their world were dying, and the dioramas were an attempt to preserve them. In *Locus Solus,* Roussel described a series of museum dioramas where dead people, revitalized through electricity, insensibly reenact the most dramatic events of their lives over and over again.

Image next spread: "Hystéro-Épilepsie, Contracture" Photograph by Régnard, Published in Iconographie photographique de la Salpêtrière, vol II, *1876–1880. Courtesy of Wellcome Library, London.*

I wanted to reference these ideas in my own museum of madness. The viewer looks into another world where patients from a hundred years ago, resurrected by electricity, reenact their traumas indefinitely.

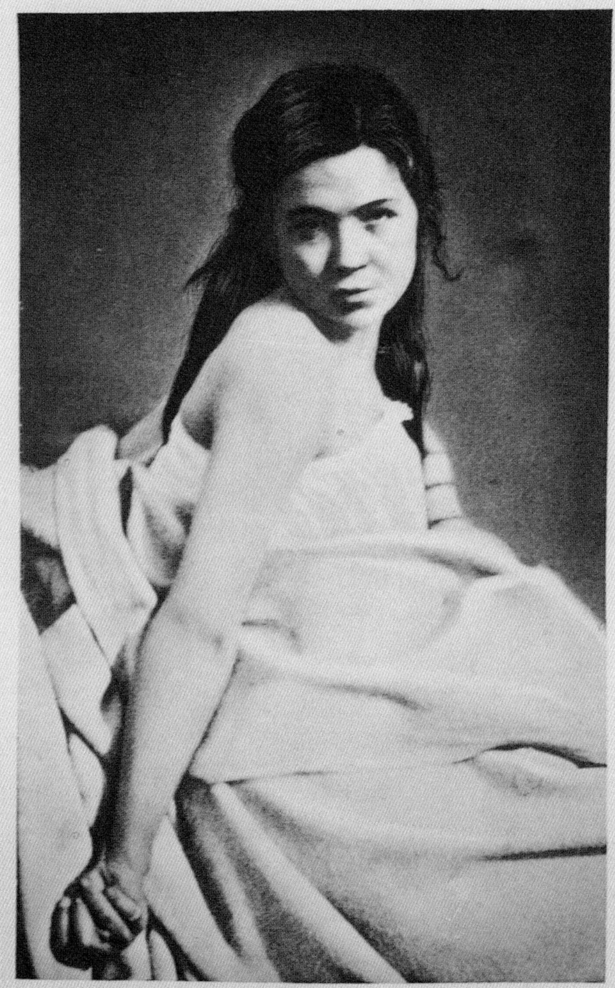

Planche XXX.

HYSTÉRO-ÉPILEPSIE

CONTRACTURE

MEMENTO MORI

Reflections on the Art of the Tableau

AMY HERZOG

I FIND MYSELF FASCINATED BY A CERTAIN TENDENCY IN STAGED tableaux such as dioramas and waxworks, one bound up in their commingling of stillness and motion. The diorama presents us with a hermetic, immobilized world; there is typically a painted background (often curved to give the illusion of boundlessness), and posed, lifeless figures (human or animal, wax or taxidermied) alongside the objects and ephemera we might imagine native to these environments. There is something profoundly fetishistic, and mildly necrophilic, at the heart of the diorama: an apparent desire to encapsulate and reanimate those items on display. This paradoxical tension between preservation and regeneration seems germane to the nineteenth-century imaginary in general, the moment at which many of the visual practices I will discuss came into being. But it is a tension that surfaces in many dioramas with a particularly powerful, and sometimes surprising, pedagogical bent.

A great deal has been written about the ways in which nineteenth-century museological practices relied upon novelty and spectacle, and the indeterminate realm between the desire to educate and the more profitable will to entertain. What I find most interesting about those displays that most fully conflate amusement

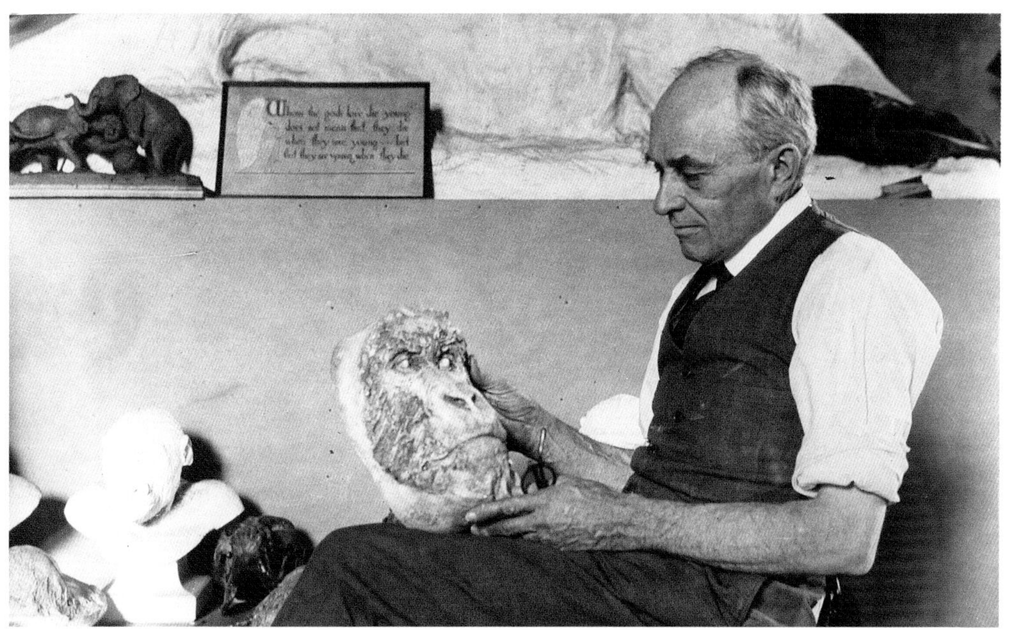

and education, however, is their reliance on a highly specific, educational mission: a directive to recognize the self through an encounter with the unknown. This moment of reflection is often compelled by a confrontation with death.

Image above: Carl Akeley with a plaster mask impression taken from one of his gorilla specimens during an expedition to Africa, ca. 1921. Image ¢ 311654, Courtesy of the American Museum of Natural History Library.

I began thinking about these questions of stillness and reanimation while doing research on Victorian postmortem photography at the George Eastman House in Rochester. The Eastman House archives hold a huge collection of memorial daguerreotypes, keepsakes that took advantage of the emerging technology of photography to capture a fleeting image of a deceased loved one that could be treasured indefinitely.

When I made my appointment to visit the collection, the archivist suggested that I wear something black. I was at first taken aback by this advice, which resonated as both strangely intimate and formal, though his reasoning was entirely practical. Daguerreotypes are captured on iodized, silver-coated copper plates. They are singular, unique images—only one is created

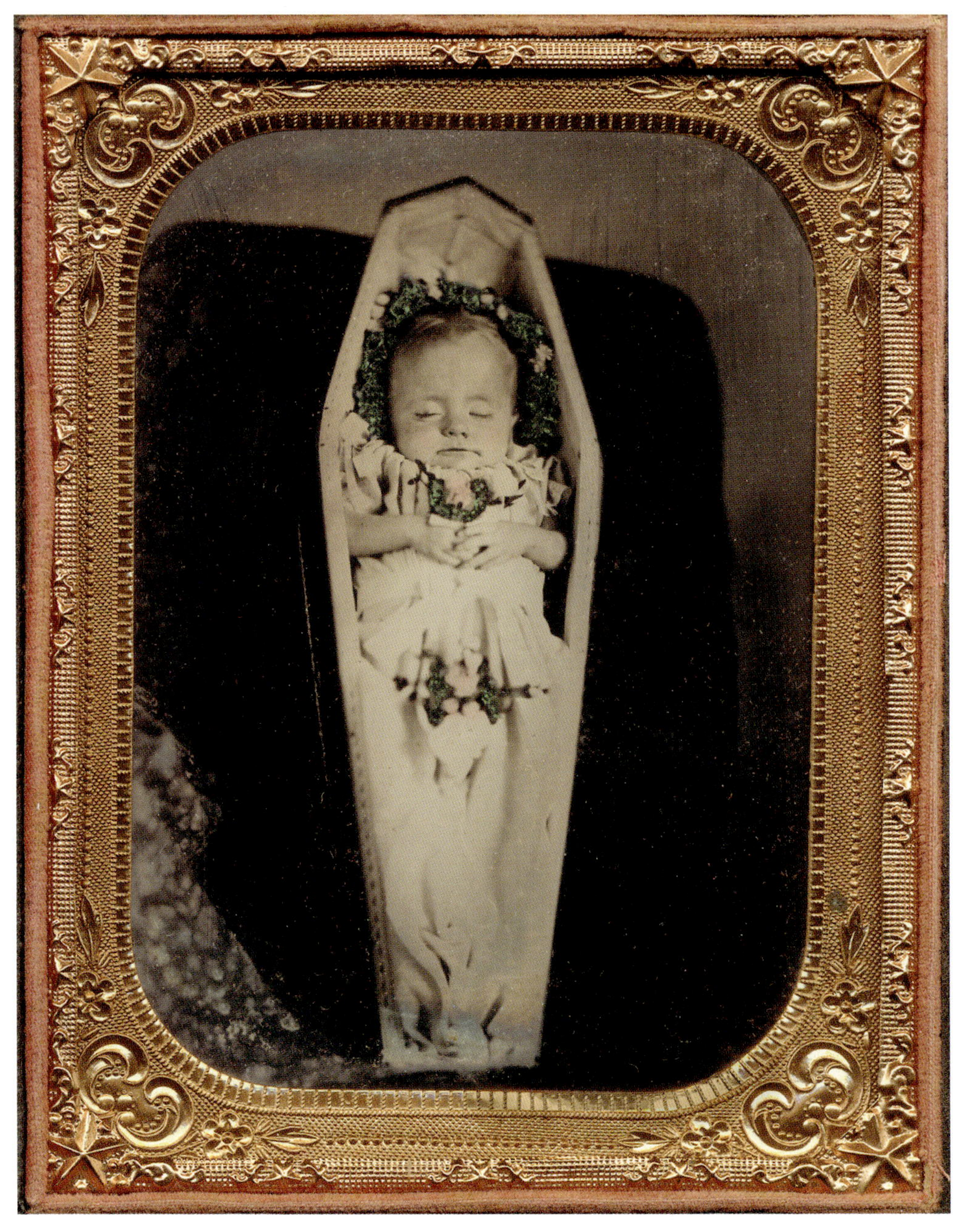

Hand-tinted ambrotype of an unidentified child, ca. 1860. Collection of Jack and Beverly Wilgus.

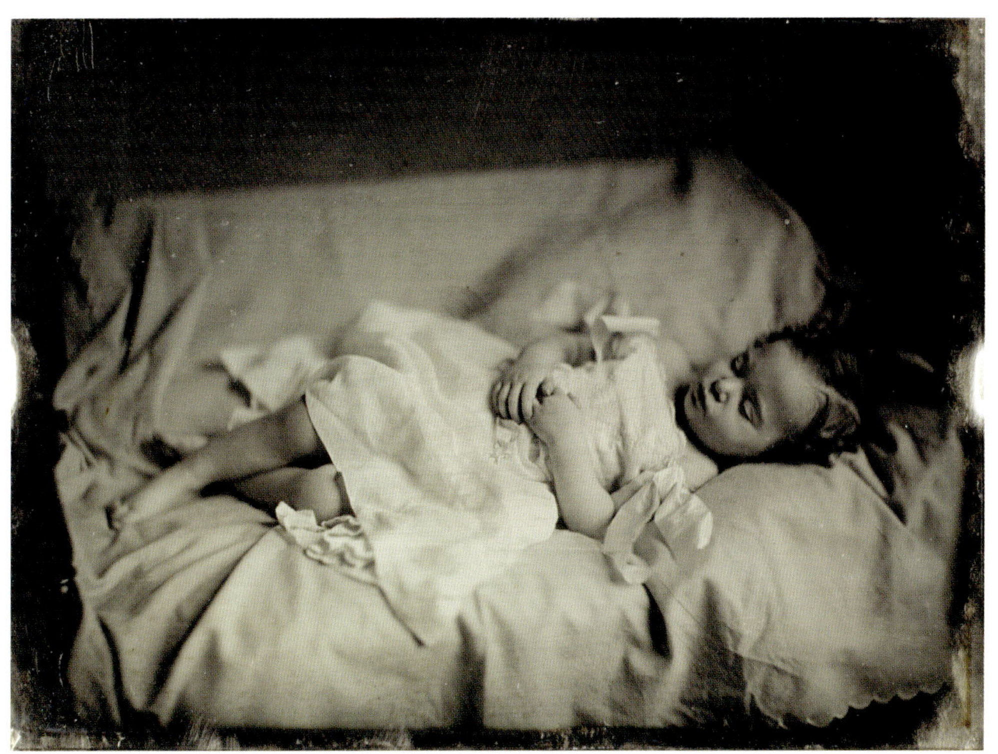

Image above: Southworth & Hawes, Post-mortem Daguerreotype of an unidentified girl, ca. 1850. Courtesy of George Eastman House, International Museum of Photography and Film.

per exposure—and they are highly reflective. Black clothing facilitates the best daguerreotype-viewing experience. Because these plates can only be seen when held at an angle, one must reflect oneself, or perhaps more accurately reflect the absence of oneself, into the mirrored image encased in one's hand.

While I had been anticipating that this research project would be challenging based on the content (many of the subjects were infants and children) I was in no way prepared for the affective experience of encountering these artifacts firsthand. Many of the images were framed in tiny velvet cases. As you tip the image back and forth in search of the best viewing angle, they begin to shimmer, fragile and specter-like, on the surface of the plate.

I was struck, too, by the range of visual approaches photographers took to this challenging task. Many of the images were straightforward and unflinching in their depiction of death. Others were almost breathtakingly beautiful; children lay in romantic repose, rosy cheeked, as if they had just drifted off to sleep. Representing perhaps the pinnacle of memorial artistry, studios like that of Southworth & Hawes engaged in acts of stunning photographic fabulation, using the deceased body to craft images of an idealized moment that might, in fact, never have existed in life.

Viewing box after box of these images, I found a complementary affinity between the more "successful," well-produced images, and those that were more awkward, morbid, or ugly. Both types of images attempt to frame for the viewer a talisman that will help them to cope with their loss, and, simultaneously, to confront their own mortality. The French critic Jules Janin wrote about his first encounter with a daguerreotype in 1839:

> Dans ce miroir magique, la nature se reflècte dans toute sa vérité naïve et un peu triste. (In this magic mirror, nature is reflected in all its truth, naïve and a bit sad.)[1]

If there is a "truth" caught in the daguerreotype's magic mirror, it arises from the unresolved contradictions of its captured moments. In the postmortem photograph, we find the comfort of familiarity (intimate objects, fabrics, the interiors of a home, the face of a beloved) at the same time we are confronted by difference and the unknown (the inaccessibility of a lost moment caught on a silver surface, that same face rendered gaunt and strange). The looking glass of the image offers just a glimpse of this intangible, uncanny, parallel world.

The link between memorial photography and the diorama might appear oblique at first glance, yet the phenomena share a certain objective: to freeze, and to reanimate, a fragment of space and time.

[1] *Jules Janin, "M. Daguerre," L'Artiste 3 (2nd series), no. 11 (14 July 1839), 181–2. As quoted in R.D. Wood,* The Arrival of the Daguerreotype in New York *(New York: American Photographic Historical Society, 1994).*

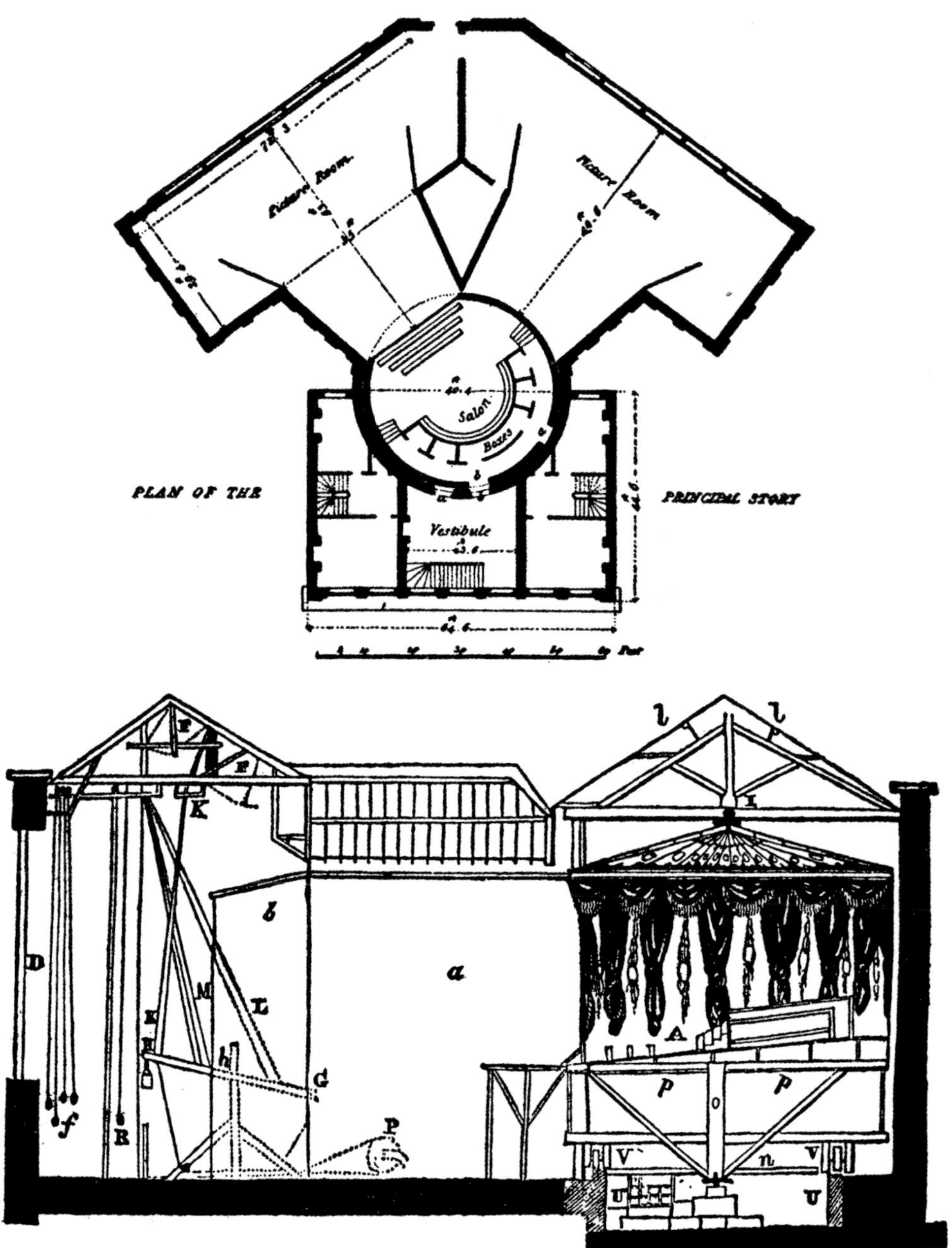

Ground plan of the Louis Daguerre Diorama building, London, by A. Pugin and J. Morgan, 1823.

Louis Daguerre, who invented the daguerreotype in partnership with J.N. Niépce, also coined the term "diorama" to refer to the immensely popular entertainment format he developed and promoted prior to the premier of his photographic experiments. In a venture with architectural painter Charles Marie Bouton, Daguerre's dioramas involved large, darkened theaters in which audiences viewed a proscenium from a rotating platform. Viewers would watch landscapes painted onto a series of layered scrims; dramatic lighting effects would create the illusion of changing times of day or seasons, sometimes with accompanying sounds and real objects. Daguerre and Bouton's diorama premiered in Paris in 1822 to great critical and commercial acclaim, spawning several international, and later traveling, venues. Popular scenes included cathedrals, alpine villages, ruins, tombs, and, in 1833, a moonlit view of the murdered bodies of the Countess of Hartzfeld and her servant lying near their still-lit fire in the Black Forest.[2]

[2] *Helmut and Alison Gernsheim,* L.J.M. Daguerre: The History of the Diorama and the Daguerreotype, *Second ed. (New York: Dover, 1968), 32.*

The term diorama, however, is more often associated with groupings of figures and objects within a stylized, scaled environment, displayed in a lit chamber, encased in glass. As Alison Griffiths has convincingly argued, museum habitat and life-group dioramas draw from the naturalistic painting styles used in panoramas or Daguerre-style moving dioramas, the staging of tableaux vivant and waxworks, and the ethnographic displays featured at the Crystal Palace in London.[3] These techniques were deployed in combination with the more modern, commercial display aesthetics of department stores, world's fairs, and advertising. Certainly the museum diorama's lineage extends to the seventeeth-century cabinet of curiosities, those treasure troves of objects and collected novelties, although the habitat display marks a significant departure from earlier groupings based on typology.

[3] *Alison Griffiths,* Wondrous Difference: Cinema, Anthropology, and Turn-of-the-Century Visual Culture *(New York: Columbia University Press, 2001), 3-45.*

With waxworks, habitat dioramas, and staged, historical displays gaining currency in dime museums and on midways, the newly established natural history museums of the late nineteenth century strove to differentiate their displays from the "hokum" peddled by less reputable purveyors. The museum diorama designers actively sought to achieve greater scientific accuracy while at the same time educating, and elevating, their urban audiences. In the introduction to *Windows on Nature: The Great Habitat Dioramas of the American Museum of Natural History*, Steven Christopher Quinn writes:

> It should be noted that, in 1868, one year before the founding of the American Museum... P.T. Barnum's entertaining American Museum in New York was completely destroyed in a fire. Barnum's museum, though it contained what was considered one of the finest natural history collections of its time, was anything but educational. New York was ready for a true museum of natural science without the show business and what Barnum called "humbug." [4]

To be certain, there is an educational component to the habitat dioramas, and an overarching mission at scientific museums that is distinct from that of the dime museum. Institutions like the American Museum of Natural History have successfully mobilized their dioramas to draw attention to issues of preservation and to generate research funding. But if the educational diorama is a fusion of art and science, as Quinn and others have argued, I'd like to suggest that this combination of approaches brings them closer to the modus operandi of all staged tableaux, including those of the "humbug" museum, than they might like to imagine.

A brief survey of minor examples from within and without the museum proper might shed light on the organizing logic of the diorama in general. The most stolidly instructive displays,

[4] *Stephen Christopher Quinn,* Windows on Nature: The Great Habitat Dioramas of the American Museum of Natural History *(New York: American Museum of Natural History/Abrams, 2006), 10.*

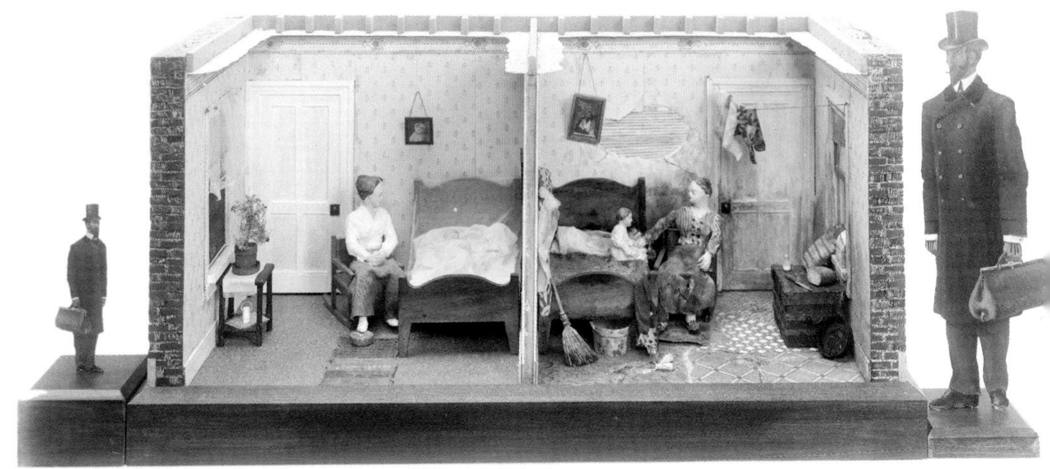

Image above: Model illustrating fly-borne diseases in screened and unscreened tenements. Photograph Kay C. Lenskjold, 1917. Image #36329. Courtesy of the American Museum of Natural History Library.

paradoxically, tend to highlight their ideological machinations most overtly. A 1917 diorama from the American Museum of American History, for example, was designed to educate audiences about the health benefits of window screens in urban environments. Yet the staging of the cross section of a tenement building clearly enacts a broader commentary about hygiene and class that has nothing to do with scientific data regarding the health risks posed by flies (following the logic of this rendering, the use of window screens allow one to hang picture frames with more precision). The decision to depict the need for health services via a scaled, doctor figure casts an ominous and paternalistic aura over the work, one that registers on an emotional rather than a rational register.

From the unabashed realm of entertainment, the dioramas featured in Lillie Santangelo's World in Wax Musee in Coney Island (in operation from 1926 through the mid-1980s) titillated audiences with effigies of important political figures and reenactments of freak births. Yet the Musee's most lurid and gripping dioramas restaged brutal murders and sex crimes as they unfolded. Santangelo described these displays as driven by a moral, educational mission:

Perez
electrocuted for the
East Side
apartment on March
25 1950.

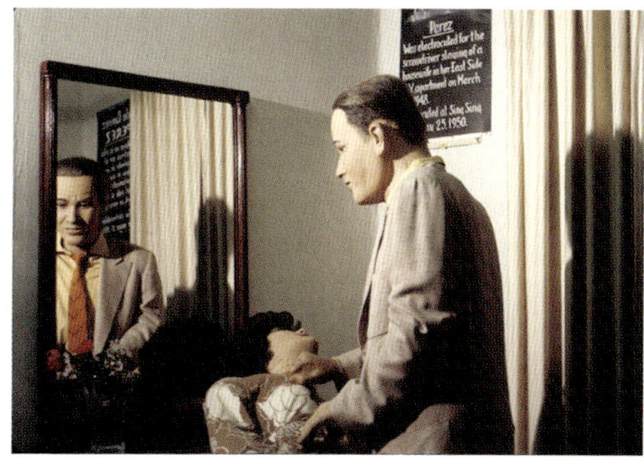

A wax show teaches the good things in life and also teaches that crime doesn't pay. What makes a person bad? What makes a clock tick, bad or good?[5]

Yet the lessons gleaned from the displays themselves are far more ambiguous. I'm particularly haunted by the image of Julio Ramirez Perez, captured in wax in the midst of strangling Mrs. Vera Lotito in 1948. Despite the passion of the crime, Perez's motionless figure seems lost in thought, his furrowed brow reflected in the mirror that forces him to contemplate his own countenance, as we contemplate him, suspended for all eternity.

In short, regardless of venue or point of origin, nearly all dioramas suggest an organizing moral or lesson. Yet these lessons are not necessarily what draw us to them, and they don't adequately describe what we learn, or what we remember.

Perhaps there is something about the mode of address of the diorama that warrants further consideration. Unlike peepshows, stereoscopes, or other single-viewer, nineteenth-century attractions, dioramas and tableaux are visible to multiple audience members. Nevertheless, these displays seem to encourage the perception of an intimate, singular experience. Like immersive spectacles such as the Daguerre diorama or the panorama, the staged diorama works to interpolate the spectator into a world

Image above: Depiction of the 1948 murder of Mrs. Vera Lotito by Julio Ramirez Perez, Lillie Beatrice Santangelo's World of Wax Musée. Photograph Costa Mantis, 1981. Courtesy of the Coney Island Museum.

[5] Lillie Santangelo, unpublished interview with Dick Zigun, 1981. Coney Island Museum Archive.

that feels crafted just for them. We are encouraged to linger, to indulge in our appreciation of each carefully crafted detail. As with the daguerreotype, we are highly aware of the diorama as a unique, auratic object. It is a public staging of a private, revelatory encounter.

Donna Haraway describes the Akeley Hall of African Mammals at the American Museum of Natural History in similar terms:

> One begins in the threatening chaos of the industrial city, part of a horde, but here one will come to belong, to find substance. No matter how many people crowd the great hall, the experience is of individual communion with nature. This is... the moment of origin where nature and culture, private and public, profane and sacred meet—a moment of incarnation in the encounter of man and animal.[6]

[6] *Donna Haraway, "Teddy Bear Patriarchy: Taxidermy in the Garden of Eden, New York City, 1908–1936," in* Social Text *11 (Winter 1984–85), 23.*

For Haraway, this encounter is enabled by the careful staging of each tableaux and the narratives they put into motion. But there is one element over all others, she argues, that holds human viewers transfixed: the gaze of at least one animal in each display is positioned to capture and hold that of the viewer through the glass. It is a meeting of looks that could never take place in nature:

> This is a spiritual vision made possible only by their death and literal representation. Only then could the essence of their life be present. Only then could the hygiene of nature cure the sick vision of civilized man. Taxidermy fulfills the fatal desire to represent, to be whole; it is a politics of reproduction.[7]

[7] *Ibid., 25.*

The art of taxidermy, like that of photography, is a prophylactic against death and decay. Each format stakes a claim in science,

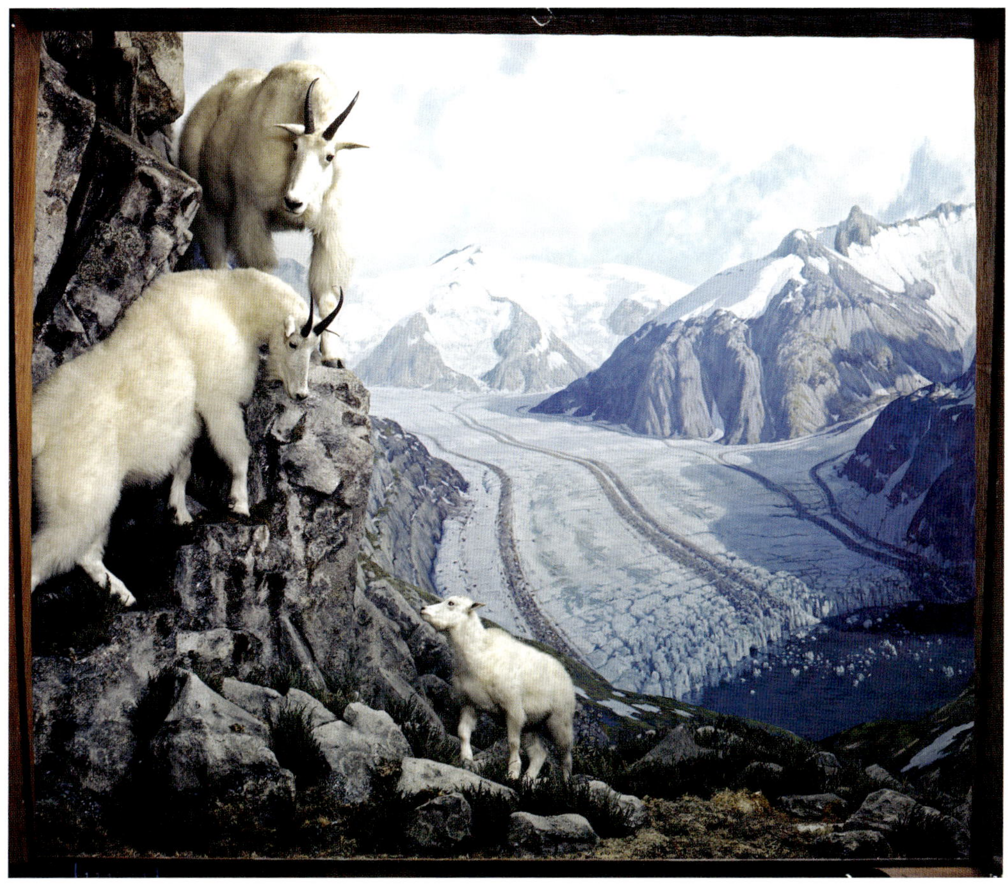

Image above: Mountain Goats, Bernard Family Hall of North American Mammals. Image #46. Courtesy of the American Museum of Natural History Library.

objectivity, and truth, forged via technology, colonialism, and the engines of capital. Each imagines a narrative, and each hails its viewers after the moment of capture has passed. Each is subject to the vision and fabrications of their creators, as well as to the accidental artifacts embalmed within their frames. And each is structured around the coincidence of multiple gazes: subject, viewer, artist. The resonances, and dissonances, between frozen and mobile looks creates a palpable tension, one in which the contemporary viewer is forced, however imperfectly, to see an image of herself reflected back.

There is an inevitable intrusion of anthropomorphism in the habitat dioramas. The idyllic family scenes in which groups of

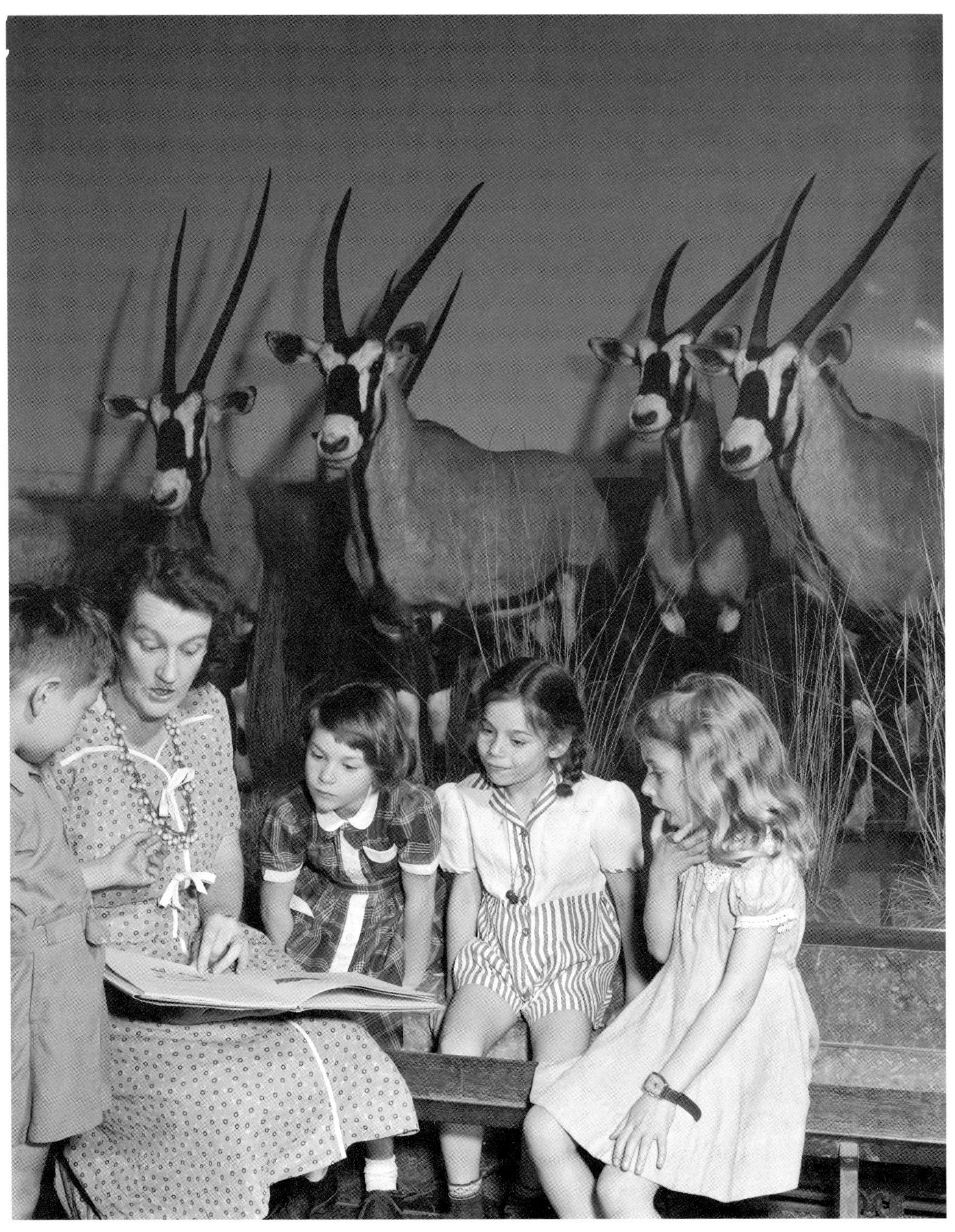

Katherine Barry reading to children at story hour. Photograph Edward Laurence Bailey, 1944. Image #298163. Courtesy of the American Museum of Natural History Library.

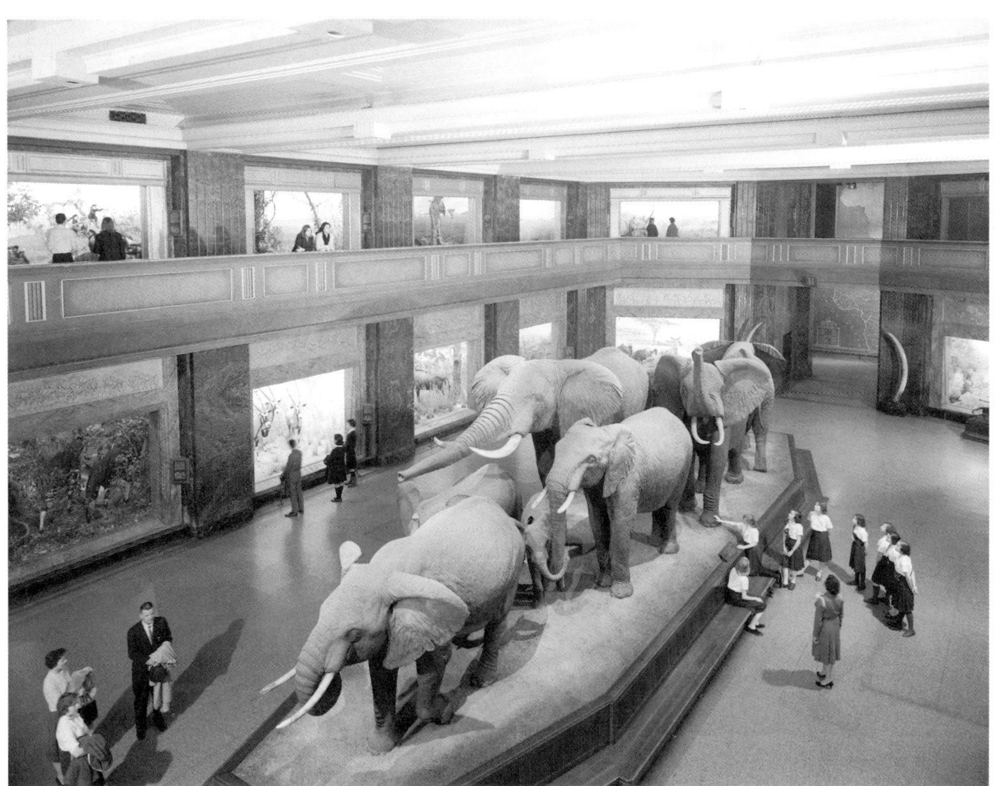

animals graze in fields unmarked by human intervention are undermined when one recalls that the real scenes that might have inspired these displays were disrupted by the violent act of gathering the "specimens" that comprise these artificially assembled herds. As we become implicated in the politically and ethically fraught relay of projection and reflection at work here, the boundaries of the framed world are revealed as porous, reality as staged, and our own constructed worlds as both fragile and alien.

Above image: Akeley African Hall. Photograph A.J. Rota, R. Sisson, and L. Boltin, 1962. Image #328663. Courtesy of the American Museum of Natural History Library.

Indeed, taxidermied dioramas delve deep into the guts of the subjects they stage, but they often tell us less about the bodies that comprise them than those who labored in their creation. Habitat diorama creators historically obtained their raw materials by going into the field to "collect specimens"—i.e.

kill live animals, bring them back to the museum setting, and reinfuse their corpses with artificial life. As with the memorial photographs, a fascination with the materiality of death often coexists with a visual denial that the death ever occurred. This duality extends not only to the body depicted, but also to those of the producer and viewer. Carl Akeley's mountain gorilla diorama manifests this paradox directly, as the scene recreated marks the spot of Akeley's own grave on Mount Mikeno, in the Democratic Republic of the Congo. The habitat diorama and the memorial photograph serve as graphic incarnations of *memento mori*, driven by the same moral reminder: remember you must die.

The dioramas created for nineteenth-century natural history museums are housed within stately monuments to Western narratives of technological mastery and cultural superiority. Here the mission to educate and to direct the undisciplined gaze of the spectator often butts up against the pure sensuality of the display, and the distracted state of the audience as they meander through the galleries. Anthropologist Franz Boas, mindful of this danger, advised that ethnographic displays at the American Museum of Natural History avoid the "ghastly impression" left by attempts at complete realism: "since there is a line of demarcation be-tween nature and plastic art, it is better to draw a line consciously than to try to hide it."[8] While Boas' motivation is surely quite different from my own, I find myself similarly drawn to those tableaux that most overtly celebrate their craft, or perhaps more accurately, those that flaunt their seams. What seems most useful to me in these circumstances is that the dioramas serve to highlight, rather than to resolve, the inherently fragmented and contradictory inclinations of their viewers.

[8] *As quoted in Griffiths,* Wondrous Difference, *24.*

Again, as with the postmortem daguerreotypes, I find a productive correspondence between "successful" and "failed"

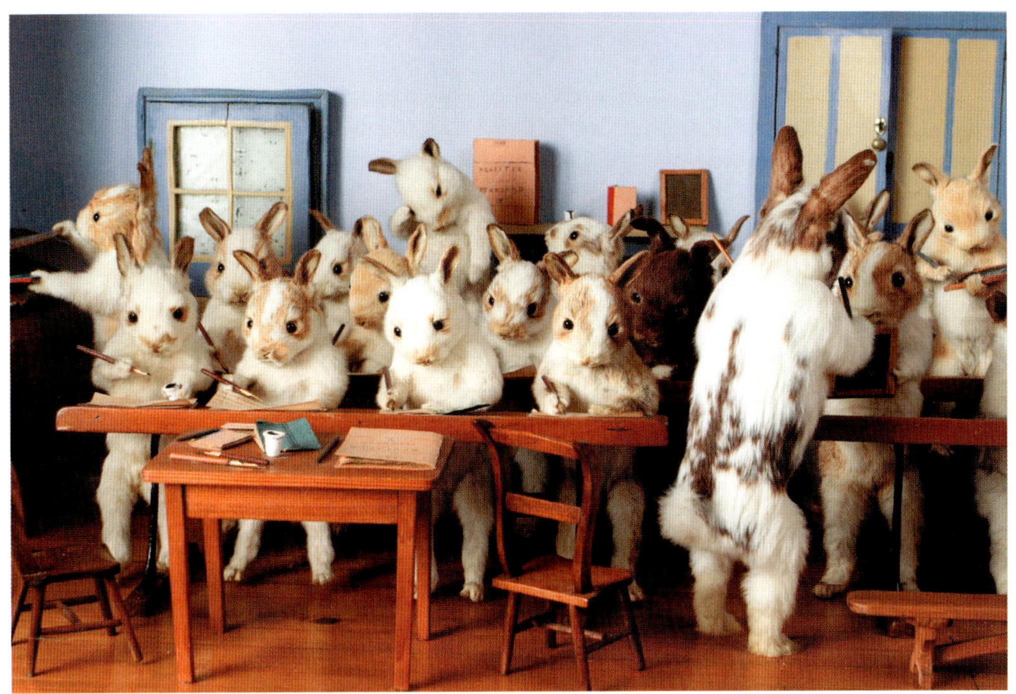

Image above: Walter Potter's The Rabbit's Village School. Courtesy of Eroll Fuller.

artistic tableaux. The awkward drape of fur stretched across a poorly crafted armature, the decrepit snout of a deer head as it hangs, neglected, on its mount—these sad siblings of the carefully tended museum display remind us of the fragility of preserved corporeal remains. Taxidermists such as Walter Potter seemed to relish drawing a firm line of demarcation between nature and art. The spectacular anthropomorphism of Potter's scenes is staggering, both for its whimsy and its utter excessiveness. *The Rabbits' Village School*, for example, features forty-eight juvenile rabbits at their various lessons in a one-room schoolhouse, peeking at each other's slates or reciting verse. There is an element of perversity and exploitation at work here, yet in its self-acknowledgement as pure human fabrication, the anthropomorphic diorama may be more honest than the righteous rationalizations of scientifically legitimized displays.

Perhaps no artist has pushed the plastic potentials of the staged diorama further than Marcel Duchamp in his final work *Étant donnés: 1° la chute d'eau / 2° le gaz d'éclairage*.... Created in secret from 1946 to 1966, *Étant donnés* is viewed through a pair of peepholes bored in a rough wooden door. Peering inside, the viewer looks through a gaping hole in a brick wall to see a nude female form, reclining with her legs splayed on a bed of twigs, her head obscured from view, holding an illuminated gas lamp in her raised hand. The back wall of the tableau features a meticulously rendered landscape of hills and trees and what appears to be a flowing waterfall. The flickering of the gas lamp and the simulated water act as counterpoint to the motionless body. The skin of the female figure was crafted using animal skin parchment stretched over a substructure of putty, lead strips and various bracing elements (metal tubing, wood, steel-wire screen).[9] The effect of Duchamp's laborious process is strikingly fleshy, although the shape of the form itself is unnerving. The proportions and angles feel off-kilter, and the exposed, hairless genitals that comprise the focal point of the piece are grotesquely, ambiguously formed.

[9] *Melissa S. Meighan, "A Technical Discussion of the Figure in Marcel Duchamp's* Étant donnés*" in Michael R. Taylor,* Marcel Duchamp: Étant donnés *(Philadelphia: Philadelphia Museum of Art, 2009), 247.*

Étant donnés is inscrutable. It is a scene that begs for a narrative, yet refuses to supply one. The body on display titillates, transfixes, and disturbs; it readily exposes its most hidden recesses, but tells us nothing of its identity or status. Even questions of gender, ironically, are vexingly uncertain, given the indefinite sculpting of the form. Is this a figure in repose? A victim of a crime? The lines between life and death, wholeness and dismemberment are indeterminate. Of even greater complexity is the perspectival structure of the tableau, which contains a room within a room, and a posed figure who returns our gaze not with the glassy eyes of the upholstered beast (to channel Haraway), but with her centrally positioned genitalia, the organizing locus of the work. As Jean-François Lyotard famously suggested about this composition,

> In this type of organization, the viewpoint and the vanishing point are symmetrical. Thus if it is true that the latter is the vulva, this is the specular image of the peeping eyes; such that: when these think they're seeing the vulva, they see themselves. Con celui qui voit. He who sees is a cunt.[10]

It is a taunt that simultaneously foregrounds and inverts the whole history of Western visual culture.

Perhaps it is an already familiar truism that we see only ourselves reflected in the world of the diorama. We create the museum to erect monuments to ourselves. We flock to the midway and the movie theater to replay our primal collective anxieties. What I'd like to suggest is that we have much to learn from those tableaux that unsettle, disturb, and expose the operations of these viewing machines. We ought to pay attention to the uncanny dissonances of the failed or awkward waxwork, of the decayed or idiosyncratic habitat display. We should trace the resonances between these marginal incarnations and the strange, but often unquestioned aesthetics of our collective cultural mythology. It is here, in the space between past and present, margin and periphery, that we can begin to excavate the visual mechanics of our old master narratives, and, perhaps, to imagine for ourselves newly transformative miniature worlds.

[10] *Jean-François Lyotard,* Les TRANS-formateurs DUchamp *(Paris: Galilee, 1977), 137-38, as quoted in Kaja Silverman,* The Threshold of the Visible *(New York: Routledge, 1995), 172. Silverman notes that* "con" *("cunt") is also used as a chiding term for men in a manner roughly equivalent to "prick" in English, making Lyotard's phrasing sympathetically ambiguous. See also Taylor,* Marcel Duchamp: Étant donnés, *192.*

THE BIRTH OF VENUS

JOANNA EBENSTEIN

The agony of a young woman is represented in her last instant of life as she abandons herself to death voluptuously and completely naked. The thorax and abdomen can be opened, allowing the various parts to be disassembled so as to simulate the act of anatomic dissection.
—Description of wax anatomical Venus from the Palazzo Poggi website

For men to be instructed, they must be seduced by aesthetics, but how can anyone render the image of death agreeable?
—Arnaud Éloi Gautier-d'Agoty (1741–1771), anatomical illustrator and son of renowned anatomical printmaker Jacques-Fabien Gautier d'Agoty (1711–1785)

...the death then, of a beautiful woman is, unquestionably, the most poetical topic in the world...
—Edgar Allan Poe, "The Philosophy of Composition"

THE ANATOMICAL VENUS IS THE CENTRAL OBJECT OF MY SCHOLARLY and artistic veneration. She baffles and intrigues; she confounds all attempts to understand, elucidate, or explain. She is, it seems to me, the departure point for a hundred paths, a thousand stories, a score of histories it would take several lifetimes to see

PHILOSOPHICAL HALL,

HUDDERSFIELD,

FOR A VERY LIMITED PERIOD ONLY.

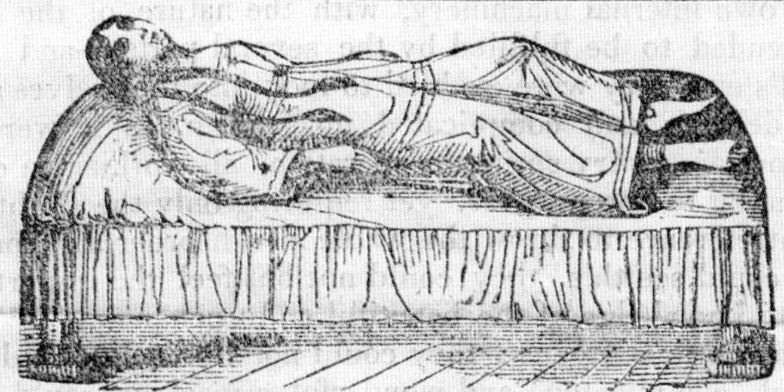

"KNOW THYSELF"

SIGNOR SARTI'S

CELEBRATED FLORENTINE

ANATOMICAL VENUS,

TOGETHER WITH

NUMEROUS SMALLER MODELS OF SPECIAL INTEREST TO LADIES,

SHOWING THE

MARVELLOUS MECHANISM OF THE HUMAN BODY,

" That small tenement in which the Soul of Man resides."

Admitted by the Lords of the Treasury free of duty, on the ground of public utility, and acknowledged by the most distinguished Medical Professors—Sir James Clarke, W. Lawrence, Erasmus Wilson, Esqrs., the late Dr. Birkbeck, &c., &c., to be faithfully correct in Anatomical Structure.

LADIES Admitted every MONDAY & THURSDAY.

Tuesday, Wednesday, Friday and Saturday, for Gentlemen.

Lectures illustrative of the sources of Health and Disease. will be given each day at the hours of Eleven, Two, Half-past Three, Seven, and Half-past Eight.

ADMISSION,........ONE SHILLING.

Open daily from TEN till FIVE, and from SIX till Half-past NINE.

N. B. Anatomical and Physiological description of the Florentine Venus, together with the causes, Symptons, and Treatment of the diseases of the principal Organs.—Second Edition, greatly enlarged and improved—Price Sixpence.

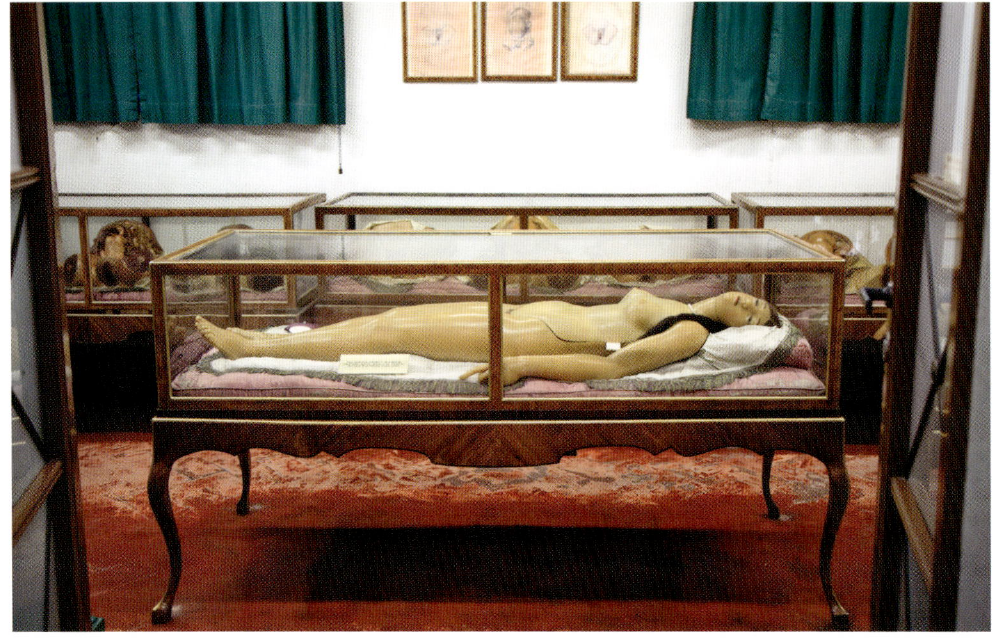

"Anatomical Venus" with human hair and pearls in rosewood and Venetian glass case probably modeled by Clemente Susini (around 1790); On view at, and courtesy of, La Specola, Zoological Section of the Natural History Museum of the University of Florence. Photo by the author.

Image previous page: Senor Sarti's Celebrated Female Anatomical Venus pamphlet. 1847. Courtesy of the Wellcome Library, London.

through to their end points. She is a Pandora's box of paradoxes revealing, in object form, a worldview at once utterly alien and yet somehow also deeply familiar. She flickers along the edges of our categories, complicating them while also drawing attention to their arbitrary nature. In her, we witness a promiscuous intermingling of eros and thanatos; life and death; science and art; animate and inanimate; kitsch and a startling beauty.

How could a creature so perplexing and peculiar to the modern eye have seemed, at one point, the perfect way to demonstrate anatomical understandings of the body? How could our cultural attitudes have changed to such an extent that she, who once seemed the perfect way of expressing anatomical understanding, now seems bizarre to the contemporary eye? How might these differences help us to better understand the historical moment of her creation as well as our own time? How can we use our own response to these confounding creatures as a way to understand how we might have changed, what we might have lost?

The Venus and Her Kin

The Anatomical Venus and her sisters—The Slashed Beauties, and the Dissected Graces—were created around 1780, by the wax workshop of the Museum of Zoology and Natural History in Florence, Italy, best known as "la Specola." Founded by Pietro Leopoldo of Lorraine, Grand Duke of Tuscany and Holy Roman Emperor in 1775, as the first truly public science museum in Europe, these spectacular life-sized wax women were the jewel on the crown of an already astounding collection of *naturalia* drawn from the former Medici *wunderkammern*; the newly opened museum contained hundreds of wax models depicting the anatomical and pathological human body as well as room after room of clumsy taxidermy, skeletons, wax animals and plants, and instruments and other elements of the Medici collection deemed scientific in nature.

The Venus and her sisters were created especially for the museum at an in-house, wax-crafting workshop established by the duke under the directorship of Felice Fontana, physicist to the court of the Grand Duke of Tuscany, and the artistic leadership of master artist Clemente Susini. These wax women were intended from their very conception to instruct, attract, and delight a popular audience and, from the moment of their public debut, they did just that, drawing a wide audience of both local Tuscans and foreigners on the Grand Tour circuit.

The life-sized, anatomically correct wax Anatomical Venus was the pinnacle of both artistic and pedagogical perfection. With the lifting of her breastplate, she could be dissected and reassembled in layers revealing the ideal female body of its time.

The final remove revealed the central mystery of the female body: a tiny glistening fetus tranquilly curled up in a bloodless womb. Her sister waxes, the Slashed Beauty and the Dissected Graces, are not dissectible but, rather, eternally fixed in a seemingly spontaneous, pain-free, and bloodless *auto*-dissection, a sort of extreme anatomical *dishabille.*

Each is far more lifelike and lovelier than seems strictly educationally necessary. Augmented with gleaming Venetian glass eyes and real human hair, they don, in turn, strings of pearls or golden tiaras, and recline or writhe rapturously in baroque Venetian glass and rosewood coffins on cascades of silk and plush, moth-eaten velvet cushions. A few of them idly finger plaits of their golden (human) hair, while others appear to writhe in uncontrollable ecstasy, clutching at their silk cushions with graceful waxen hands. They seem to be, all at once, incorruptible saints, anatomical visualizations, and provocative and slightly perverse artwork. They remind one of the wax "saints in boxes" which fill the churches of Italy; of reclining Venuses seen in paintings at the Uffizi; of *ex votos*—or wax body parts commemorating or imploring a saints intervention on the behalf of one's body. They also suggest life sized *memento mori*—objects intended to remind the beholder that they, too, will die, and thus implores them to live a moral life for which they would be eternally rewarded in heaven—or sexy dolls intended, perhaps, for unspeakable use.

In their catalog for the exhibition *Spectacular Bodies,* Martin Kemp and Marina Wallace shine light on the confusing nature of early anatomical representations by pointing out that

> The purpose of anatomical images during the period from the Renaissance to the nineteenth century had as much to do with what we would call aesthetic and theological understanding as with the narrower intentions of medical

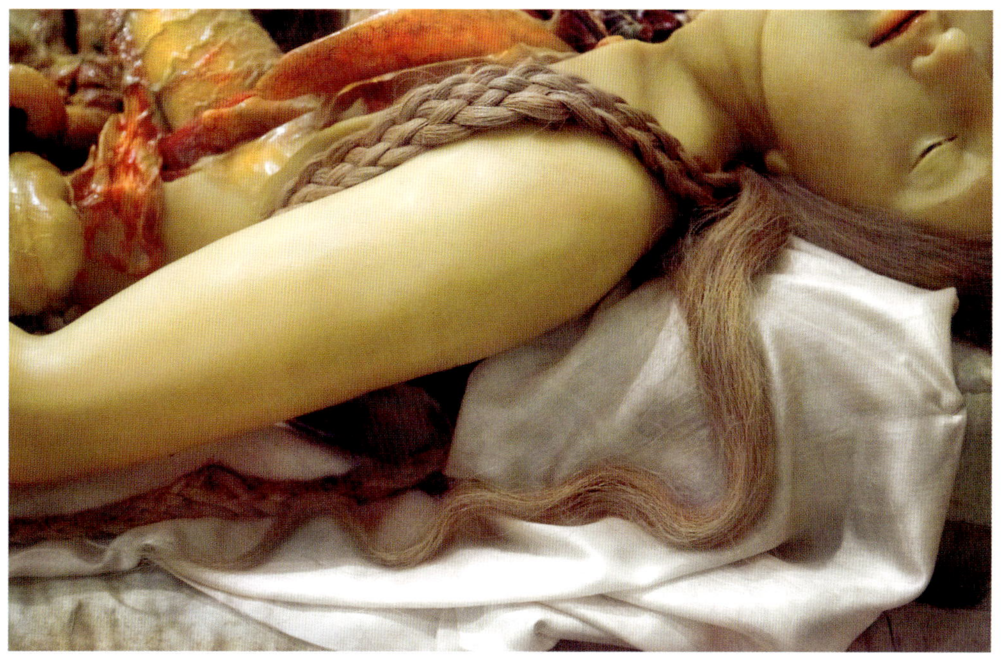

The wax statue was made in 1794 by Clemente Susini in Florence. Courtesy of the University Museum System of Pavia, Museum for the History of the University; Photo by the author.

> illustration as now understood.... They were not simply instructional diagrams for the doctor technician, but statements about the nature of human beings as made by God in the context of the created world as a whole. They are about the nature of life and death...[1]

Indeed, at the time of their creation, science as we now think of it did not yet exist; the Venus and her sisters are products of the more heterogeneous worldview of natural philosophy, which sought to understand the natural world in ways we would now term "scientific" along with ways we might now term occult, mystical, and magical. The human body in particular held special significance; if humankind was understood to be created

[1] *Martin Kemp and Marina Wallace,* Spectacular Bodies: The Art and Science of the Human Body from Leonardo to Now *(Berkeley: University of California Press, 2000), 11, 68.*

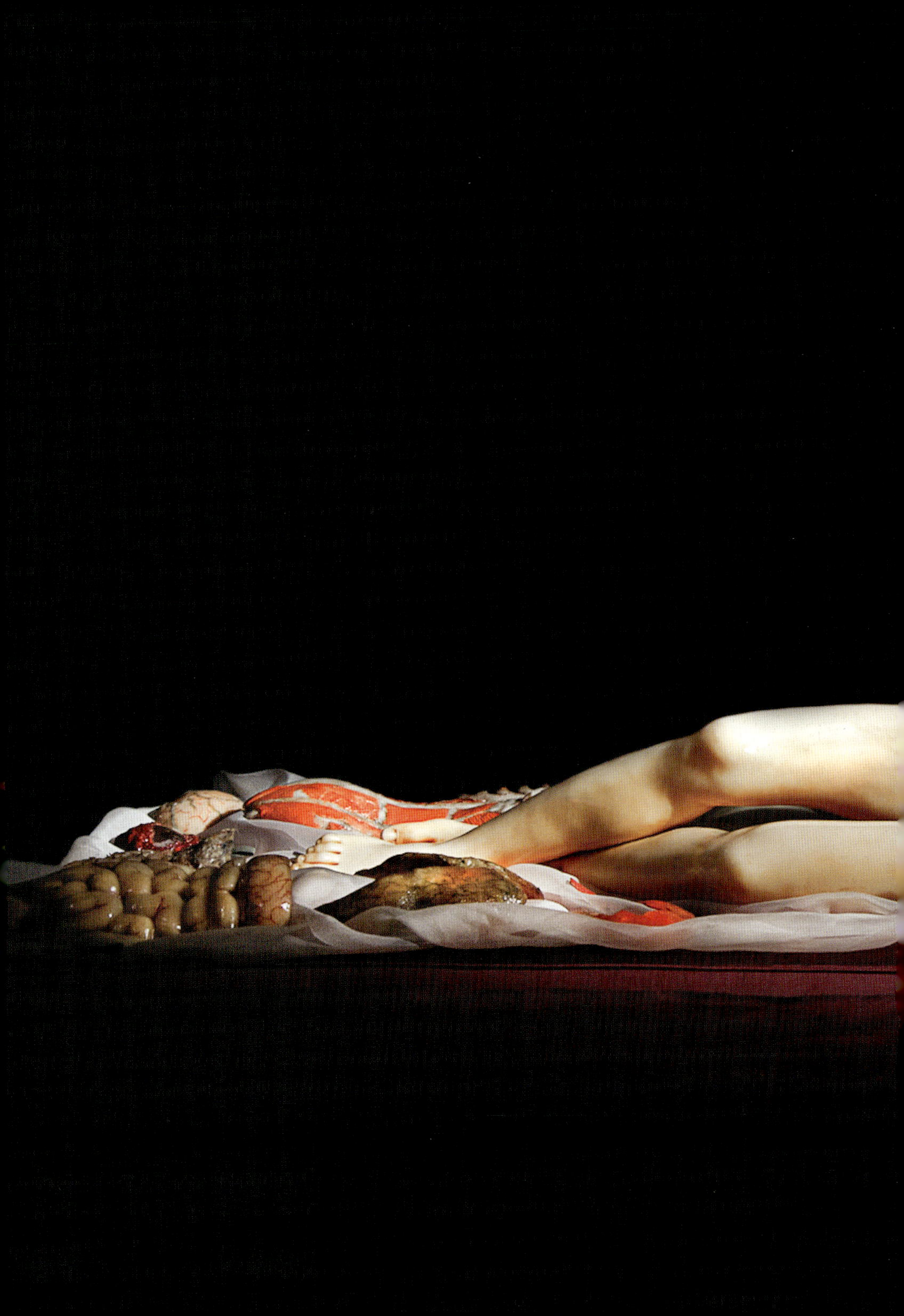

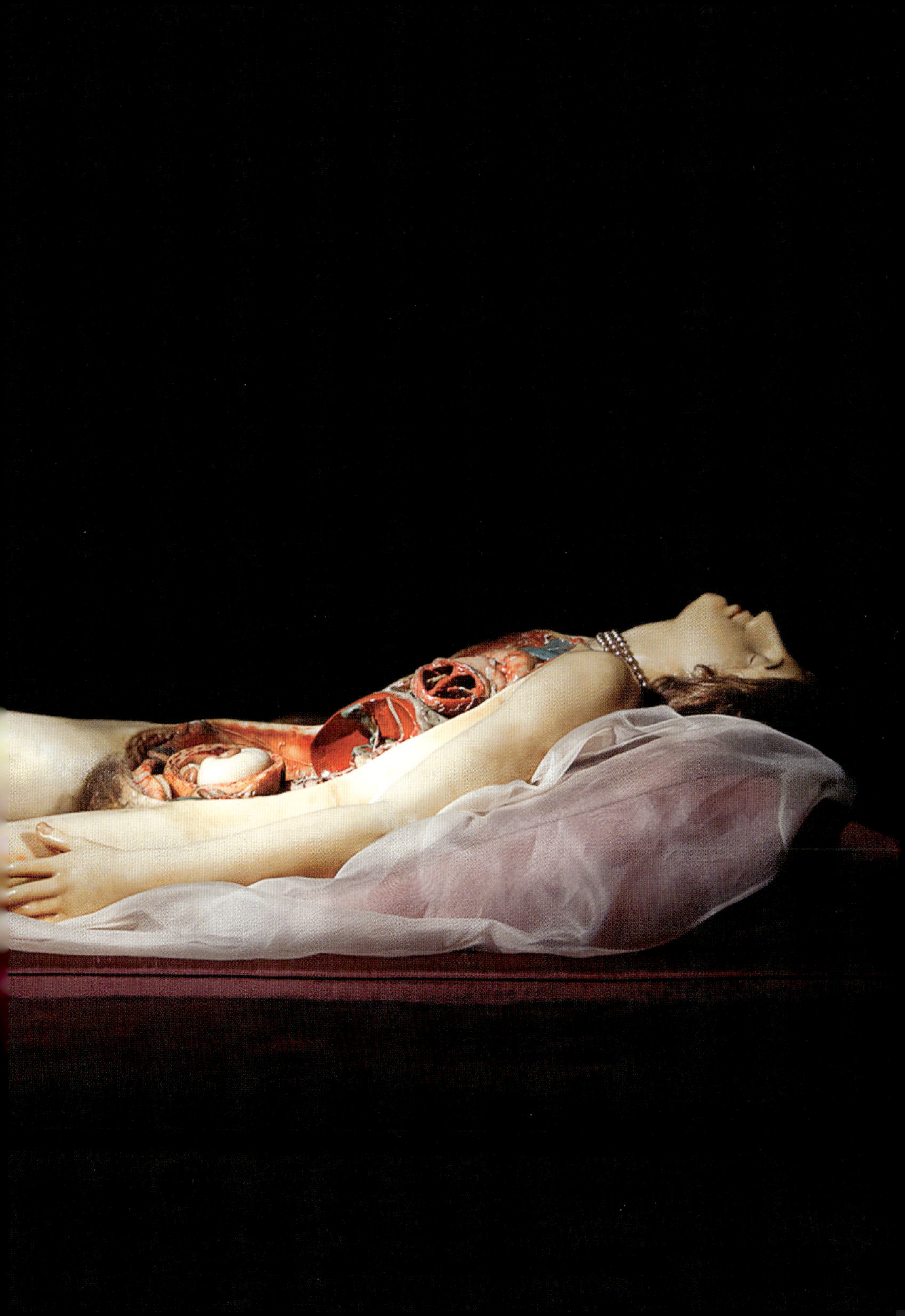

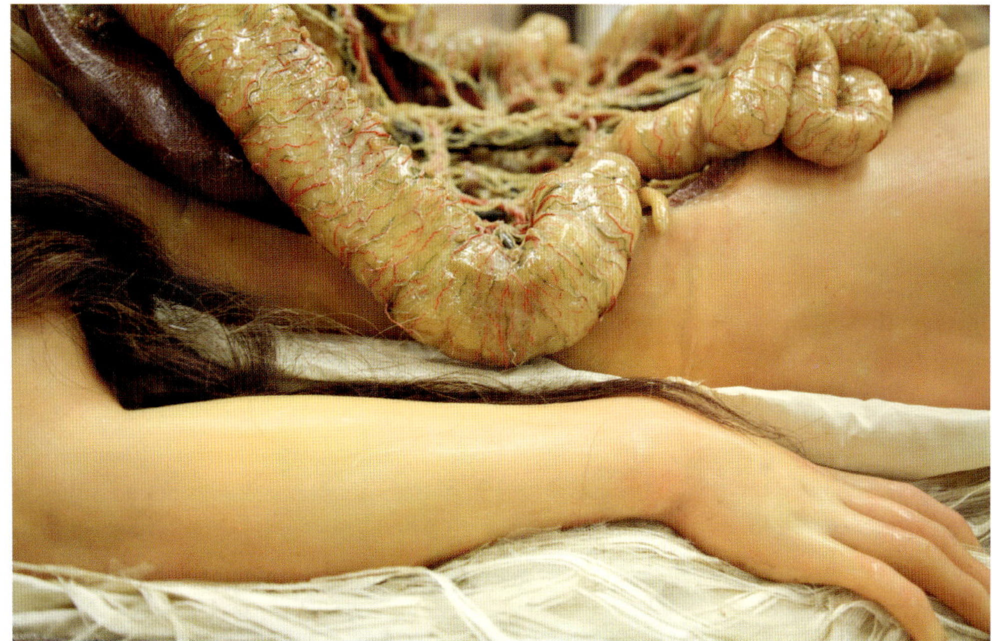

"The Slashed Beauty" with human hair and pearls in rosewood and Venetian glass case, probably modeled by Clemente Susini (around 1790); On view at, and courtesy of, La Specola, Zoological Section of the Natural History Museum of the University of Florence. Photo by the author.

in God's image, then certainly to know the human body was to know the mind of God, and the pursuit of the secrets of the human body must be sacred in nature.

The Anatomical Venus and her dissected sisters were, then, an idealized reflection of this universal notion of the human form; they were also the realization of the noble dream of an end to the need for human dissection, a way to teach anatomy without having to resort to the ethical and logistical troubles implicit in the practice. Unlike an actual cadaver, these models revealed their secrets and mysteries to all, layman, student, and physician alike, in a clear and *beautiful* way, transforming the body into an easily readable cipher. The immaculate, peaceful and bloodless nature of these models—who seem so far removed

Image previous page: The "Venerina" or "Little Venus" anatomical model by Clemente Susini, 1782. Courtesy of the Palazzo Poggi, Bologna, Italy. Photo by the author.

from death and pain, engaging the viewer with calm glass-eyed gazes as they offer forth their viscera like so many glisteningly pristine jewels—made them attractive to, and appropriate for, a non-specialist audience. They also disguise the violence behind their creation, and, indeed, all anatomical knowledge, which relied on scores of the unfortunate dead in order to create just one single demountable model.

The Allure of the Venus

With her evocative and appealing *frisson* of sexuality and rationality, it is perhaps no surprise that the Susini/Fontana Anatomical Venus was neither the first nor the last of its kind produced in order to delight, educate, titillate and attract a popular audience. In 1719—years before our Florentine Venus—the French anatomist Guillaume Desnoues publicly exhibited a dissectible wax woman with a newborn child still attached to its umbilical cord. In 1733, the Paris-trained anatomist, surgeon, and modeler Abraham Chovet exhibited in London a "representation of a woman big with child chained upon a table; supposed to be opened alive. In the face there is a lively display of the agonies of a dying person, the whole body heaving and the hands clinched, the action suitable to the character of the subject." This ingenious piece demonstrated the circulation of the blood during pregnancy via a network of blown glass tubes filled with claret, and was later purchased and shown as a centerpiece by Benjamin Rackstrow (proprietor of a popular eighteenth-century London museum) in 1772.[2] Around the same time, Marie Marguerite Biheron, a French anatomical modeler, exhibited a full-size body of a woman that could be opened up and taken apart like those at La Specola.[3] Bologna's open to the public anatomical collection—which served as inspiration for the one at La Specola—featured a wax-

[2] *Matthew Craske, "'Unwholesome' and 'pornographic': A reassessment of the place of Rackstrow's Museum in the story of eighteenth-century anatomical collection and exhibition,"* Journal of the History of Collections *23, no. 1 (May 2011): 75-99.*

over-bone "Anatomical Eve" with her Adam flanked by human skeletons posed with scythes like personifications of death; these went on display in 1747 in a collection established by Pope Benedict XIV as part of his campaign to reduce superstition through education and enlightenment values.

The famed La Specola Venus herself also inspired a variety of knockoffs: dozens of "Florentine" or "Medician" Venuses crafted to draw customers to the popular anatomical museums and touring anatomical displays popular with audiences up from the eighteenth until the early twentieth century in Europe and the United States. A particularly famous example was the automated *breathing* Venus showcased by the Musée Spitzner, a typical popular anatomical museum of its time. Opened in Paris in 1856 by self-styled "doctor" Pierre Spitzner under the banner "Science, Art, Progress!," it resided at a permanent location in Paris until the 1880s when it took to the road, traveling the great fairgrounds circuits of France, Britain, Germany, Holland and Belgium until finally closing its doors during World War II.

The Spitzner Collection is unique in that it remained a viable business for so long, and also in that it still exists—as part of a larger medical museum—in a relatively intact state, with its remarkable pieces in excellent repair and looking much like they must have to early viewers. It is also remarkable for the cultural ripples it left in its wake. Surrealist Paul Delvaux cited Spitzner's breathing Venus—clearly already strange to the twentieth century eye—as a life and art-changing moment, and the inspiration for the somnambulant women who peopled his paintings; in his own words: "All my Sleeping Venuses originate there.... [They are] an exact transcription of the Sleeping Venus of the Spitzner Museum, but with Greek temples or with models—anything you like. It is different, but the understanding is the same."[4] Also, despite a lack of citation,

[4] *Paul Delvaux,* Paul Delvaux 1897–1994 *(Brussels, 1997), 18.*

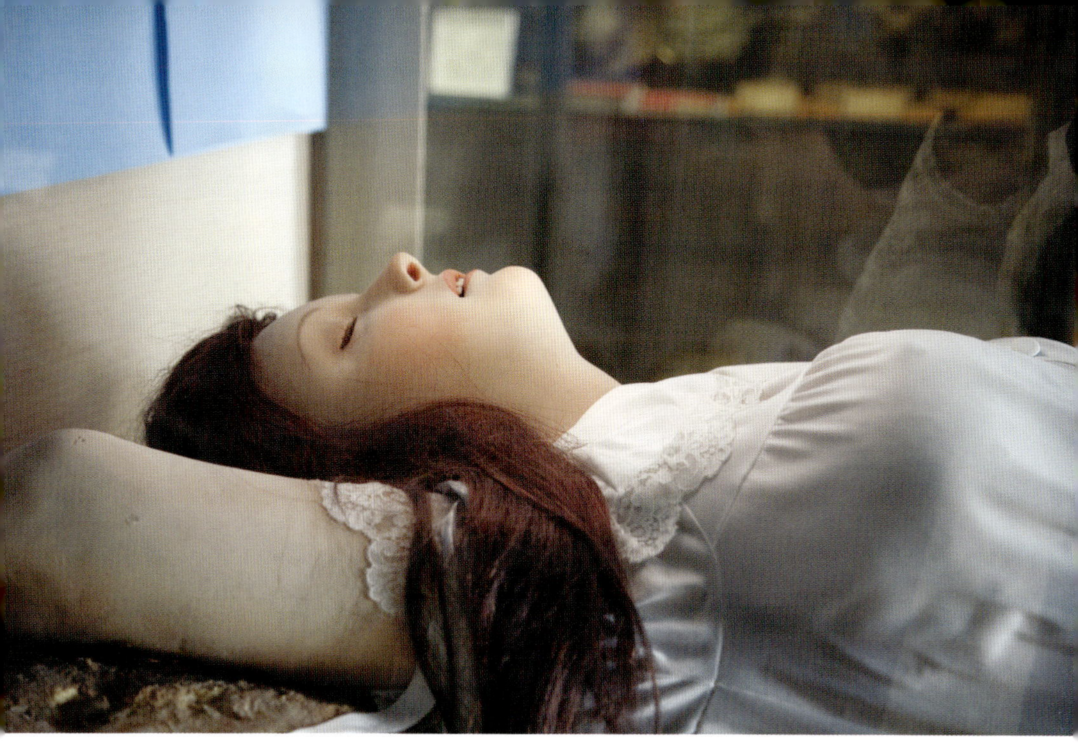

Venus Endormie (breathing wax model), Spitzner collection Collection Spitzner, Musée Orfila; Courtesy of Musée Orfila, 45 rue des Saints Pères, Paris 6ème FranceCourtesy of the Université Paris Descartes. Photo by the author.

I am intuitively certain that Marcel Duchamp was directly inspired by, if not this very collection, then a very similar one, when creating his enigmatic and haunting Étant donnés.[5]

[5] *See Amy Herzog's essay in this volume.*

Wax

Another element of the special resonance of the Venus is the material of wax itself. Wax has long been linked to death—at least as far back as ancient Rome, where wax portraits of the dead were displayed in the atria of homes and carried in funerals. Magical properties have also long been attributed to wax as in its use in the fashioning of dolls for casting dark magic on one's enemies. It was also used for a host of Catholic magical objects, including the *Agnus Deis* (discs of wax impressed with the figure of a lamb and blessed at stated seasons by the Pope) and especially, due to its uncannily skin-like appearance, for sacred stand-ins

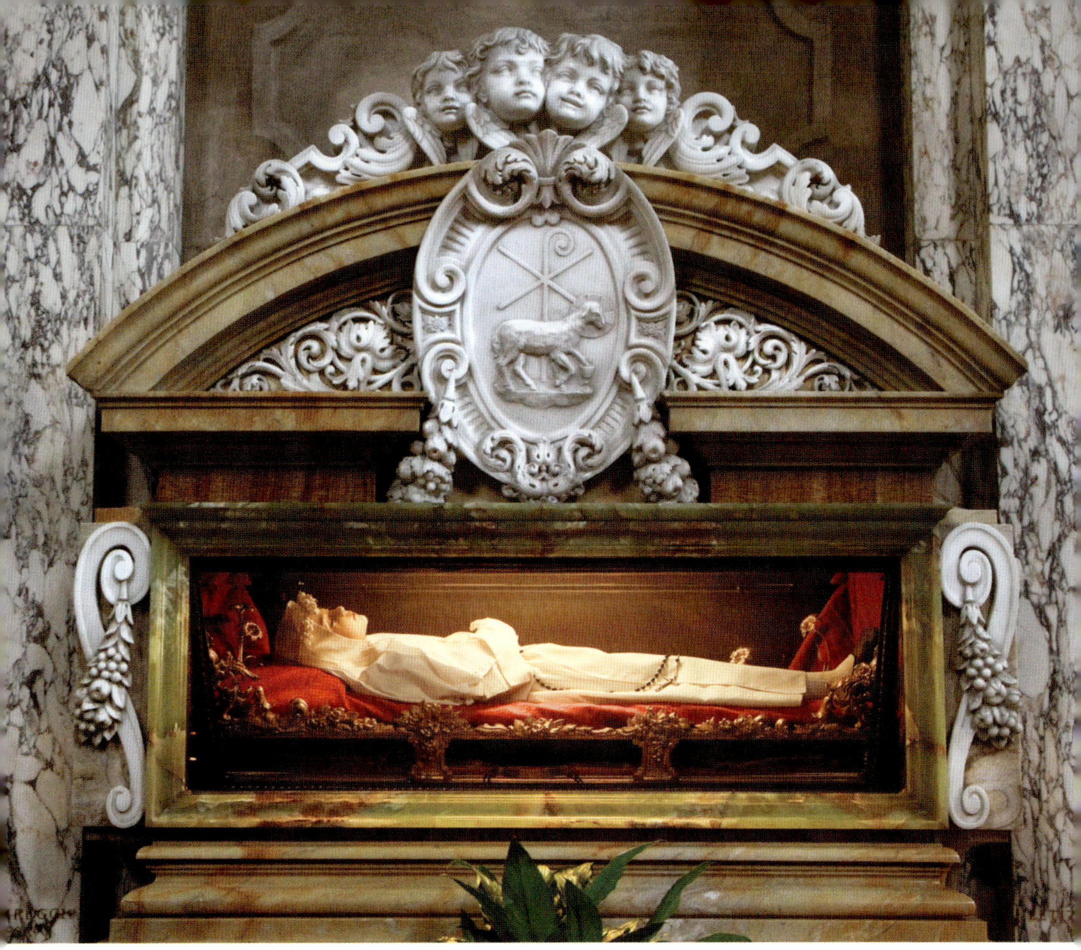

Image above: Wax effigy of "Blessed Imelda Lambertini," an adolescent who fell into a fatal swoon of overwhelming joy at the moment of her first communion with Jesus Christ, as seen at a church in Bologna, Italy. She is now the patron saints of first communions. Photo by the author.

for the human body including *ex votos,* effigies of saints, and the care and touch ups of "incorruptibles," the corpses of saints whose lack of decomposition prove their sanctity.[6]

Florence, the home of La Specola, had, indeed, been a famed center of wax crafting since the thirteenth century, specializing in votives and effigies serving the pilgrims who flocked to the Florentine church of Santissima Annunziata. In this church was a painting of the Virgin Mary said to provide miraculous healings; pilgrims would offer wax *ex votos* or leave behind life-sized wax statues dressed in their own clothes as acts of commemoration and sacred offerings. At one point, there were so many *ex votos* and effigies hanging from the church that, it is said, every available space was covered, and it was not unheard of for waxworks to fall on and harm the worshippers below. This veritable museum of votives was destroyed as part of a larger series of policy changes instituted by Pope Benedict XIV to discourage superstition in the church by, among other things, discouraging the practice of votive offerings and the use of the wax *Agnus Deis*. Hand in hand with these policy changes—and part of the same aim—was the establishment of the first scientific museums, with the torch being passed from religion to medicine, via the continuum of wax simulacra of the human body.

[6] *Roberta Ballestriero, "The History of Ceroplastics/Wax Modelling," in* Flesh and Wax: The Clemente Susini's Anatomical Models in the University of Cagliari, *ed. Alessandro Riva (Nuoro, Italy: Ilisso, 2007), 17-34.*

Much of the intrigue in these waxes, then, their enchanting incongruity, the nature of their flickering, perhaps stems from the fact that both realities are still very present and strongly resonate in the wax form of the Anatomical Venus. Florence was, after all, famed for the expertise of its wax workers in the creation of lifelike human bodies and body parts, in a sacred context; the skilled artisans put out of work by the new Catholic guidelines must surely have found work in the new studios dedicated to *scientific* waxes. Clemente Susini, creator of the Venus himself, is known to have created at least one religious wax—a poignant dying Christ—while a wax effigy of Saint Imelda Lambertini was created by a wax worker best remembered today for his anatomical works. There were surely many other examples of artists working on both religious and anatomical works, and, in a sense, the broad approach to knowing the natural world that characterized natural philosophy cultivated this overlap, combining ways of understanding the body and, indeed, the world that ranged from cosmology to the nature of death and disease to what we now think of as medical science.

The genesis myth of wax anatomical modeling beautifully illustrates these overlaps and this ontological confusion. The first anatomical waxwork in the modern sense was created by a Sicilian abbot named Gaetano Giulio Zummo, or Zumbo, around 1700, the product of what could be described as a sort of mystic marriage between the nascent science of human anatomy and the centuries old art of *memento mori*. Before the first anatomical model, Zumbo was well known as a master wax worker who created obsessive, wax miniature *memento mori*-themed tableaux he called his "Theaters of Death;" they bore such names such as "The Plague," "The Transience of Human Glory," and "The Triumph of Time," and featured exactingly rendered dead, decomposing and exquisitely tortured bodies. His work drew the attention of both the Grand Duke Cosimo of Tuscany—who became Zumbo's patron—and the Marquis de Sade, who said of one of his pieces: "So powerful is the impression produced by this masterpiece that even as you gaze at it your other senses are played upon, moans audible, you wrinkle your nose as if you could detect the evil odours of mortality.... These scenes of the plague appealed to my cruel imagination: and I mused, how many persons had undergone these awful metamorphoses thanks to my wickedness?"[7]

[7] *Jane Eade, "The Theatre of Death" in* Oxford Art Journal *Special Issue: Theorizing Wax: On the Meaning of a Disappearing Medium 36, no. 1 (2013): 109-125.*

Around 1700, Zumbo was approached by the French surgeon Guillaume Desnoues to use his renowned skills to create a likeness in wax of an important medical preparation which was beginning to decompose. The product of Desnoues' and Zumbo's collaboration was the first wax anatomical teaching model; it also established the tradition of an artistic/medical partnership in the creation of such tools.

On Death

The Anatomical Venus, then, is the enchanted predecessor of contemporary, more seemingly neutral forms of bio-medical visualization, sleeping beauties from a previous era. Her visual incongruity, the nature of her categorical flickering, can be

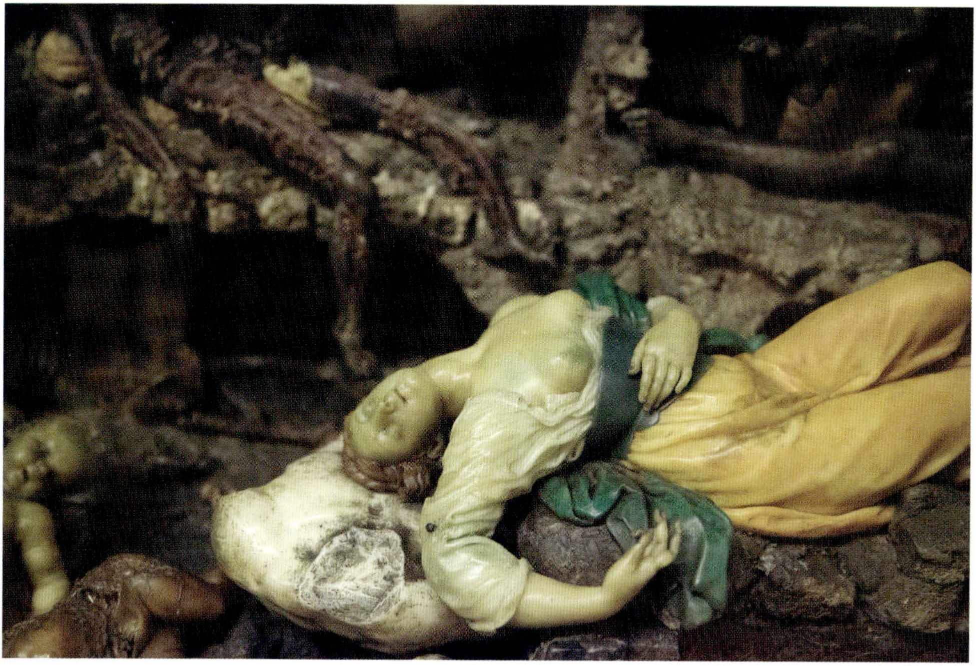

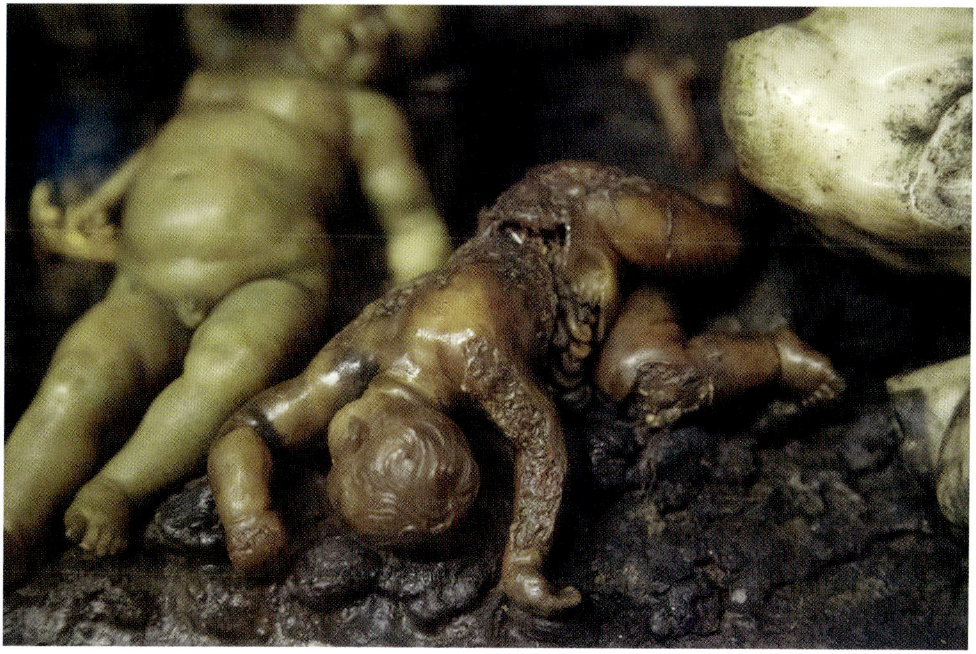

Details from Zumbo's Theatre of Death entitled "The Triumph of Time" circa 1690; On view at, and courtesy of, La Specola, Zoological Section of the Natural History Museum of the University of Florence. Photo by the author.

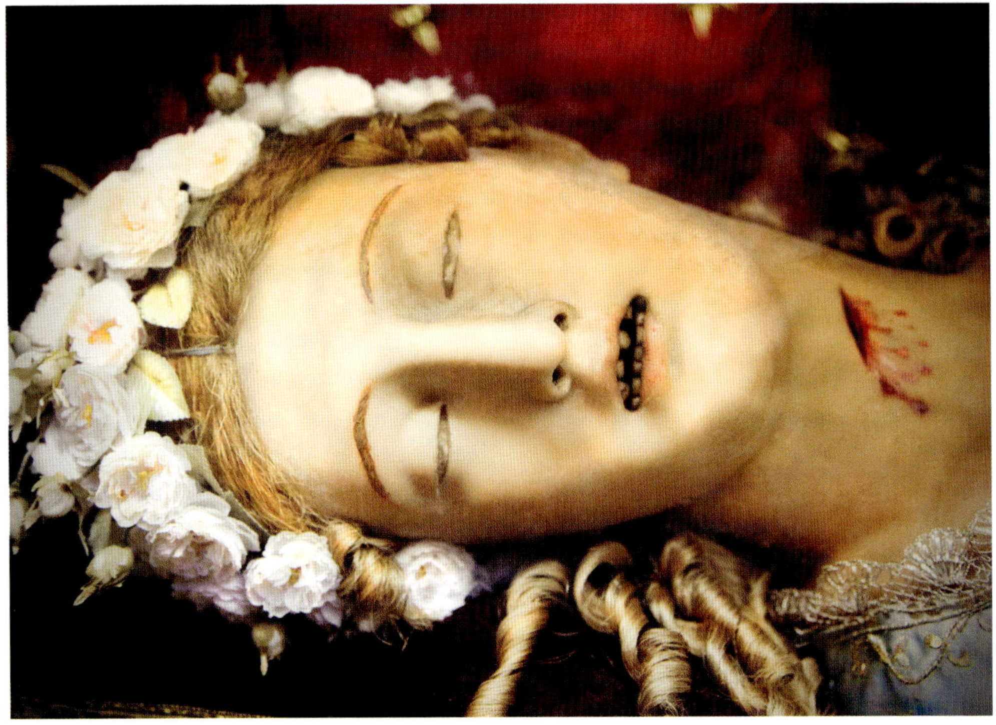

Wax effigy containing the bones and teeth of Saint Vittoria, or Victoria, on view in the church of Santa Maria della Vittoria, directly across from Bernini's masterwork "The Ecstasy of Saint Theresa." Photo by the author.

understood by the historically loaded materiality of the wax, the tangled web of their creation merging *memento mori* with medicine, and the universalistic approaches of natural philosophy.

Perhaps this complication alludes also to the nature of death itself, and the formal and functional similarities between religion and medicine, which both seek to keep death and disease at bay. If *ex votos* and wax saints represent God's intervention on our behalf against death and disease, medicine seeks *science's* intervention. What is medicine, after all, but the latest (and arguably most successful) of a long line of strategies intended to cheat death, and ensure our personal survival, regardless of "fate," "destiny," or God's will?

This is all a reminder that the divisions we have between death and beauty, eros and thanatos, religion and medicine, spectacle and education are products of our own contemporary perspective; our discomfort with the material culture of the past reveals more about us than about them. Perhaps the draw of the Venus comes from an unspoken, intuited but completely understood resolution of our own divided nature, as an unconscious comprehension that she might suggest another avenue abandoned, one in which beauty and science, religion and medicine, soul and body, might be one.

[This article is indebted to the scholars who have worked with and translated this material from the Italian, especially Roberta Ballestriero, Anna Maerker, Rebecca Messbarger, and Lucia Dacome. It is also indebted to the work of Michael Sappol, Ludmilla Jordanova, and Mark Dery. Special thanks is also due to Amy Herzog who invited me to write—and generously edited—the article on which this was based: "Ode to an Anatomical Venus," published in WSQ Journal *(Volume 40:3 & 4), 2013]*

[BIBLIOGRAPHY]

Ballestriero, Roberta. "Anatomical models and wax Venuses: art masterpieces or scientific craft works?" *Journal of Anatomy* 2010 February; 216(2): 223–234.

Ballestriero, Roberta. "The history of ceroplastics." *Flesh and Wax: The Clemente Susini's anatomical models in the University of Cagliari.* [Nuoro, Italy]: Ilisso, 2007.

Barnett, Richard. "The art of medicine: Lost wax: medicine and spectacle in Enlightenment London." *Lancet.* 372, no. 9636: 366-7, 2008.

Burmeister, Maritha Rene. Popular Anatomical Museums in

Nineteenth-Century England. Thesis (doctoral)—Rutgers University, 2000, 2001.

Craske, Matthew. "'Unwholesome' and 'pornographic' A reassessment of the place of Rackstrow's Museum in the story of eighteenth-century anatomical collection and exhibition," *Journal of the History of Collections.* Oxford, U.K.: Oxford University Press, 23 (1): 75-99, 2011.

Dacome, Lucia. "Waxworks and the Performance of Anatomy in Mid-18th Century Italy." Endeavour 30(1): 29–35, 2006.

Daninos, Andrea. *Waxing eloquent: Italian portraits in wax.* Milan: Officina Libraria, 2012.

Dery, Mark. *I Must Not Think Bad Thoughts: Drive-by Essays on American Dread,* American Dreams. Minneapolis: University of Minnesota Press, 2012.

Düring, Monika, Georges Didi-Huberman, Marta Poggesi, and Saulo Bambi. *Encyclopaedia Anatomica: A Complete Collection of Anatomical Waxes : Vollständige Sammlung Anatomischer Wachse : Collection Complète Des Cires Anatomiques.* Köln [etc.]: Taschen, 1999.

Hoffmann, Kathryn. "Sleeping Beauties in the Fairground: The Spitzner, Pedley, and Chemisé Exhibits." *Early Popular Visual Culture* 4(2): 139–159, 2006.

Jordanova, Ludmilla. *Sexual Visions: Images of Gender in Science and Medicine Between the Eighteenth and Twentieth Centuries.* Madison: University of Wisconsin Press, 1993.

Kemp, Martin, and Marina Wallace. *Spectacular Bodies: The Art and Science of the Human Body from Leonardo to Now.* London:

Hayward Gallery, 2000.

Maerker, Anna. *Model Experts: Wax Anatomies and Enlightenment in Florence and Vienna, 1775–1815*. Manchester: Manchester University Press, 2011.

Messbarger, Rebecca Marie. *The Lady Anatomist: The Life and Work of Anna Morandi Manzolini*. Chicago: The University of Chicago Press, 2010.

Panzanelli, Roberta, Julius Schlosser, and Julius Schlosser. *Ephemeral Bodies: Wax Sculpture and the Human Figure*. Los Angeles, Calif: Getty Research Institute, 2008.

Riva, Alessandro Gabriele Conti, Paola Solinas, and Francesco Loy. "The Evolution of Anatomical Illustration and Wax Modelling in Italy from the 16th to Early 19th Centuries." *Journal of Anatomy* 216 (2): 209–22, 2008.

Sappol, Michael. *Dream Anatomy*. Bethesda, Md: U.S. Dept. of Health and Human Services, National Institutes of Health, National Library of Medicine, 2006.

Susini, Clemente, Alessandro Riva, and Luigi Cattaneo. *Flesh & Wax: The Clemente Susini's Anatomical Models in the University of Cagliari*. [Nuoro, Italy]: Ilisso, 2007.

Sato, Akira and Nahoko Kametsu. *Anatomica Barocca*. Tokyo: Editions Treville, 1995.

PART II

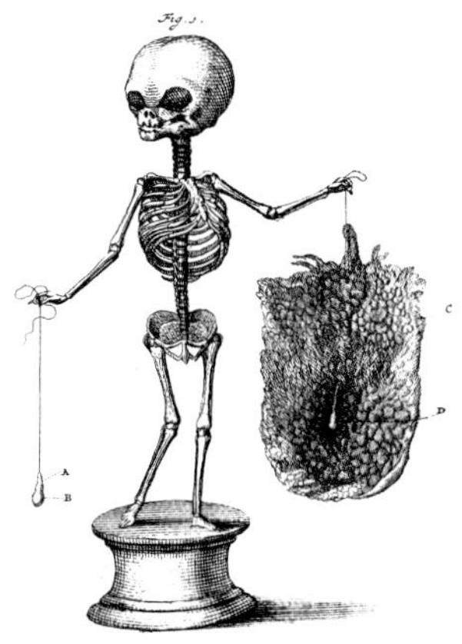

TOUGH

CARL SCHOONOVER

OY VEY, THE *DURA MATER*, BANE OF ALL STUDENTS OF THE CENTRAL nervous system, sworn enemy of neurobiological investigation. *Dura*, we curse under our breaths: that thick, leathery, protective sheath that envelops the brain, keeping goodness within and evil without—a category to which we, arguably grey matter's greatest fans, have inexplicably been relegated without so much as a fair hearing. "Tough mother," indeed.

But we get in. We slash our way in.

We ram delicate electrodes—the tool of choice to study the activity of rodent brains—like so many ships battered against the rocks by a storm. When this strategy fails, we recant, set out once more with the reverence (and secret optimism) of those who have not yet been systematically disappointed. We subject the dura to the firm, controlled and yet somehow tender manipulation of our finest microsurgical instruments, only to be rebuffed once again. It is now late at night, we can almost hear the dura laughing at us. To which, needless to say, we react with mounting frustration, which varies inversely with that hotshot surgical confidence. Soon enough the entire surgery is bungled, a spectacular failure, the experiment a wash—the unified theory of the nervous system further delayed.

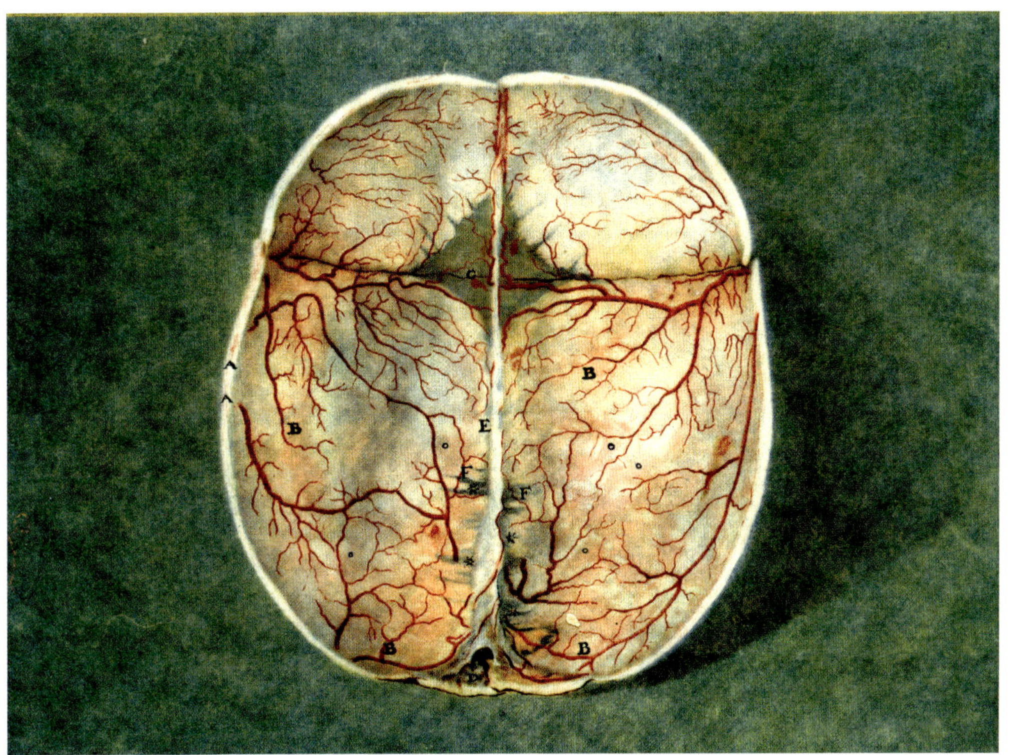

A recent visit to the New York Academy of Medicine puts this whole business into perspective, when Arlene Shaner digs out a color mezzotint by Jan Ladmiral based on a preparation by the legendary seventeenth-century Dutch anatomist, Frederik Ruysch.[1] In this image we stand inside the dome of the skull looking up at a breathtakingly intricate preparation of the *dura mater* of an eight-month-old human fetus. For a structure this beautiful all must be forgiven.

The accompanying text sings the praises of the illustrious professor who, employing methods that remain mysterious to this day, succeeded in filling even the extremities of the fetus' delicate blood vessels—in some places "thinner than fibers of cotton"—with red wax.

[1] *Jan Ladmiral,* Icon durae matris in concavâ superficie visae... *(Amstelodami: Jacobus Graal & Henricum de Leth, Lugduni Batavorum, Theodorum Haak,* 1738*). Courtesy of the New York Academy of Medicine Library.*

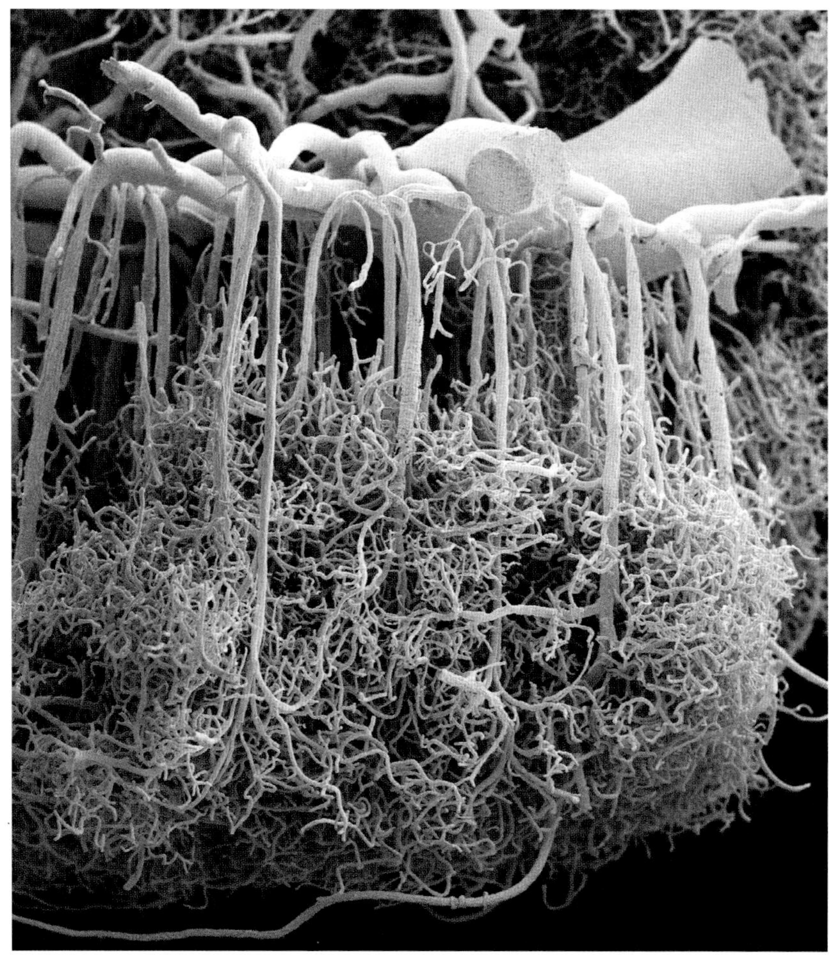

Alfonso Rodríguez-Baeza and Marisa Ortega-Sánchez, 2009.

But how, Professor Ruysch, did you produce this object? A question Tsar Peter the Great asked the aging master to the tune of 35,000 eighteenth-century guilders,[2] with Ruysch's collection of anatomical preparations bundled into the deal—now on display in St. Petersburg's Kunstkamera collection, many in surprisingly good shape.[3] In spite of a muscular contract

[2] *Jozien Driessen-van het Reve,* De Kunstkamera van Peter de Grote. De Hollandse inbreng... *(University of Amsterdam,* 2006*).*

ensuring the transfer of the anatomist's trade secrets—to some excessively secret—the apogee of the art more or less died with him. Obsessive attempts by lesser mortals followed over the ensuing decades but it gradually emerged that he must have left something out of the recipe. So much for that.†

[3] *http://www.kunstkamera.ru/en/*

And yet all is not lost. You might even say that the spirit of Frederik Ruysch is alive and well in contemporary anatomy. Witness this relatively recent cast, here not of the *dura mater*, but of the microscopic capillaries of the human cortex, prepared in a manner that would have made the master proud: delicately inject a liquid resin in a postmortem subject, wait a bit for it to harden, dissolve the surrounding brain tissue with a basic solution, examine under the microscope, *et voilà*.

[With thanks to Arlene Shaner, Reference Librarian & Acting Curator of Rare Books & Manuscripts at the New York Academy of Medicine, for locating the print by Jan Ladmiral, and to Dániel Margócsy (see next essay), assistant professor in the Department of History at Hunter College, for expert guidance.]

† *For an entertaining account of a contemporary reenactment, based on a Thomas Pole's Anatomical Instructor* (1790)*—eighteenth-century DIY at its finest—see the appendix of Marieke Hendriksen's PhD dissertation* Aesthesis in Anatomy. Materiality and Elegance in the Eighteenth-Century Leiden Anatomical Collections *(Leiden University,* 2012*).*

A PHILOSOPHY OF WAX
The Anatomy of Frederik Ruysch

DÁNIEL MARGÓCSY

Cartesian Lines

Throughout his distinguished career, the French philosopher René Descartes repeatedly came back to the problem of images. As he observed with wonder and amazement in his *Optics*, engravings tended not to fully resemble the objects that they represented:

> It is enough that the image resembles its object in a few respects. Indeed the perfection of an image often depends on its not resembling its object as much as it might. You can see this in the case of engravings: consisting simply of a little ink placed here and there on a piece of paper, they represent to us forests, towns, people, and even battles and storms. [1]

It is no surprise that Descartes chose prints as his pet example of why we might not want to fully trust our senses. To produce an engraving, the printmaker scrapes thin lines into a copperplate, which are then inked and pressed against a sheet of paper. The clever use of hatched lines brings into life the sad face of the Virgin Mary, dappled flowers in bloom, or the cloudy sky with its delicate interplay of light and shadows. The fine, linear texture of a print creates in viewers the illusion of reality.

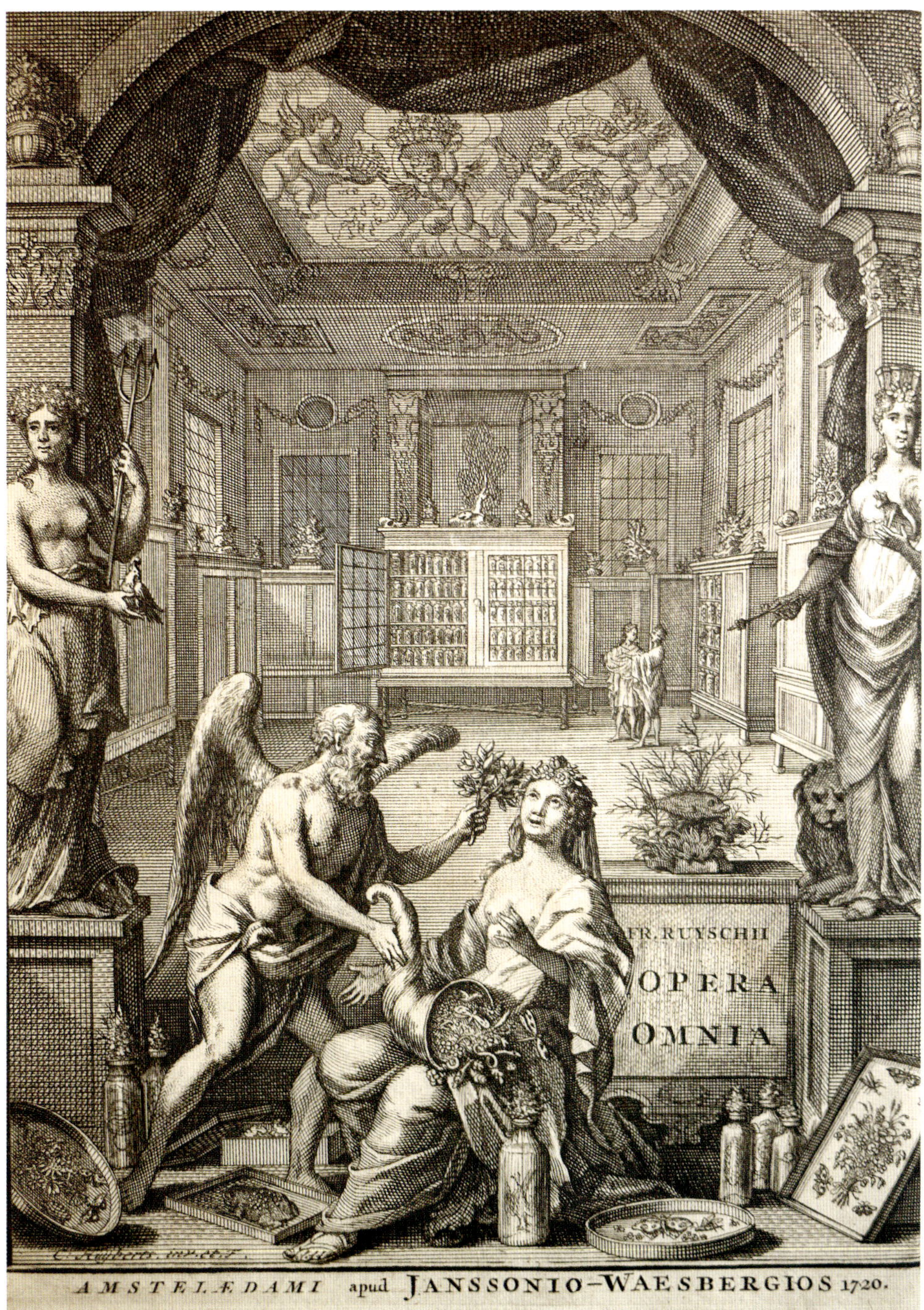

Image previous page: Ruysch's museum, from Frederik Ruysch, Opera omnia..., *Amsterdam: Janssonius Waesbergen, 1721-1727. Courtesy of the New York Academy of Medicine Library.*

Such illusions were dangerous from Descartes' perspective because they broke down the trust you had in your senses. A philosopher as he was, Descartes quickly came to an abstract generalization from his particular point about engraved lines. If we could not trust prints, there was also no guarantee that our visual perceptions resembled the objects out there in the world. He famously began his *Treatise on Light* with the boisterous claim that "for although everyone is commonly convinced that the ideas that we have in our thought are completely like the objects from which they proceed, I know of no compelling argument for this."[2]

[1] *René Descartes,* Selected Philosophical Writings, *trans. by John Cottingham, Robert Stoothoff and Dugald Murdoch (Cambridge: Cambridge University Press, 1988), 62.*

[2] *René Descartes,* The World and Other Writings, *trans. and ed. by Stephen Gaukroger (Cambridge: Cambridge University Press, 1998), 3.*

Descartes' philosophical speculations, and his *cogito ergo sum* (I think therefore I am), are closely related to his distrust of the senses. How can I trust my perception, and how can I trust what I know, if my eyes or a malicious demon can deceive my understanding at any given moment? Much of Descartes' career was devoted to answering this very question. He cooked up complex philosophical arguments, he dissected sheep and cows, and he even devised a machine to grind hyperbolic lenses, only to find a solution to this conundrum. By the end of his life, he was convinced that he had found certain knowledge. Thanks to his clear and evident reasoning, he could prove that God existed, that human consciousness resided in the pineal gland, and that the heart served like a furnace to warm up blood.

We all admire Descartes and his groundbreaking philosophical enterprise, yet few us believe that our inner self hides in the pineal gland. Seventeenth-century physicians were similarly ambivalent about Cartesian philosophy and its bold claims about human physiology. What if you could actually have certain knowledge, but not based on Descartes' metaphysical foundations? Or, if such philosophical heights made you feel vertiginous, what if you could simply create an image that actually resembled nature? Or, if you thought nature was too big a word, what if you could at least create a trustworthy picture of the human body? Such a modest aim drove the macabre physician Frederik Ruysch. Born in 1638, just a year after the publication of the *Discours de la méthode*, Ruysch grew up in the Netherlands, the adopted home of Descartes in those years. Although he rarely discussed Descartes in his writings, Ruysch was surely aware of the French philosopher's ideas. He received his medical education in the university town of Leiden, where his professors vigorously debated Cartesian philosophy and medical theories, and then went on to make a career in Amsterdam, the bustling hub of seventeenth-century world commerce.

Ruysch was a physician with diverse interests, equally at hand in making drugs, growing exotic plants, advising midwives, and most importantly, investigating human anatomy. He combined these scientific activities with a passion for the arts, and excelled at drawing, painting and engraving. He appears to have been a good and caring father, too. His son, Hendrik, was a promising naturalist, only to be destroyed by alcohol and then the plague; while his daughter, Rachel, became one of the best-selling flower painters of the early eighteenth century. Yet even Ruysch's versatility had its limits. He was ignorant of the ancients, at least by the standards of his age. His writing style was cramped, his temper was volatile, and he could only think of himself in superlative terms. He welcomed adoration in unhealthy doses, but lashed back malevolently at any attempt of criticism. Throughout his career, he rejected the Cartesian cocktail of philosophical theory and dissection, replacing it with an experimental anatomy injected with a dash of art. Certain knowledge could only be achieved by the careful observation of human bodies, and he was certainly the best observer in the field of anatomy; or so he thought.

Posterity remembers Ruysch for his idiosyncratic anatomical museum, which offered a morbid combination of his artistic and scientific sensibilities. This museum was the largest collection of wet and dry anatomical specimens in contemporary Europe. By the mid-1710s, Ruysch had created and exhibited over two thousand specimens, which he then sold to the Russian Czar Peter the Great. Not to leave empty the walls of his museum, the octogenarian anatomist decided to make evermore preparations. By 1732, the year of his death, he had successfully built a new museum with over 1,200 preparations. No wonder that every tourist wanted to drop by Ruysch's in Amsterdam, from poor Hungarians to rich English aristocrats, and leave an admiring comment and a signature in his guest book.

Ruysch's anatomy collection filled up five rooms, where thousands and thousands of bottles lined densely packed shelves, offering a stunning sight to all the visitors who flocked to see these collections. Thanks to the surviving catalogs, one is able to reconstruct his museum shelf by shelf. In one of his cupboards, for instance, a bottle with an infant's auditory organs was standing next to a bottle that held another infant's monstrous lips that looked like velvet. On the same shelf one could also find another bottle with an infant's head, with the top of the skull removed so that one could observe the brain from above. Next came a bottle filled with intestines, two bottles with brain membranes, a bottle with an adult spleen, a dissected testicle displaying the spermatic vessels, and the sexual organ of a young girl. A startling sight for eighteenth-century onlookers, and a stunning sight for those who visit the surviving specimens in St. Petersburg, Russia, today.

Ruysch's cupboards also held exotic plants, fish and other little-known creatures, as well as his richly decorated, famous anatomical *tableaux*. These *tableaux* were complex sculptural

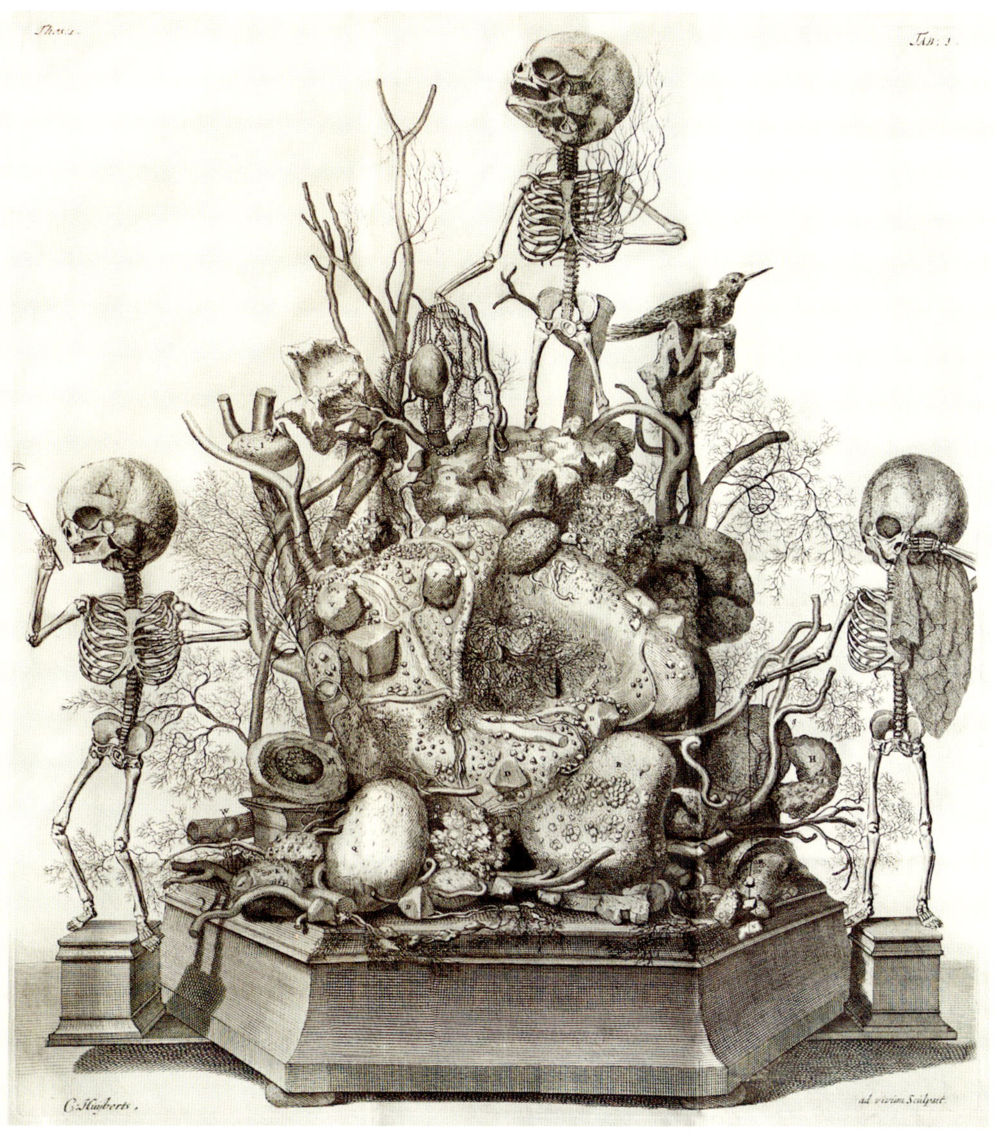

Tableau with Three Skeletons, from Frederik Ruysch, Opera omnia..., *Amsterdam: Janssonius Waesbergen, 1721-1727. Courtesy of the New York Academy of Medicine Library.*

installations, assembled from skeletons, bones, and kidney and gallstones. They conveyed a deeply Christian, and often deeply depressing, message of the futility of human life. Look at the illustration of the *tableau* with the three skeletal infants, for

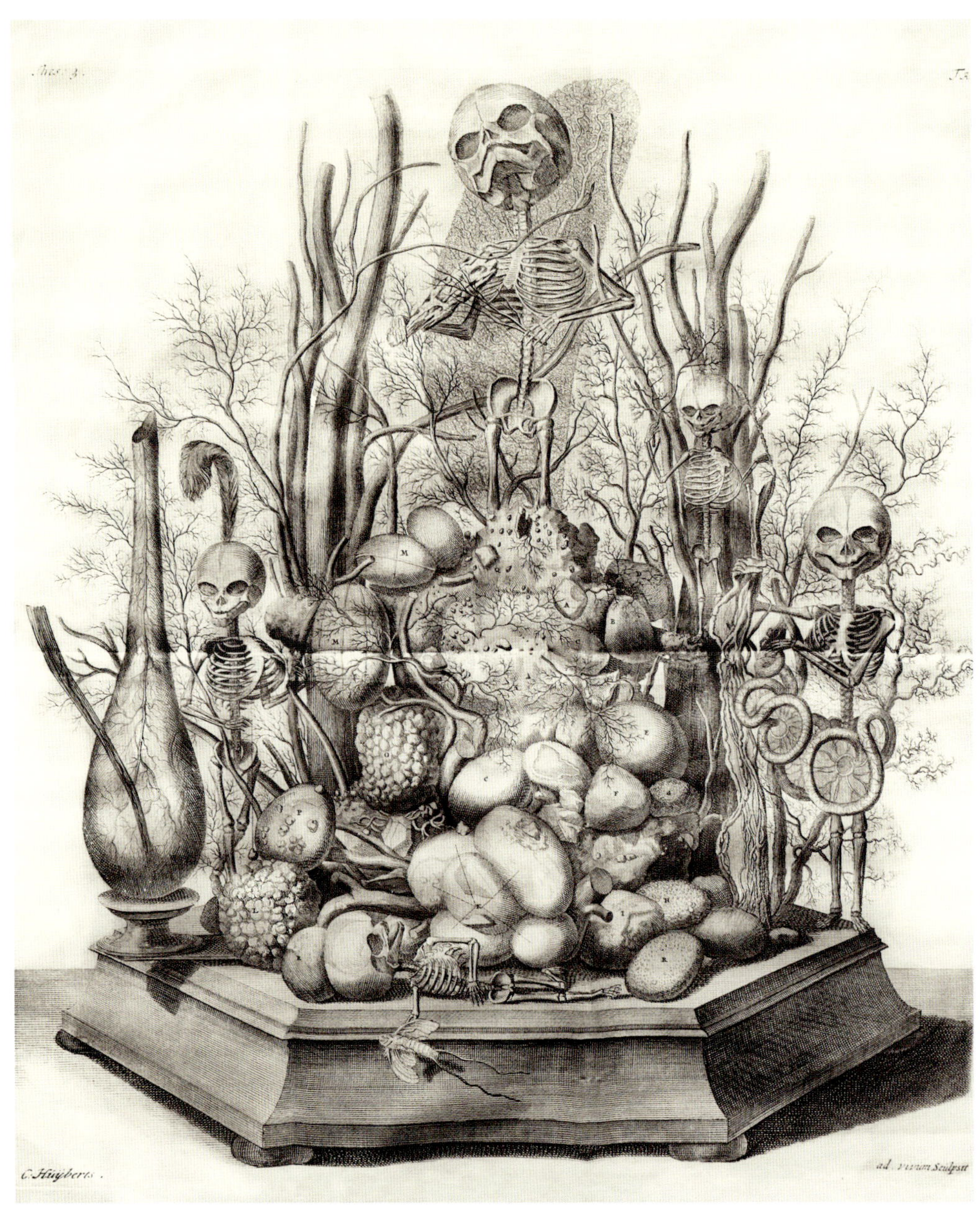
C. Huijberts.
ad. vivum Sculpsit

instance. These strangely lively skeletons stand on a mountain of kidney and gallstones, amidst a forest of prepared blood vessels. One of them holds a sickle in his hands, reminding viewers of their impending death. The other one holds a napkin, crying over humankind's fate. What is the worth of wealth and expensive jewelry (like the ones the third skeleton holds in the hands) if we are soon to die? Mortals can find rejoice only in admiring God's miraculous creations, Ruysch seems to suggest.

Experimenting with Circulation

It was exciting to be an anatomist in the seventeenth century when the discipline was fresh with new energy. Anatomy theaters were opening across Europe, with about a dozen established in the Netherlands itself, offering demonstrations of human anatomy to the larger public. Dutch artists made the discipline popular for wider audiences by portraying physicians in the act of dissection, including Rembrandt's renowned *Anatomy of Dr. Tulp* (1631). English, French and Dutch anatomists were excited to engage with William Harvey's recent discovery of blood circulation, a finding that prompted Descartes to develop an alternative theory. Ruysch also threw himself into the investigation of circulation. Not necessarily the circulation of blood, though. His first research focused on the lymphatic system, which had been discovered a few years earlier. Soon after he graduated from Leiden, he found out that, like the veins, the lymph vessels also possessed valves. This was not just a curious fact; it helped him determine which way the lymph flowed, a much-debated problem amongst contemporary physicians. Ruysch remained faithful to circulation throughout his very long career, up to his death at age 92. Together with his fellow students in Leiden, he developed a new and revolutionary technique to trace the flow of the bodily fluids. The new

Tableau with Five Skeletons from Frederik Ruysch, Opera omnia..., *Amsterdam: Janssonius Waesbergen, 1721-1727. Courtesy of the New York Academy of Medicine Library.*

invention relied on the injection of colored, molten wax into the blood vessels of a cadaver. The hot liquid quickly filled up the veins and the arteries. Once it solidified, it showed with unparalleled clarity the meandering routes that the vessels had taken in the organs. And, if only slowly, it led to a major revelation for Ruysch. The Dutch anatomist gradually came to realize that, if one looked carefully, vessels were the only building blocks of the human body: blood vessels, lymphatic vessels, and the nerves.

He gave an intimation of this idea in his letter on the spleen. As he wrote to a forgotten colleague, the closer he looked at the spleen, the more he was convinced that it contained nothing but "arteries, veins, lymphatic vessels and nerves." [3] While earlier physicians had thought that the spleen contained a number of glands, upon closer examination, these glands turned out to be intricately interwoven nets of vessels, held together by a thin membrane. Then he probed further. Next came the brain, and its white matter. When Ruysch injected molten wax into the vessels of the brain, it became crystal clear, at least for him, that the white matter consisted exclusively of nerves and blood vessels. As the blood vessels branched into tiny arterioles, they began to resemble the intricate structure of moss. The white matter's strange consistency resulted from the messy and mossy mishmash of blood vessels. From the brain, it was only a quick step to female breasts. While earlier (and later) physicians thought that the breast was filled with milk-producing glands, this was clearly an error, Ruysch declared. What looked like glands, he argued, was a complex web of blood vessels, of course. As the blood vessels branched right and left, they separated the various ingredients of blood. The red particles of blood went left, while the white particles went right, and turned into milk. One did not need glands to explain the production of milk, the

[3] *Frederik Ruysch,* Alle de werken *(Amsterdam: Janssoons van Waesberge, 1744), 260.*

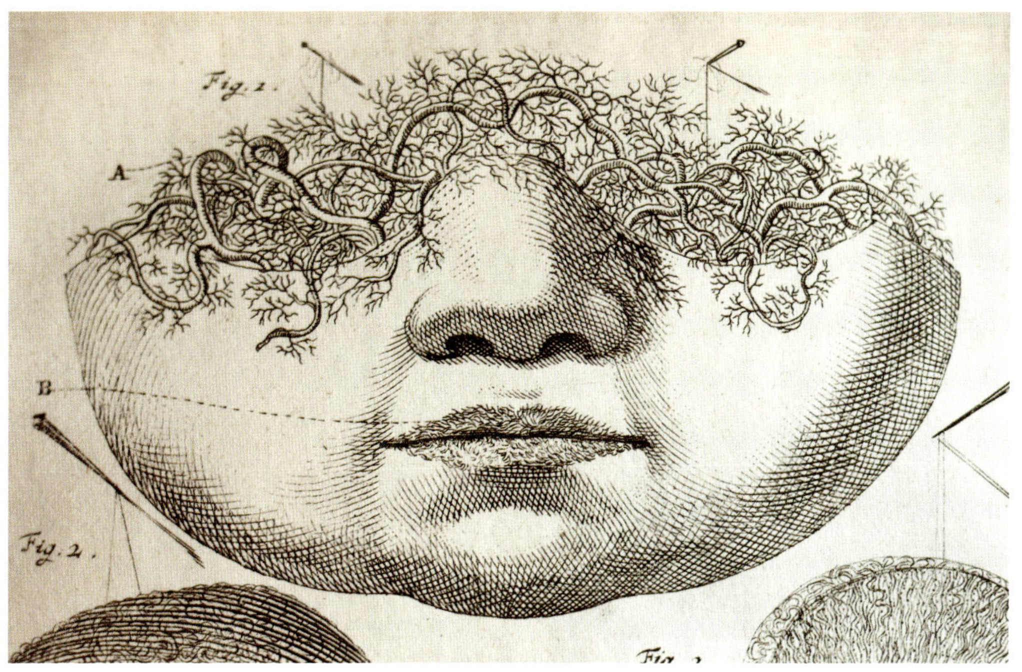

Image above from Frederik Ruysch, Opera omnia..., *Amsterdam: Janssonius Waesbergen, 1721-1727. Courtesy of the New York Academy of Medicine Library.*

vessels did it on their own. And once the breasts were done, it took only a leap of imagination to believe that the whole body was a network of vessels that circulated the vital fluids. Humans were the early modern Internet.

Ink as Blood

What does the body look like if it is made out of vessels? How can you best picture it? Ruysch did not compare the human body to the Internet. Instead, as the historian Bert van de Roemer points out, he compared it to textiles, woven or knitted together from long threads. Like the glands of the spleen, clothes appear to have a solid structure at first sight. If you look closer, though, you will notice their threaded texture. Ruysch's *tableau* nicely illustrates this analogy. Weeping over the fate of humankind,

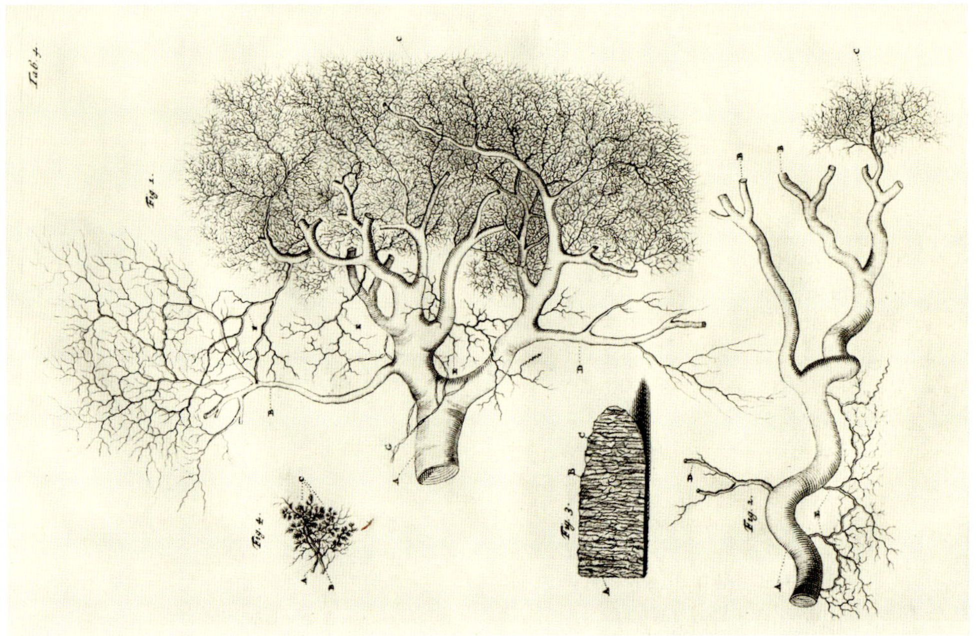

The Spleen (above) and The Pleura, the Scrotum, the Breast and the Pericardium (above right), from Frederik Ruysch, Opera omnia..., *Amsterdam: Janssonius Waesbergen, 1721-1727. Courtesy of the New York Academy of Medicine Library.*

the infant skeleton cleans his eyes with a handkerchief. Not a silk handkerchief, though, but a handkerchief made of a human membrane filled with the blood vessels.

Yet, if the body had a textile texture, could you also compare it to engraved images? Maybe, just maybe, no Cartesian metaphysical doubt was needed about pictures if engravings actually resembled the bodily organs. If humans consisted entirely of tiny vessels brimming with blood, lymph and semen, they were surely similar to an engraving plate whose engraved lines, carved into copper with a burin, were not unlike a vein, filled with the printmaker's ink, Ruysch may have thought. When one carefully examines his illustrations, it is indeed striking to see how the engraved lines serve as the equivalent of blood vessels. Look at the spleen for example, with its meandering and crisscrossing linear structure. On the left,

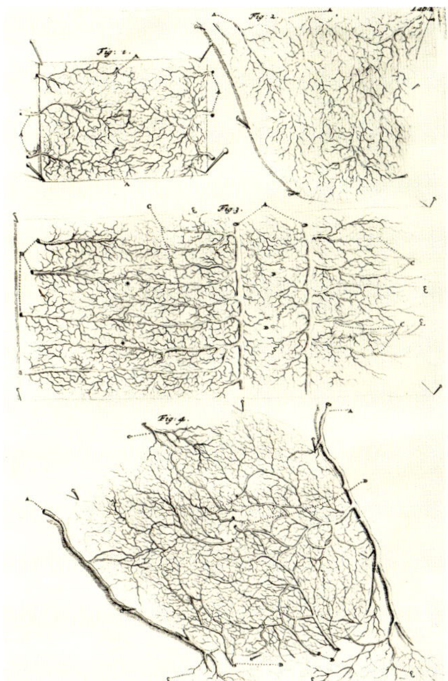

the circular shape of the large artery is indicated by the rounded lines of shading. Yet, as the arteries branch into the smaller arterioles, each engraved line comes to represent an individual blood vessel. A forest of tiny strokes recreates the forest of vessels that we call the spleen.

Ruysch's equation of engraved lines with tiny vessels resulted in strangely uniform illustrations for the body's various parts. Take a look at the illustrations of the pleura, the flattened out scrotum, of the breasts, and the pericardium, juxtaposed on one sheet. If you focus on the small details, would you be able to say what differentiates the arterioles of these organs? It is not easy to tell the difference, and this was Ruysch's precise point. For him, all body parts were built up from the same building blocks. Vessels were vessels, regardless their location in the body. His composite engraving was a strong visual argument to prove

Image right: The Heart, from Frederik Ruysch, Opera omnia..., *, Amsterdam: Janssonius Waesbergen, 1721-1727. Courtesy of the Countway Library of Medicine.*

his point. Each engraved line represented the brutal simplicity of human anatomy.

Yet Ruysch's strategy had its drawbacks. If you identify engraved lines with vessels, how do you create the effect of light and shadows? How can you tell whether a dark area on paper represents shading, or, instead, an intricate web of vessels? Take another look at Ruysch's illustration of the spleen to realize the limitations of his visual strategy. The overlapping vessels, the shading, and the meandering lines create a rather chaotic image. When two engraved lines cross each other in this image, are you able to tell what they represent? Do the two blood vessels merge into each other, exchanging blood, or does one blood vessel pass in front of the other one, without merging together, instead? By equating lines with vessels, Ruysch fell into a trap. He could no longer adequately represent the human body's three dimensions in two.

And there were other problems, as well. As Ruysch came to realize, engravings did not have a high enough resolution to represent the body. Despite his best efforts, he could not picture the tiniest blood vessels on paper. He asked his illustrator Jan Wandelaar to observe the body's structures through a microscope, and, when that was not enough, he took up the engraver's tools himself. Even then, he had to admit, it proved too difficult to create a faithful image of all the coronary arteries of the heart. His intricately-detailed illustration appears certainly impressive for today's lay viewer, yet Ruysch was dissatisfied. As he wrote, "it is to be noted that the arteries, spread across the heart, are much more numerous in number, and are divided into finer branches than what I could print in the illustration."[4] Similar warnings also appeared in his other writings, alerting readers that his image was "crippled." This did not mean that his illustrations were useless. They were still better than his rivals'

[4] *Frederik Ruysch,* Alle de werken *(Amsterdam: Janssoons van Waesberge, 1744), 243.*

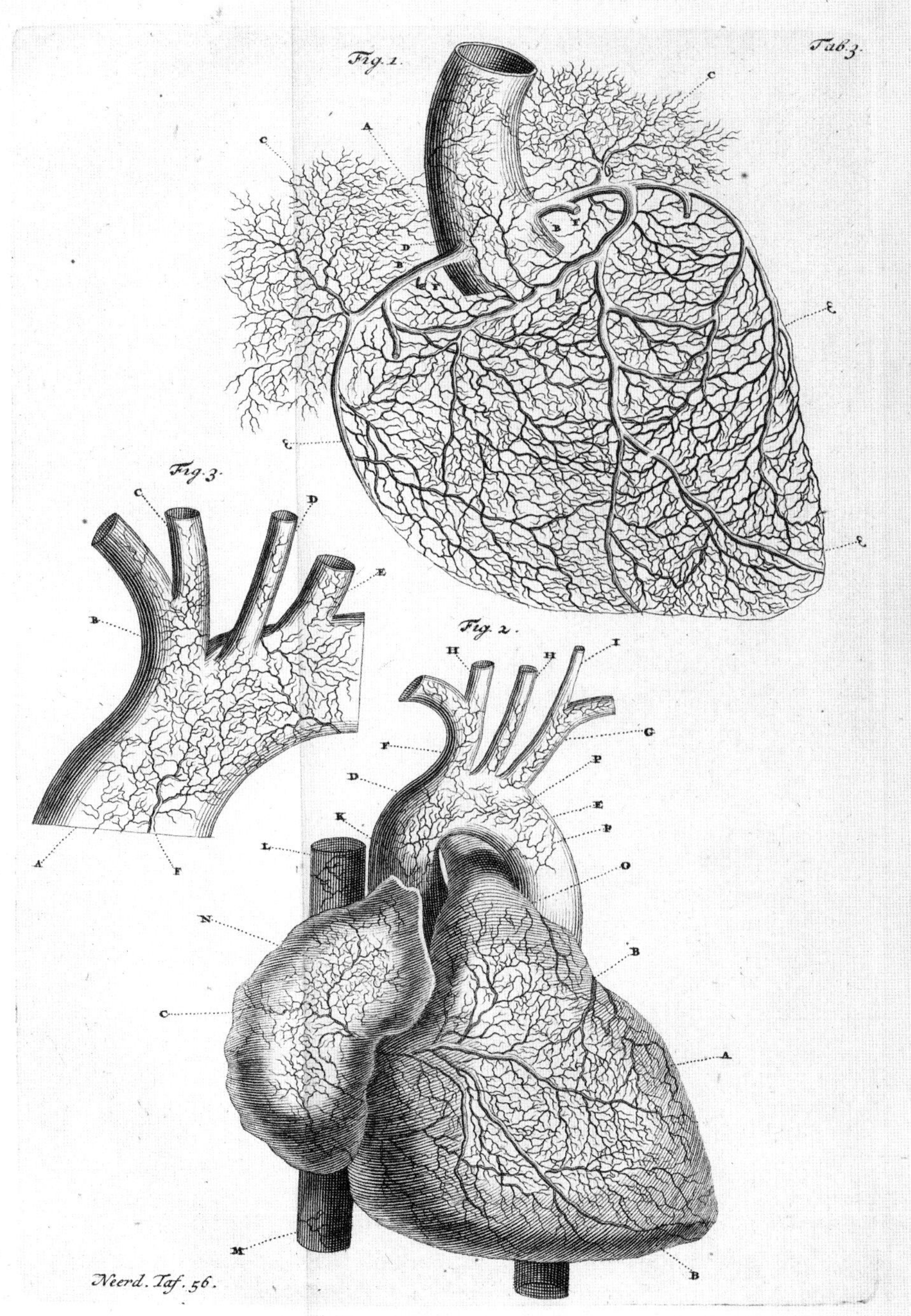
Fig. 1.
Tab. 3.
Fig. 3.
Fig. 2.
Neerd. Taf. 56.

images, and offered clear and evident proof that Ruysch was the best anatomist. But these images failed at resembling nature itself. So, maybe, Descartes was correct. It was enough that the image resembled its object in a few respects.

Auto-Sculptures

For Ruysch, though, the quest was not over for making the perfect image. Instead of focusing on faulty engravings, he came to argue that his anatomical specimens offered a perfect image of the human body. These were, after all, the body parts of a deceased person. Not just representations, but the real thing itself! Moreover, the preserved specimens did not rot, and did not even look dead. While one can easily make a distinction between a cadaver and living being, Ruysch's specimens blurred this boundary. As he filled the collapsed blood vessels of the body's parts with wax, the injected organs regained their natural shape and color. While the skin of a dead person appeared pale, Ruysch's preparations did not. He dyed his wax with cinnabar so that the injected blood vessels were just as red as if they had been filled with blood. The illusionistic effect of these preparations was considerable. Famously, when the Russian czar came to a visit, he mistook the prepared body of a young infant for a sleeping baby. The rosy cheeks of the girl looked so lively that the czar decided to shower kisses on them.

Yet Ruysch did not use wax injections only to trick traveling emperors. He truly believed that, by making his corpses look alive, he was able to show to tourists, students, and fellow anatomists the intricate structure of the living human body. His museum became the ultimate site where perfect resemblance was achieved between preparations and human life, erasing any doubt from the minds of the viewers. Because the body was nothing but an intricate network of vessels, and the injected, colored wax visualized all these vessels in their natural shapes, the resulting specimens revealed the body to the viewers in all its glory, without a fault. Remember this if you visit the Kunstkamera in St. Petersburg today, where the specimens are still preserved in a mint condition. Ruysch's specimens might appear macabresque. They might appear to be the products of a death-obsessed anatomist, who used the infant skeletons and fetuses to remind you about the futility of human efforts. Yet, back then, they primarily served scientific purposes to picture life, and to reverse the process of decay that sets off after death. Throughout his life, Ruysch remained convinced that his preparations succeeded in doing just that. They truly resembled living human bodies, and correctly represented anatomical structures. Whenever he engaged in a debate with another anatomist, he referred his sparring partners to his museum. There, they could see his specimens. There, they could be convinced that Ruysch was right. In the Ruyschian museum, Cartesian suspicions were suspended and truth was revealed.

The story appears too good to be true, and it was too good to be true. In one crucial case, Ruysch was forced to acknowledge that even his preparation method was imperfect. In his study of circulation, our anatomist came to believe that the arteries were connected to the veins through tiny, extremely thin capillaries. It was probably at the level of these capillaries that blood came in contact with other materials. Within the lungs, for instance, the capillaries facilitated the exchange of air and blood between the lung's pipes and the circulatory system. Yet nobody knew how such exchanges happened. Did they happen in tiny little glands? Did the blood vessels simply end, releasing blood into the flesh? Ruysch was convinced that neither of these explanations was correct. Since vessels were the ultimate building blocks of life, the capillaries surely connected arteries

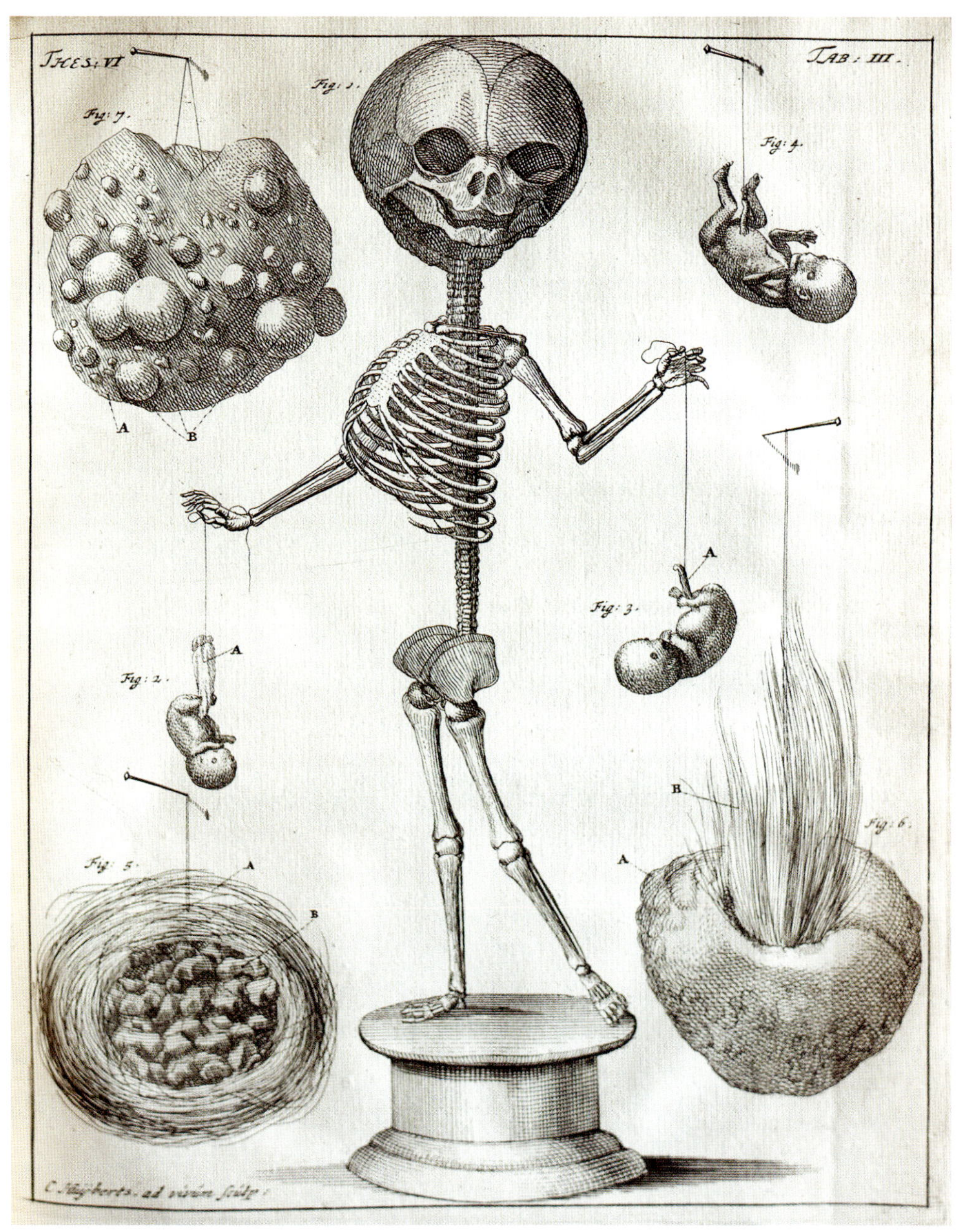

Illustration from Frederik Ruysch, Opera omnia..., *Amsterdam: Janssonius Waesbergen, 1721-1727.*
Courtesy of the New York Academy of Medicine Library.

to the veins. Yet, he thought, these capillaries must have had some holes, which allowed blood and air to mix. This was surely the right explanation, but Ruysch had no evidence to back it up. He could not see the holes of the capillaries, and he could not even see the capillaries themselves. Thanks to his injection technique, Ruysch could pump molten wax into the arterioles, but not into the capillaries. They remained invisible to him. He could only say that, when he pumped red wax into the arterioles, they surrounding tissues also became slightly red, which suggested that the red wax escaped from these vessels. For him, this indicated that there were holes in the capillaries. But, of course, other explanations could also have worked. Maybe, the injection technique was too invasive, and punctured the tiniest vessels. Or, alternatively, there were no capillaries. The small arterioles emptied blood into the tissues, without any direct connection to the veins.

Ruysch was not really shaken by the shortcoming of his technique. He treated it as a minor problem that would surely be repaired when, with the passage of time, his preparation methods would improve. It did not invalidate the many, many experimental results that he obtained thanks to his specimens. He was the best anatomist, and his preparation technique was the best. Yet I wonder whether Descartes would have nodded in agreement, or if he would have ridiculed Ruysch's confidence. At a philosophical level, after all, Ruysch's failure to visualize the capillaries was damning. It showed his inability to visualize all the vessels of the human body. He could not prove how circulation worked, nor could he not prove that the body was made out of pipes. While he claimed to be an experimental anatomist, a major premise of his visualization technique turned out to be a pure hypothesis. Yes, his anatomical preparations represented the human body. But they did not necessarily resemble it in all

Image following spread: Illustration from Frederik Ruysch, Opera omnia..., *Amsterdam: Janssonius Waesbergen, 1721-1727. Courtesy of the New York Academy of Medicine Library.*

aspects. A kernel of doubt remained that, maybe, at the level of capillaries, you could not use wax injections to picture the anatomy of the human body. And, for Descartes, you needed only a kernel of doubt to build up a whole metaphysics. There was no escape from philosophy.

[In writing this essay on what Ruysch might have thought about Descartes and engravings, I found the publications of Rina Knoeff, Evan Ragland, Hans-Jörg Rheinberger & Bert van de Roemer especially helpful. Many thanks to the New York Academy of Medicine's Rare Book Room for the permission to use the illustrations, and to the Countway Library of Medicine for the illustration of the circulatory system. While working on this essay, I was the Birkelund Fellow at the Cullman Center for Scholars and Writers at the New York Public Library.]

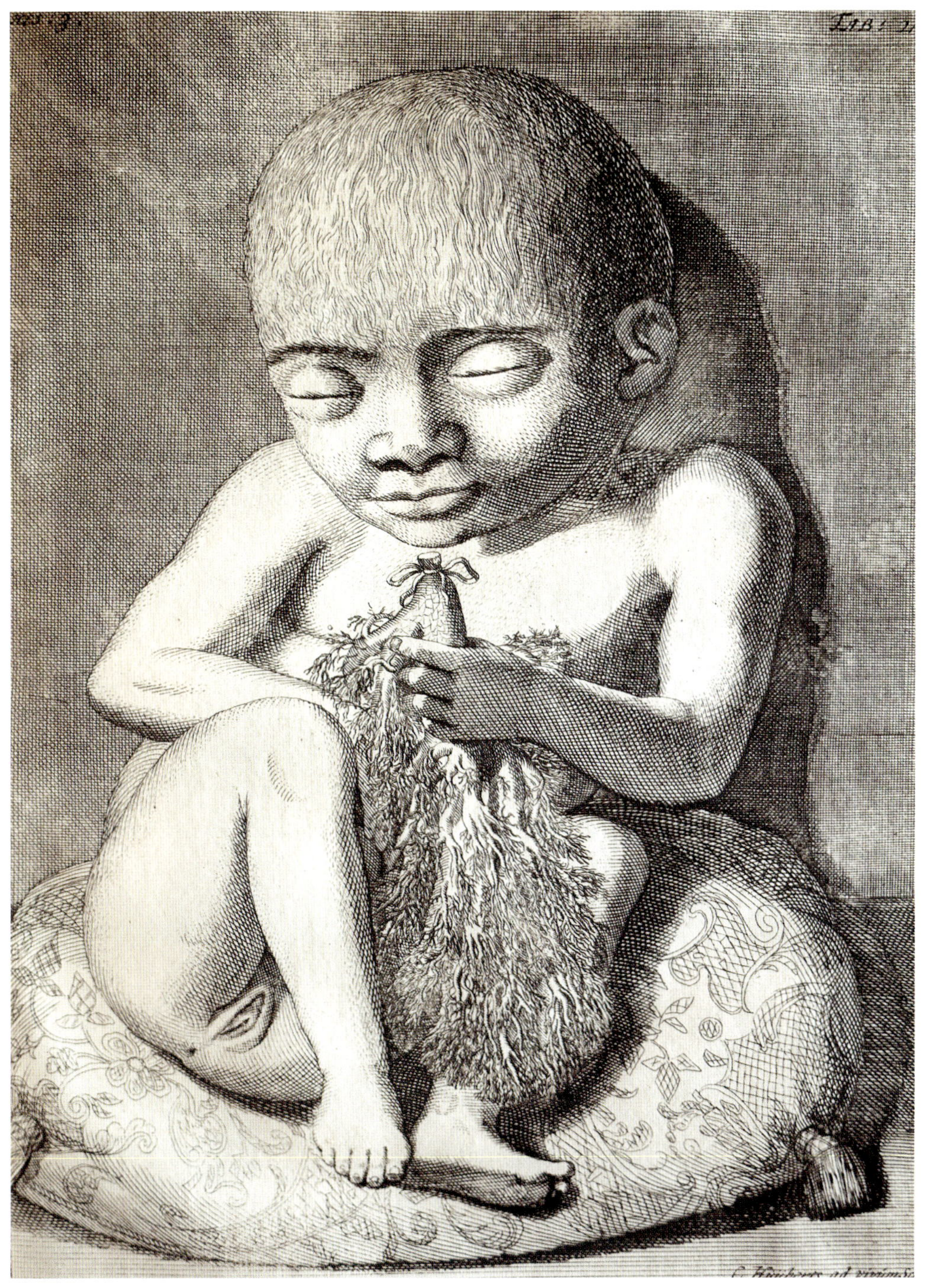

NAPLES
In the Court of Miracles

CHIARA AMBROSIO

The city stirs, volatile land ruled by myth and the elements.

IF NAPLES WERE A PERSON, IT WOULD LOOK DESTITUTE: A WEATHERED old man, resting under a creased cloak of stony rags, stretching its awkward limbs between the mountain and the sea, a shiny brooch, worn with pride and curiously out of place, pinned to its torn and dirty rags.

Just like the volcano at the foot of which it lies, its myriad eyes and manifold paths appear veiled in slumber under the nursing warmth of a midday sun. But its entrails are molten, and what courses through its damp body of brick and moss is ebullient and wild, as irreverent and incongruous as its adorned rags.

The narrow streets that unravel like an intricate web of veins and arteries from its tangled heart cut through the debris of different epochs with the same casual familiarity of fingers stretching from the palm of a hand. They all lead toward impossible directions—not only across, but more often upward and downward, transcending matter and decency, facilitating journeys that are more appropriate for nighttime and dreaming along unpaved trails where only spirits are expected to venture, and apparitions. All along these crepuscular paths, without fanfare, the living will defiantly step across those

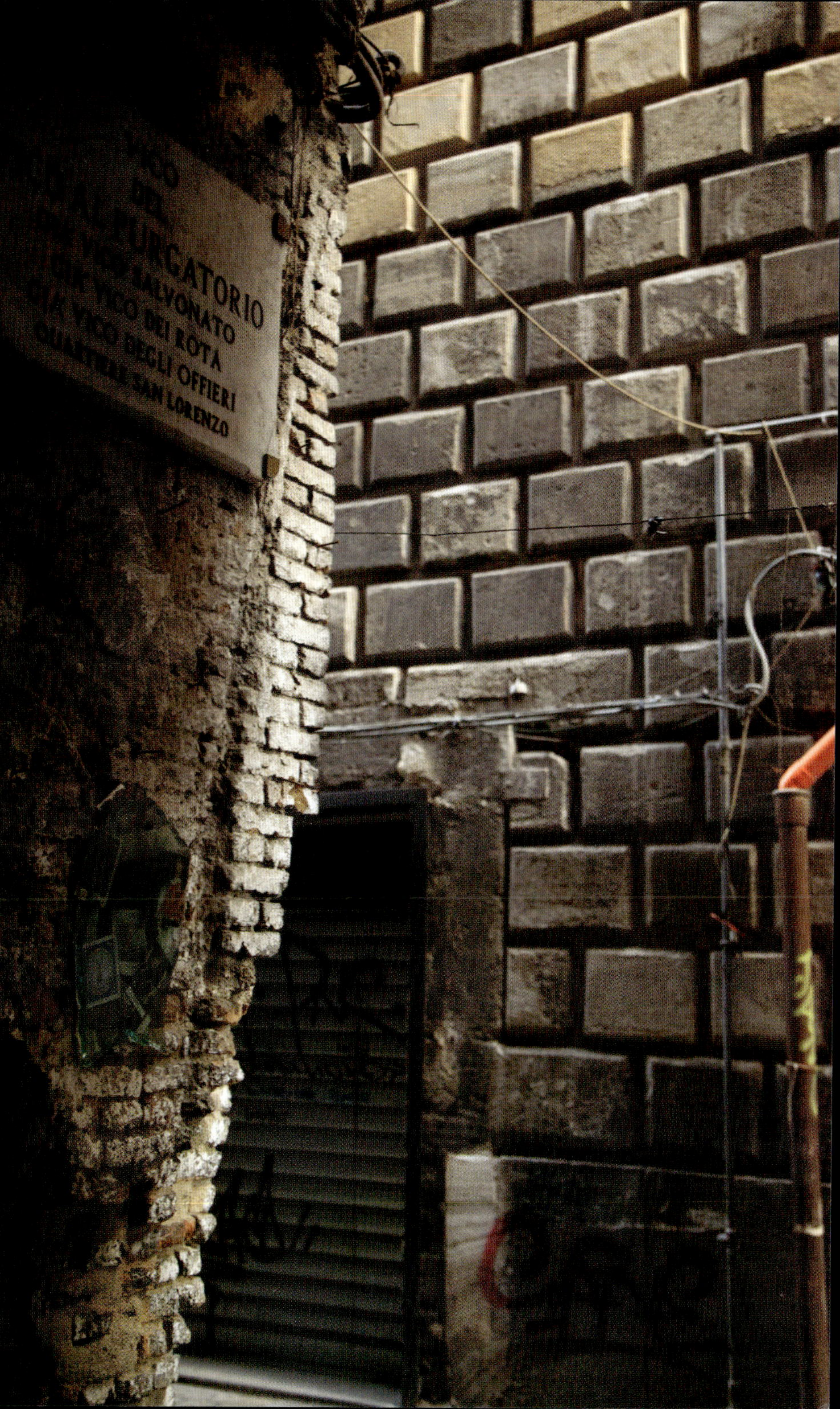
DEL
PURGATORIO
SALVONATO
VICO DEI ROTA
VICO DEGLI OFFIERI
SAN LORENZO

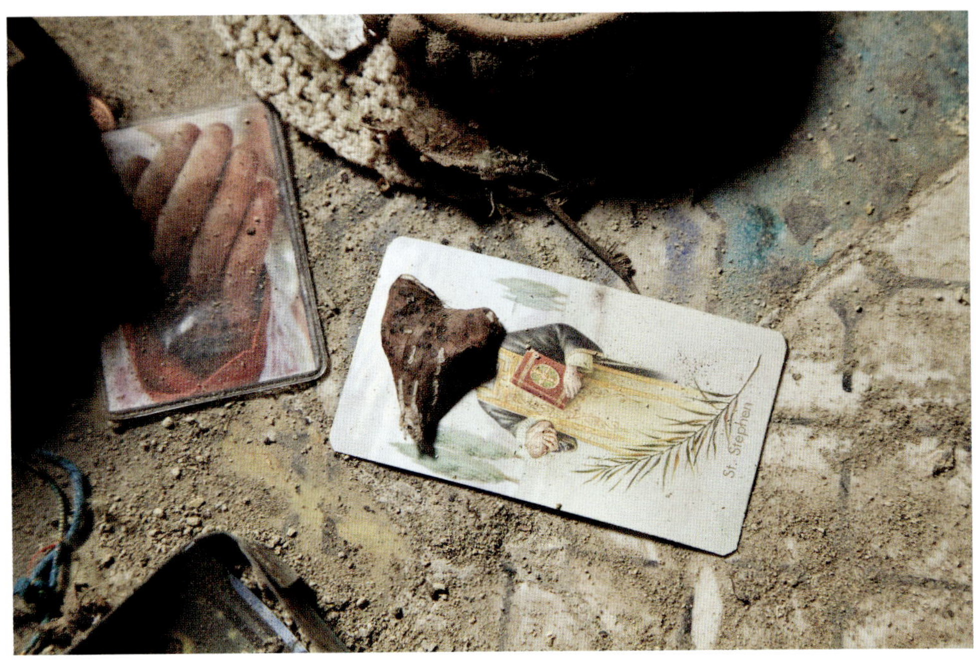

All photos by Joanna Ebenstein, taken in Naples, 2012–2013.

thresholds that are impassable elsewhere, and with great ease travel between life and death, through time and space, spinning at each step and with supreme confidence all the disparate fragments of a secular collective memory into a cacophonous, often humorous tale of hope, memory, freedom and subversion.

Naples occupies a distinctive psycho-geographical position, framed by natural, historical and literary thresholds (the sea, the volcano, the crater lake Avernus, mythical gateway to Hades, the ruins of Pompeii and Herculaneum, ravaged by the great eruption of Mount Vesuvius in AD 79, and the entrance to the Cumaean Sibyl's cave, to mention but a few) and rising above a specular, labyrinthine "other" city that stretches beneath a large portion of the historic center—one that has grown to represent a physical manifestation of a complex and troubled collective unconscious.

Any coherent, rational attempt to understand and synthesize a life that might grow and sustain itself on such mercurial terrain is literally undermined by the shape and consistency of the soil, of the landscape and of the city itself, that by its very persistence and survival subverts and challenges all facile preconceptions or rules of reason. To understand such a place and its many inscrutable moods, one must embrace paradox and contradiction fully, entering an uninhibited and spirited stage where life resembles theater.

Everywhere in Naples life and death are inextricably bound.

The torrential noise that spills out of its perpetually open windows decorates an overwhelming silence that erupts from the mountain as a sinister premonition of its dormant fire, a heavy shadow never far from the minds of those who move and shout raucously through the bustling streets.

The volcanic soil within which its foundations are laid is fertile and rich, and it yields fruit and flowers whose colors and scents lace the stench of indigence that emanates from the towers of rubbish bags abandoned to rot like grotesque totems watered by neglect, rattling and swaying in the suffocating heat amidst buildings of exceptional grace.

All around it, a landscape of ravishing beauty crowns with gold a head that is neither hallowed nor pure, but still worthy of all honors that may be bestowed upon it. Mount Vesuvius sits calmly while its guts rumble menacingly, and although no sound is heard, everyone can feel its sinister, subterranean pulse vibrating the ground beneath their feet day and night, relentless and near. On its flank, temporary shelters once carved out of the naked rock have swelled into small towns where people awake and count their blessings as they open their eyes each

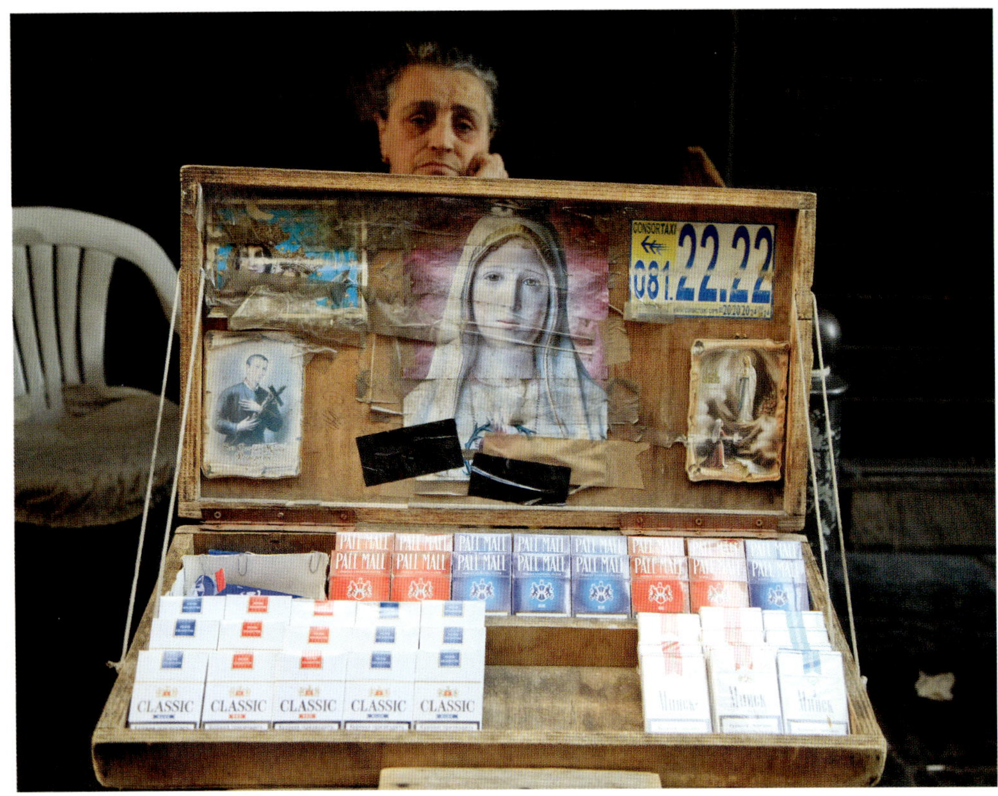

morning, while the mountain yawns with an acrid, sulphuric breath, an invisible *memento mori* that is etched in the landscape and carried on the breeze. Light washes the slumber from the limbs and hearts, and life creaks into motion, at once defiant and respectful of that constant promise of inexorable death.

Under this sword of Damocles, of imminent and inevitable loss, the relationship that has developed between Neapolitans and their faith is a peculiarly pragmatic one, born out of a sense of urgency and a unique understanding of personal freedom and responsibility. A devotional caution towards the mysteries of everyday life and death is intertwined with a spirit of

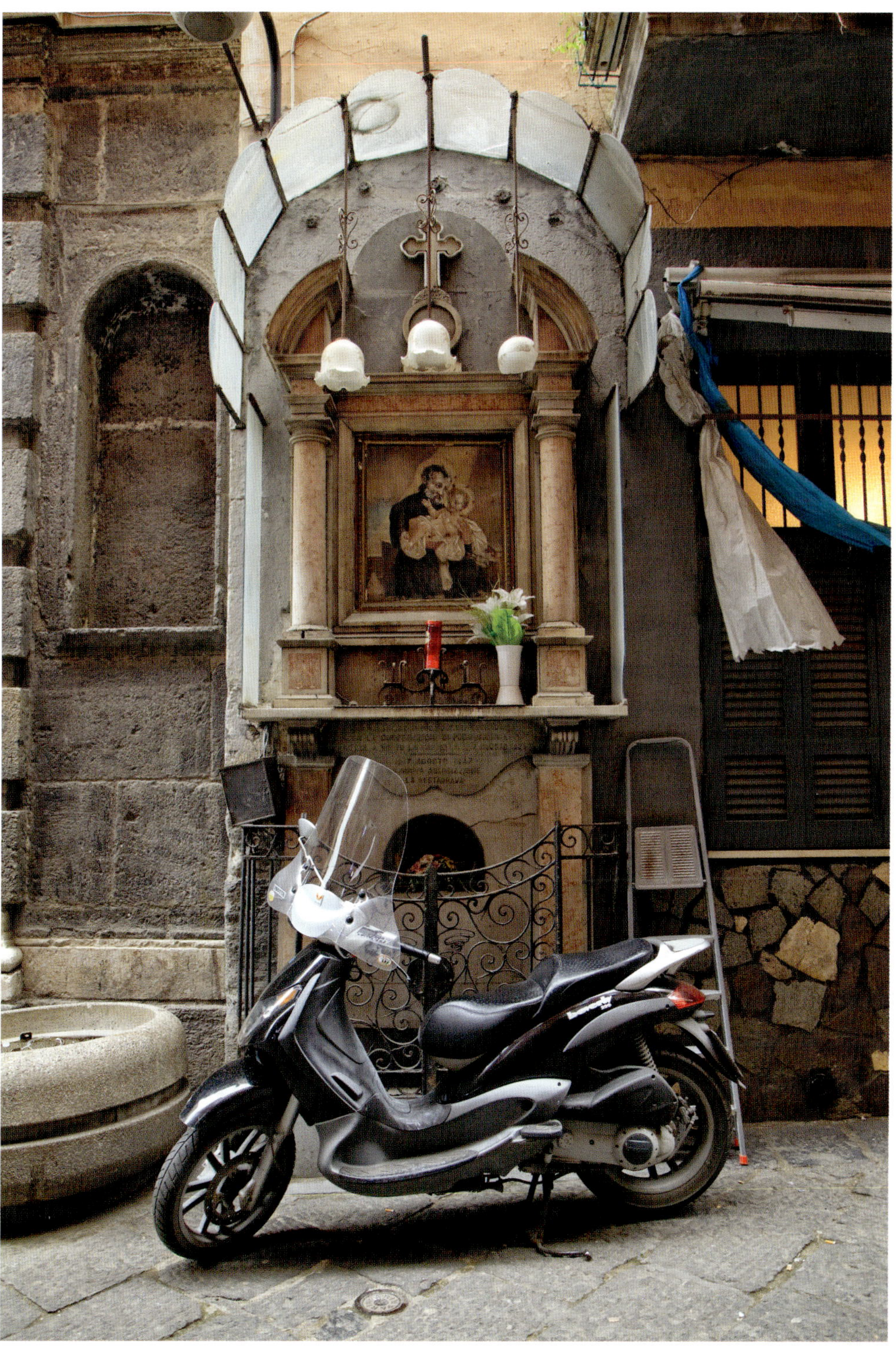

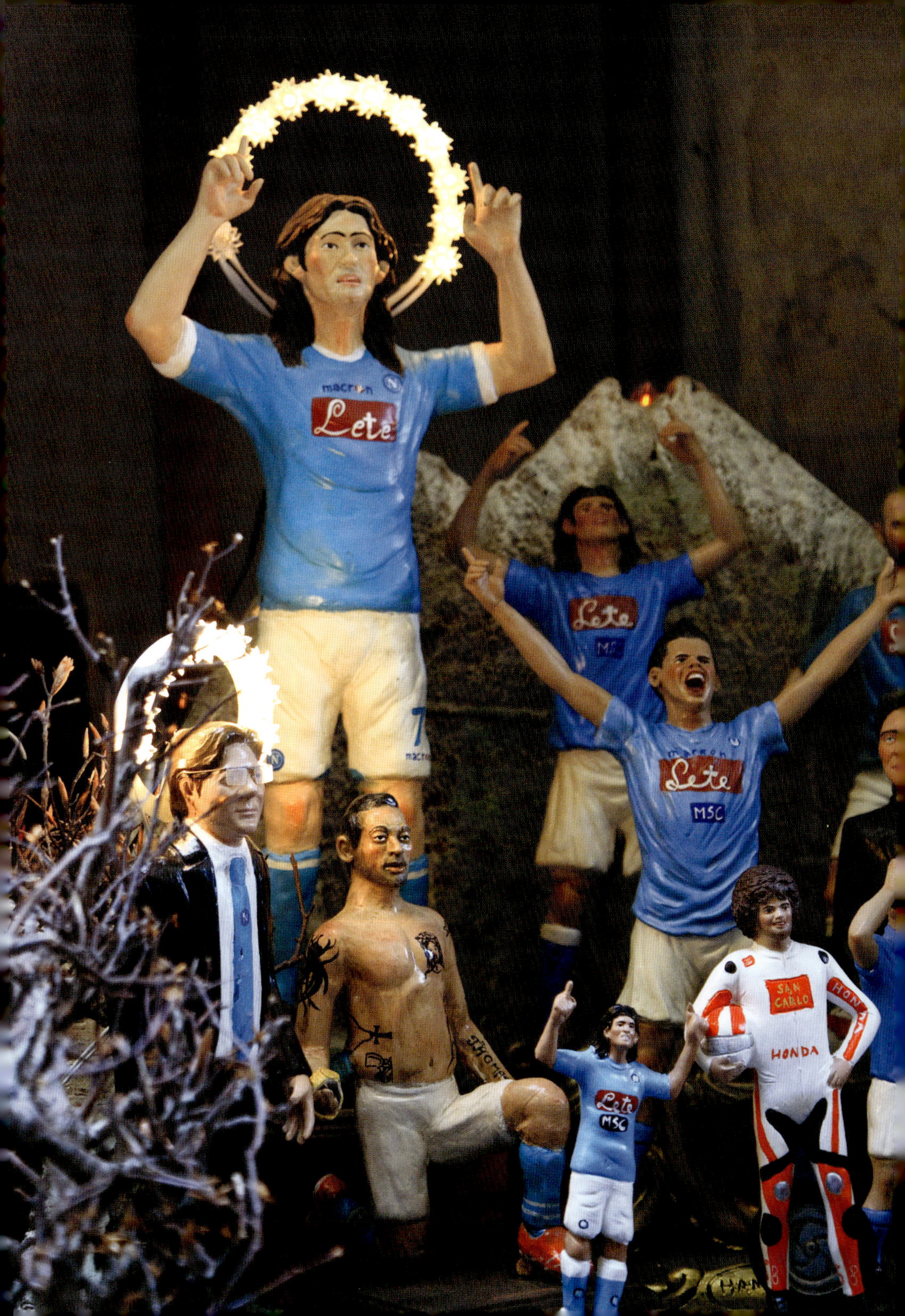
macron
Lete
Lete
MSC
Lete
MSC
Lete
MSC
SAN CARLO
HONDA

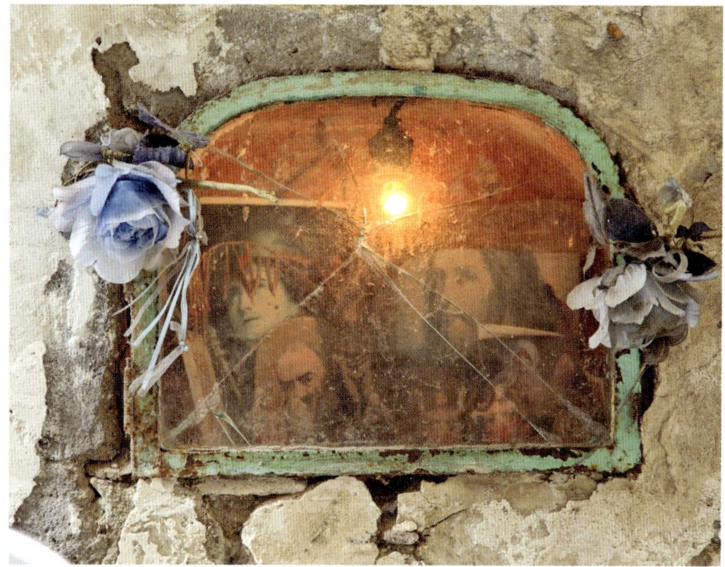

insubordination that allows them to transgress all boundaries and stare without fear or hesitation into the very eye of that paradox that the simple fact of being alive poses to all. They are ruled by impermanence and, just like the quickened earth on which they are delivered, their existences are transitory, volatile and unpredictable; here the veil that separates myth from reality, dream from wake, is permeable, malleable, and so is any material possession, social structure, individual heritage, or any understanding of collective past, present or future.

Prayers are the only currency available to all, without distinction of provenance, class or status, with which graces and miracles can be sought, through which survival may be beseeched or granted, both the momentary survival of the body and the eternal one of the soul.

The sooty, sweaty streets of the historic center overflow with commerce, gossip and crime, life and death in all their conflicting and discordant aspects. The open doors that line the streets lead to the bassi (lows), so-called tiny, crammed interiors

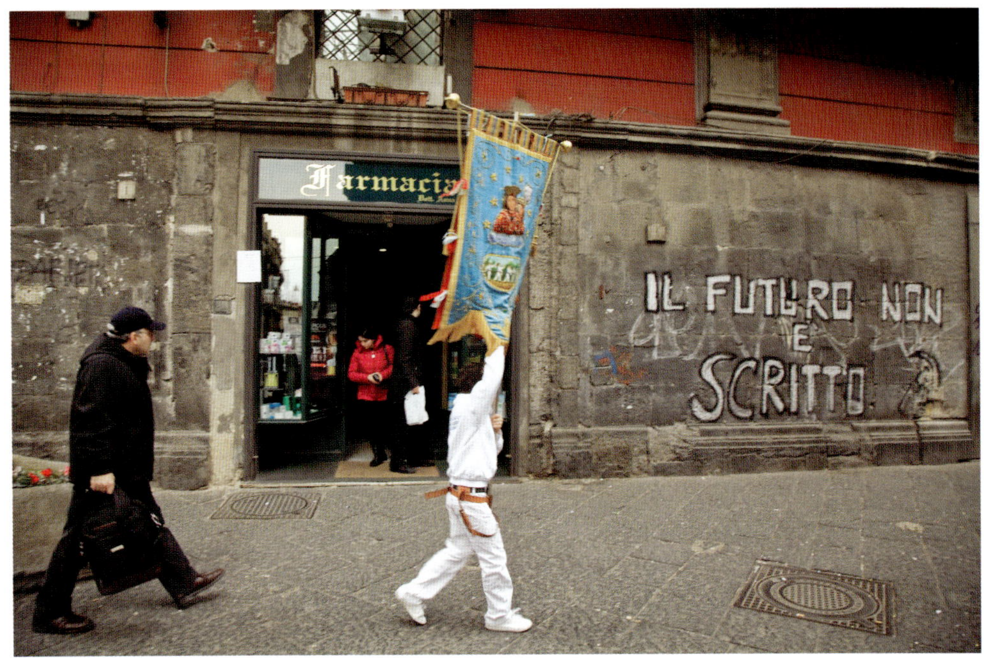

where lives are played out publicly even in the intimate privacy of grief and desperation. Behind the goods laid out for sale one will always glean the familiar shape of a bed, a cooker, and a shrine to the dear departed: a faded photograph surrounded by votive candles and fresh flowers, damp with whispered prayers, kisses and tears.

Thus the space between the living and the dead shrinks to that between two sides of a very narrow threshold, and to cross it is never a taboo. In the numerous niches carved out of stone walls and dotted around the city, the painted faces of the saints rest amiably next to those of the victims of organized crime (the Camorra), staring out of creased and faded photographs and surrounded by a hoard of nameless, faceless figurines, wrapped in flames, their arms extended pleadingly above their heads; these are lovingly referred to as the *aneme perse* (lost souls), *aneme poverelle* (poor souls), *aneme pezzentelle* (beggar souls), the souls that belong to those equally nameless, faceless multitudes of dead whose unclaimed bones have accumulated in the hidden bowels of the city since the great plagues of the seventeenth century, and for whom nobody could pray, whom nobody remembered.

They are the souls who are condemned to purgatory, that liminal waiting room of suffering that can only be transcended with the intervention of the living, who may offer the souls a mass, a thought or a prayer to help them rise a little closer to the *refrigerio*, the refreshing, cool air of heaven. That they should be placed next to those other lost souls, the victims of the Camorra (in itself a veritable plague that has ravaged the city for decades and is still gathering numberless dead today) are a testament to the complex role that faith holds within the unique, often impenetrable (and equally as complex) cultural and social landscape of the city.

Like the city itself, faith in Naples is multifaceted and seemingly incongruous, almost absurd, although when considered from a more humanistic perspective it reveals a great deal more sense than any other organized religion might, drawing close to its natural, pagan identity. Like in most places in Italy, the Catholic religion reached the unruly southern regions as an infrastructure imposed at the time of the Holy Roman Empire to reign in and supervise a wealth of diverse and insular local cults, mostly inherited from the Greeks, through which all matters of life and death had been interpreted and understood thus far. The natural belief in a transcendence in the matters of the earth, nature and its gods, amongst people whose lives were ruled so unabatedly by the weather, the seasons, and a primal, often brutal, but always fundamental relationship with their environment, was slowly displaced and reframed through the lens of an organized religion that appropriated the language and lexicon of these cults. In the process, though, this cultural legacy was stripped of any individual meaning, reinstated instead as a supervised, cleansed and hierarchical system—based on a single, unified story—that sought to rule over the subconscious of each community (in a way similar to how politics attempts to rule and reconcile often widely diverse social and economical matters and interactions).

In a city like Naples, where the role of dreams and the subconscious, with all its complexities and contradictions, overrules that of reason, this has precipitated a rift within systems of belief and the rituals and manifestations of faith itself. Above ground is the theater where the "official" ritual plays out, the one connected to the saints and performed in consecrated spaces and under the supervision of the Catholic Church. Naples wears its congregation's faith proudly on the walls of its many churches; the Chiesa del Gesu' on *Spaccanapoli*, the street that is the neuralgic center of the old quarter, is drowned in countless *ex votos*, silver familiars in the shape of hands, feet, eyes, lungs, bellies, and any other part of the body, or signifier of life, that might be the object of the saint's benevolence and for which he is being thanked.

Each saint has a name, an identity and a past that is distinct and unique and is irrevocably removed from the condition of the nameless crowds. There is an obvious, unbridgeable gap that separates the living from the hallowed, inviolable space occupied by the saints, whose extraordinary and pious conduct in life has granted them such veneration after death. The gilded altars, the holy light falling in rays from the stained windows, the marble effigies resplendent in their size and polish—all are a world away from the poor, the criminals, the orphans, the loud-mouthed widows, the legions of flawed and unremarkable individuals who shuffle daily through the aisles, falling on their knees in prayer or crowding the confessionals to unburden themselves of their sins, sins that one can almost taste in the

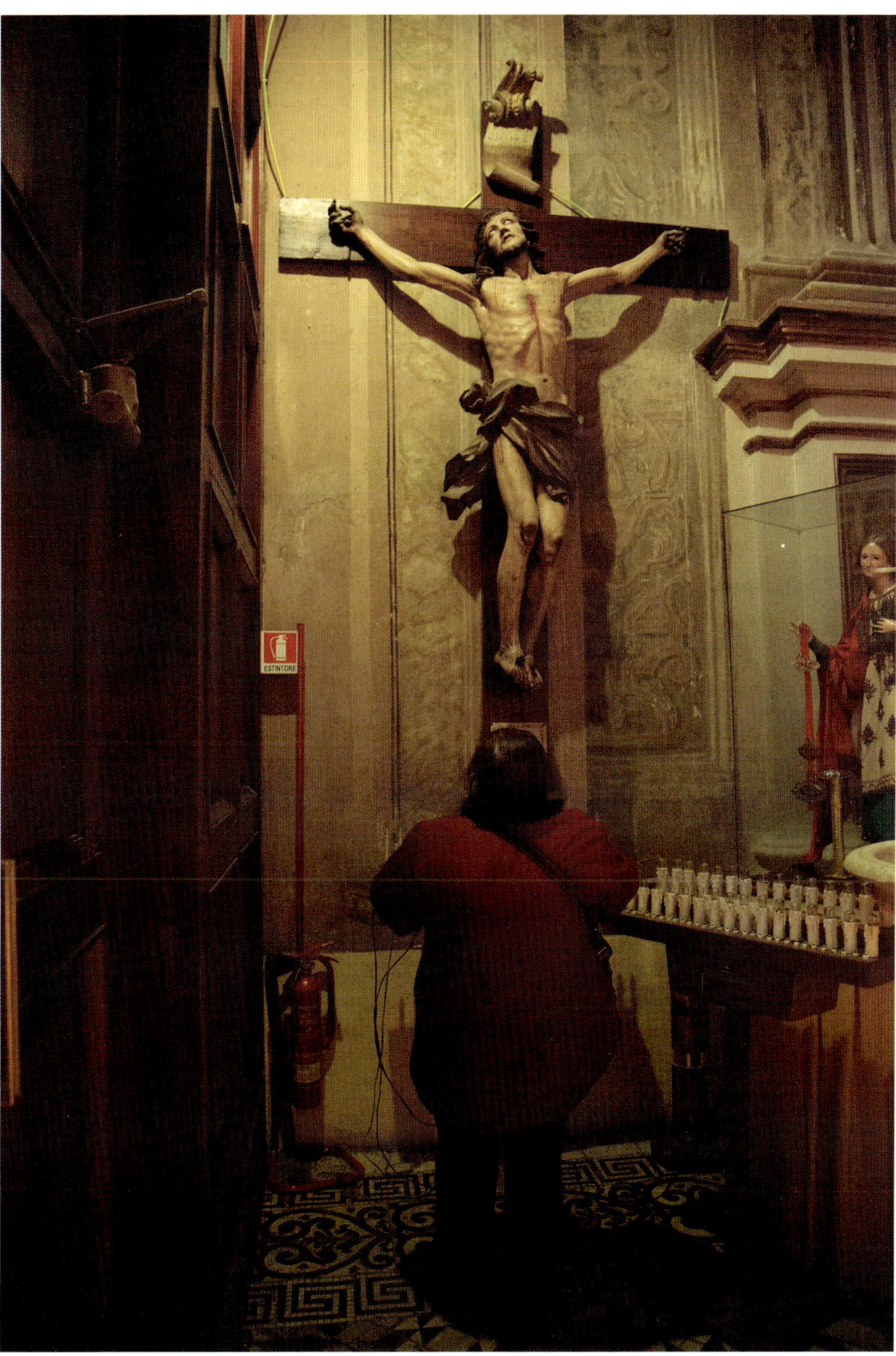
ESTINTORE

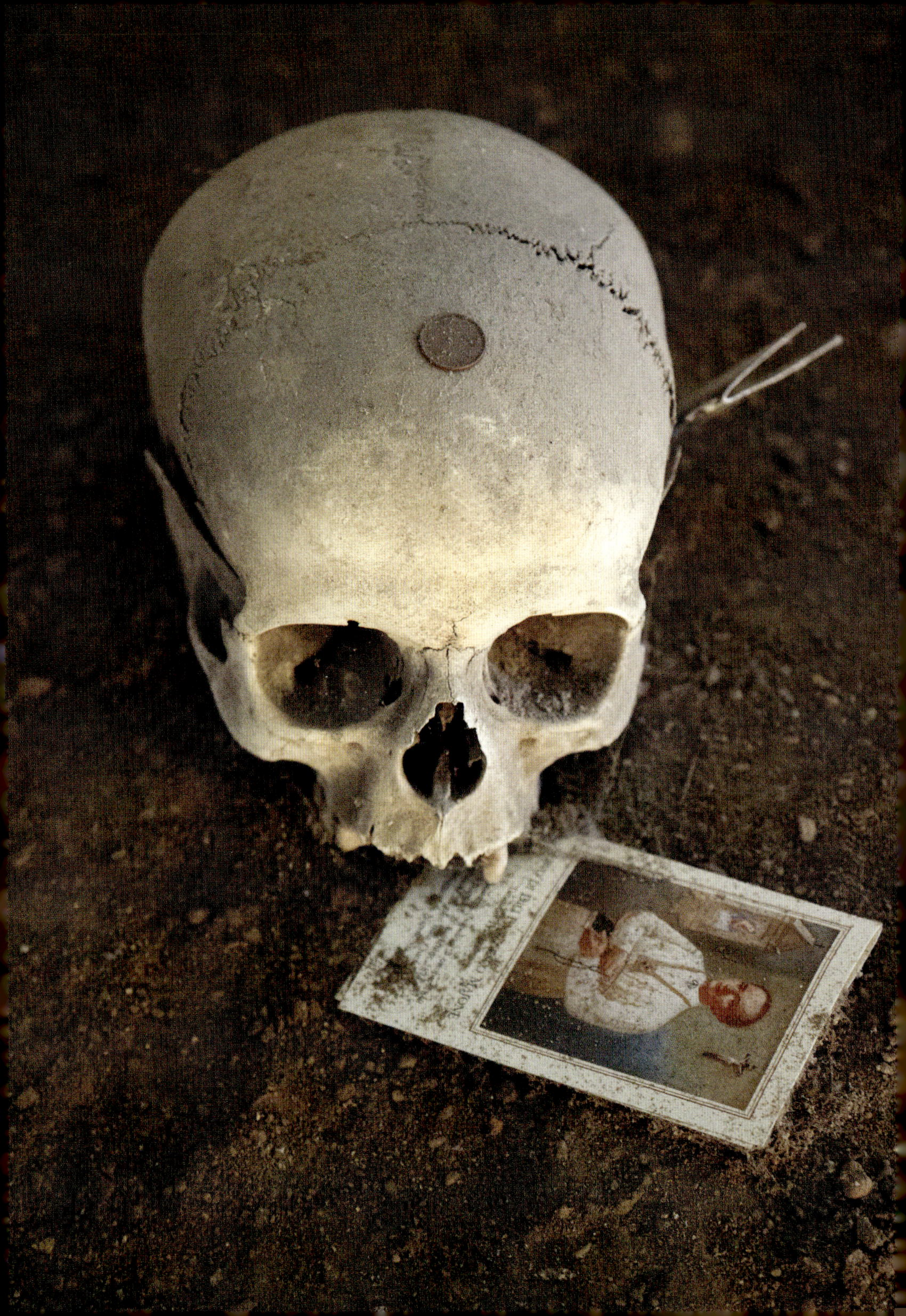

air and that no saint could ever have known first hand. These confessions are reserved for the priest, himself a reluctant member of the crowd, and surely not a stranger to sin.

Neapolitans approach the saints directly only at times of great need, imploring them for a specific miracle or grace that might help the individual through an exceptionally difficult circumstance, one that only a saint could have the power to affect, like grave illnesses, accidents or natural disasters. The saints, when welcomed into the homes, are guests of honor and are referred to with a reverence that keeps them apart from the people for whom they intercede. They inhabit the lofty heights of heaven, and only their benevolent gaze crosses the distance to descend benignly on the lives of those who pray to them.

Underground, in the *ipogei*, the dark and musty rooms below the earth, buried underneath the splendor of sainthood, another, unofficial ritual unravels. This hollow city is where Neapolitans gather to pray for the souls of purgatory, those very same crowds of abandoned souls whose toil after death mirrors so closely their everyday suffering. It is believed that this cult, although with some variations in form, has been kept alive since its inception in the 1600s, following the great plagues of that century. Hundreds of thousands of bodies were buried with great haste in communal graves beneath the city, without ceremony and with no time or resources to keep track of names and burial locations.

The bones, and in particular the skulls of these *male morti* (badly dead), lovingly referred to as *capuzzelle* (little heads), became the silent and reluctant inhabitants of the underground and, once rediscovered, the pivot of this very peculiar cult. As

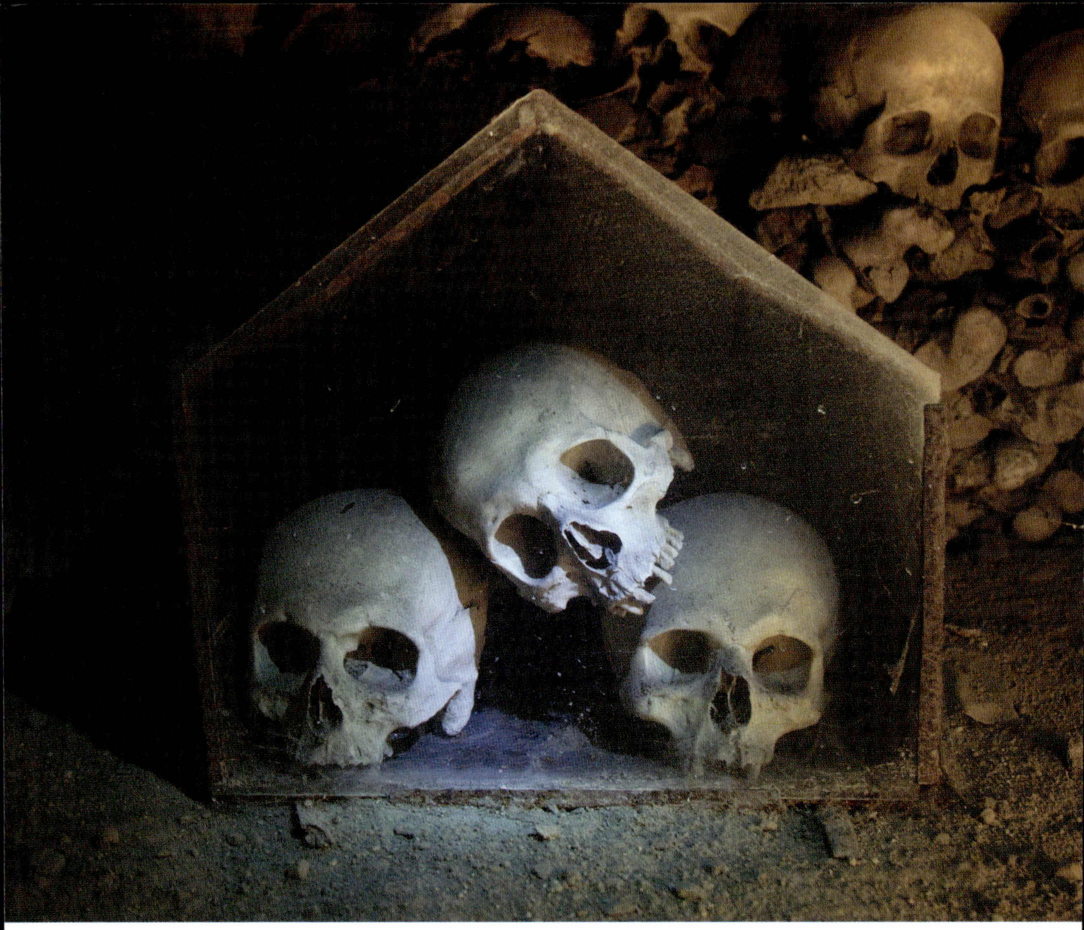

Stefano De Matteis explains,

> The skull is a symbolic synthesis of the idea of death, or it represents a memento mori, a reminder of that crossing that nobody can avoid. But within this cult, the two elements—both the presence, and the passing—are unified and placed in a physical space that is separated from the world of the living, an edge-land. In such places there appears to be a particular understanding of liminality: this edge-land is inhabited by those who don't belong to life anymore, whose remains we can see and touch, but who are not considered to be properly "dead" due to their inhabiting a space of passage, of transition, Purgatory—that third space between life and death: this

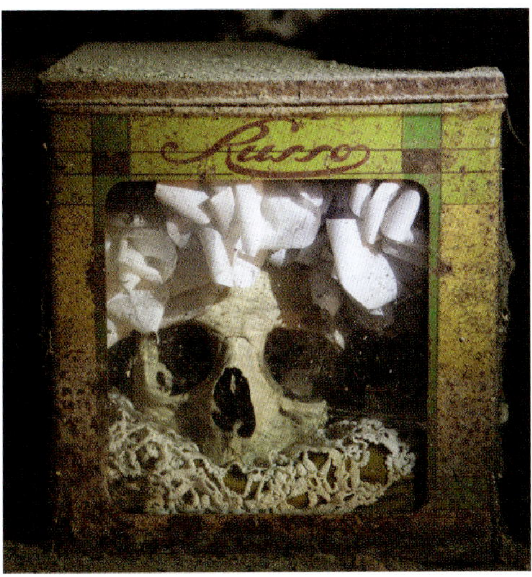

> becomes a place for waiting and hoping, very similar to life itself. It is in this very same place that social actors establish a system of communication aimed to create a dialogue with the otherworld, taking as their starting point an equivalence of liminal positions: that of the souls damned to Purgatory, and of the devouts, damned to the margins of society. [1]

The first encounter between the living and the dead happens in a dream, where a lost soul manifests itself to the devotee for the very first time and shares with them his story and the circumstances of his death. Following this first encounter, the devotee will be guided through the underground tunnels of one of the three epicenters of this cult—the Cimitero delle Fontanelle in the old historic Sanita quarter, Santa Maria del Purgatorio in Arco, or San Pietro in Aram—until the specific skull is found amidst the piles of bones; once located, the skull will be cleaned, polished, and placed on a small white pillow, and offerings will be brought to it.

[1] Stefano De Matteis, *Antropologia delle anime in pena* (Argo, 1993).

Unlike with the saints, there is a direct equivalence between these souls (once lost, now found and reunited with their name and history) and the poor people who pray for them: their circumstances, although on opposite sides of the ultimate threshold, are very similar, and the contract established between them through prayers and offerings is one of mutual succor. The devotees will offer prayers to grant the soul (and through a single soul, the nameless multitudes of purgatory) a swift crossing into heaven, while the soul will in turn look over the living and their families and grant them a normal, untroubled journey through life, following the natural steps of existence that may be considered as given but that for many are a luxury: growing into adulthood, marrying, having a child, occasionally winning a lottery—all humble milestones that shape and embroider a person's life and allow them to become a part of the mystifying order of the universe, vast and unknowable.

Once the first graces are received, the devotee will build a structure, often a simple marble, stone or tin cabinet in the shape of a small house (not unlike the bassi, where the living reside), in which the skull will be placed. This marks an official adoption: the soul has now become a recognized member of the family and will intercede for them until the time comes for it to finally pass on. From then onwards a relationship flourishes between the living and the dead, who will keep meeting and conversing in dreams, and grow accustomed to one another, exchanging interactions that echo those between the living, until the obvious distinction between them becomes but a small detail in a rather more important and fulfilling picture.

Naples is, by its very nature and appearance, an accurate representation of purgatory on earth, both geographically and metaphorically, and this hidden cult (outlawed for a short portion of the twenty-first century by the Catholic Church that feared the repercussions of what they deemed to be just a superstition, but otherwise accepted as a fundamental aspect of Neapolitan culture) fosters a strange kind of empathy amongst its conflicting and divided classes. Its poor are an idiosyncratic court of miracles that shares the same condition as that of the souls of purgatory, condemned to a marginal life of suffering and hardship as they wait to transition to a better state (the *refrigerio* of a happy death). Alongside the spiritual help that they seek from these souls, they often rely on the tangible help of the wealthy or of local charities to survive their daily lives. Against the backdrop of the city, they are the actors that play the part of the lost souls, and are identified with them to such an extent that they cannot be denied the help they need, as that would also mean denying that the souls be freed from their suffering.

Everyone in Naples is familiar with the catastrophic consequences of refusing the requests of the dead. It is a strange contract that has been honored for centuries and that contributes to a non-hierarchical structure of both society and belief that invests Naples with its peculiar and mythical intensity.

The cult of the dead weaves a strong and unbreakable line of continuity between different times and fragmented, traumatized histories, placing the multitudes of abandoned dead at the beginning of a collective past, inviting them back, through the ritual of naming and adopting, to inhabit a present that is shared by the living, inherently granting them the possibility of doing the same when their turn comes to join the otherworld. The multitudes of skulls are the tangible manifestation of a shared destiny, and people from all classes and backgrounds are sensitive to their plight: they remind the city of its traumatized heart (plagues are those events that not even saints can avoid, and that are bound to repeat themselves through history), a heart that nevertheless pumps nervously and defiantly through layers of sediment, both physical and temporal, committed to the perpetuation of an existence that is cherished and jealously escorted along its entropic drive towards the otherworld.

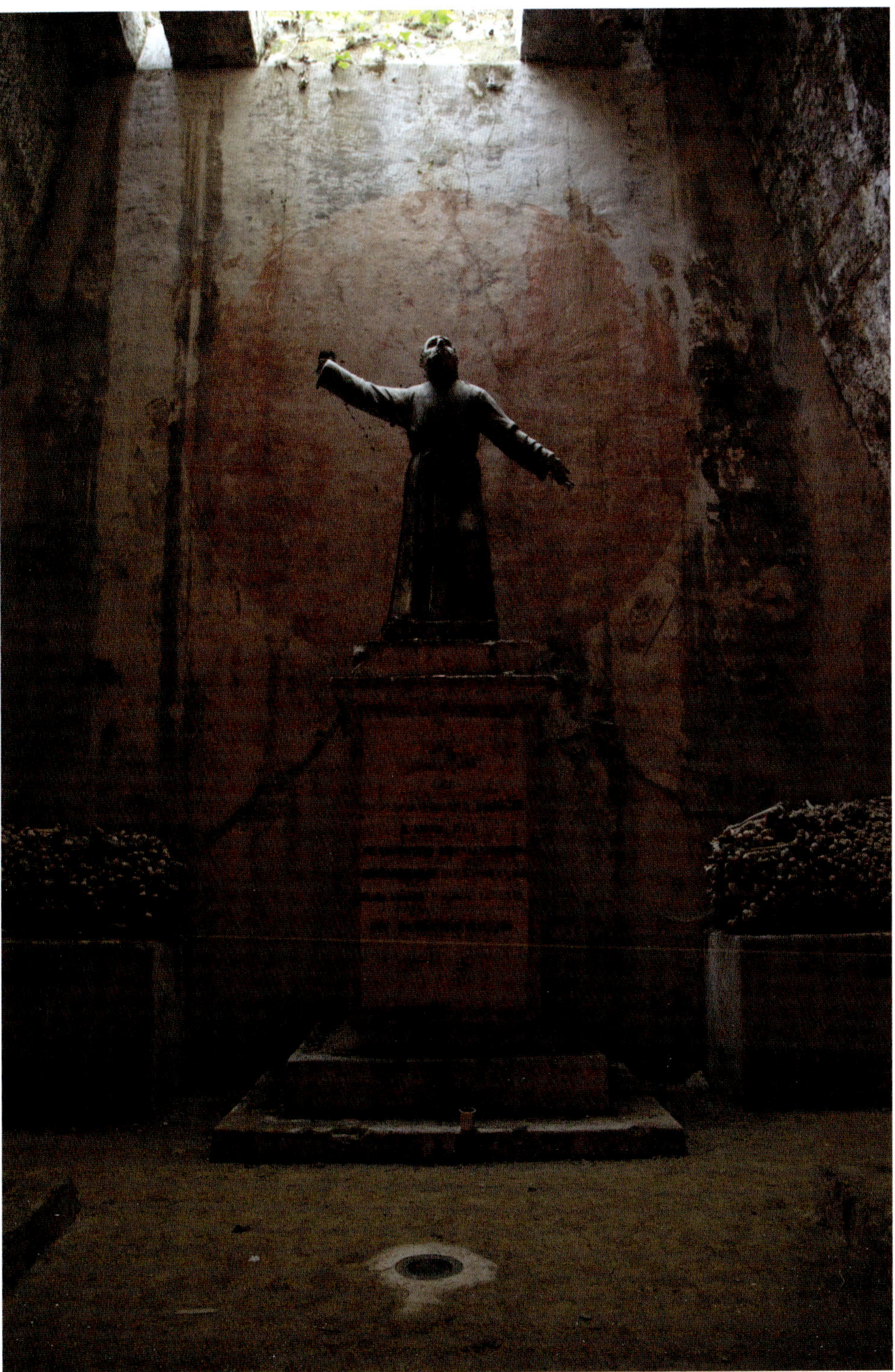

GHOST IMAGES

The Curious Afterlife of Postmortem Photographs

MARK DERY

Grace Stewart: Do you have any idea what this might be?
Mrs. Mills: 'Tis a photograph album, ma'am.
Grace Stewart: Yes, but look: they're all asleep.
Mrs. Mills: They're not asleep, ma'am; they're dead. 'Tis a book of the dead. In the last century, I believe that they used to take photographs of the dead in the hopes that their souls would go on living through the portraits.
Grace Stewart: They're in group portraits. [gasps] And children! Oh, it's macabre! How could these people be so superstitious?
Mrs. Mills: Grief over the death of a loved one can lead people to do the strangest things.
— *The Others* (2001, directed by Alejandro Amenábar).

As time passes by and you look at portraits, the people come back to you like a silent echo. A photograph is a vestige of a face, a face in transit. Photography has something to do with death. It's a trace.
—Henri Cartier-Bresson

The traffic in dead babies is booming, on Ebay.

There are daguerreotypes of dead babies, ambrotypes of dead babies, tintypes of dead babies, cartes de visite of dead babies, cabinet cards of dead babies; dead babies from the Victorian era, the Edwardian era, the roaring '20s.

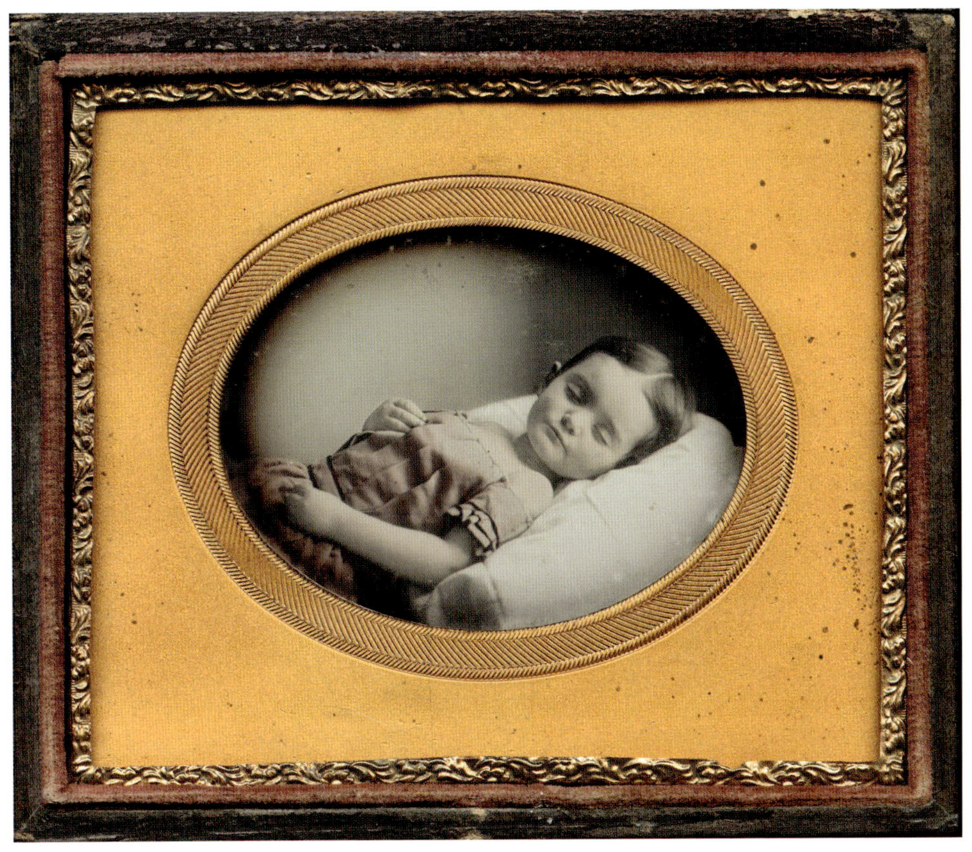

Nineteenth century post-mortem photograph. Courtesy of The Thanatos Archive / Thanatos.net.

Here's a listing for a daguerreotype of an "Exquisite Post-Mortem Girl," accompanied by a description that strikes an uneasy balance between graveside elegy and auctioneer's patter: "The young girl is surrounded by blankets and quilts. Very dramatic poignant image. Excellent!"

"Poignant" is a pet word in the collectible postmortem photo category. As in: "POIGNANT POST MORTEM BABY," an antique photograph of an infant, asleep forever in her toy casket.

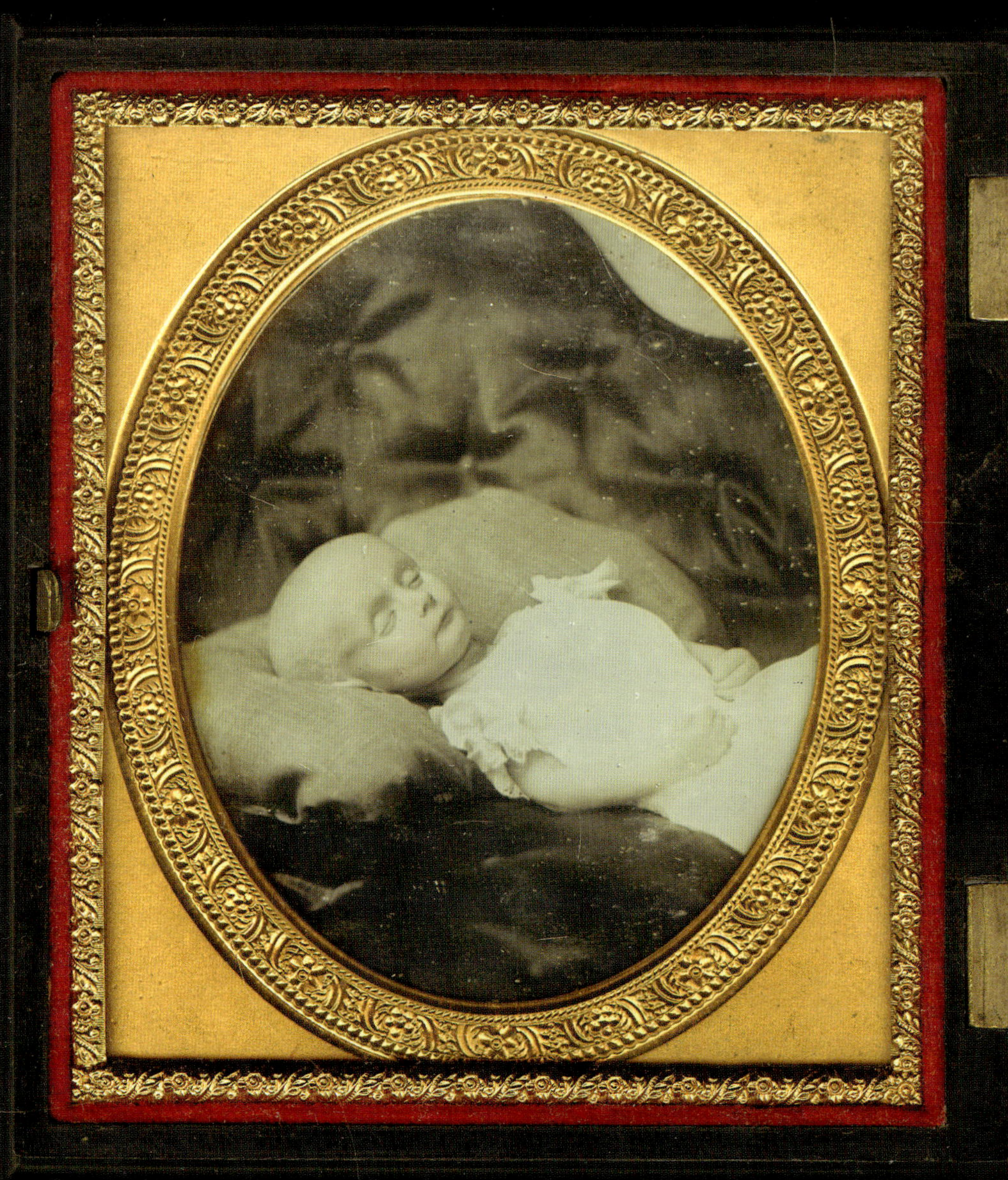

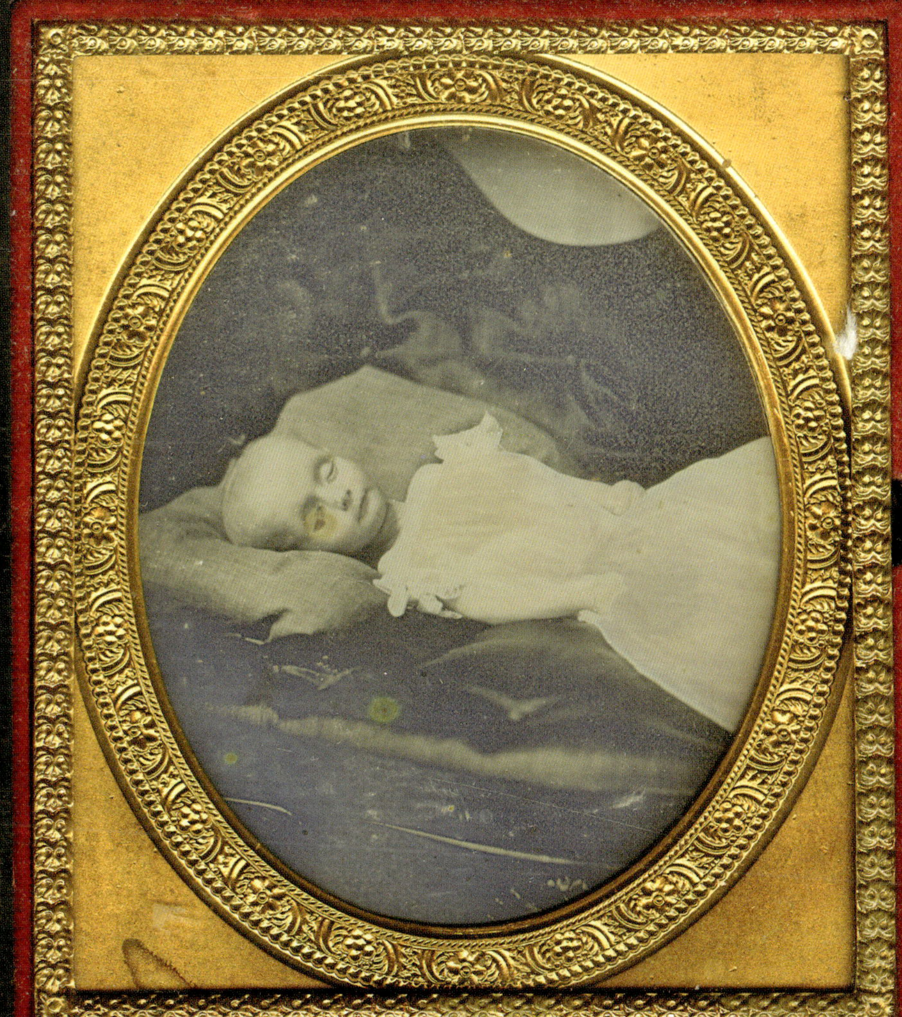

Image previous page: Nineteenth century post-mortem daguerreotypes. Courtesy of The Jeffrey Kraus Collection, www.antiquephotographics.com.

Her arched eyebrows give her a fretful look, querulous but a little quizzical, as if she's startled to realize that death, unlike gas, doesn't pass. "Heartbreaking postmortem photo," notes the item's description, conceding the obvious. Should we read this as a moment of silence—a brief halt in the hum of commerce, in recognition of the fact that this lugubrious curio memorializes the last, precious glimpse someone had of her child, before the undertaker dropped the lid? Or is it a lucky charm against the charge that buyers and sellers of such artifacts are trafficking in tears? Or just more of the mawkish morbidness that characterizes the "American Way of Death"?

> Fittingly, some sellers court the goth bidder. Eschewing Forest Lawn sentimentality, they accentuate the macabre: "Haunting Open Eyes Original Post Mortem Cabinet Card"; "EERIE POST MORTEM MAN Cabinet Card"; "1910s PHOTO! POST MORTEM DEAD WOMAN in GLOWING CASKET!"

Demand for postmortem images is sufficiently high that some sellers, fresh out of dead people, do their best to drum up business for dead-*ish* people, as in the unwittingly hilarious listing for a carte de visite of "CIVIL WAR ERA 2 WEIRD CADAVER-LOOKING MEN." Despite their baleful stares and unsmiling rigidity, the two men in the photo are victims of photographic technology in its infancy, nothing more: the long exposure times required by the daguerreotype process—up to 10 seconds, depending on the light—compelled subjects to assume a rigor mortis-like stiffness.

—⁂—

In his seminal study, *Secure the Shadow: Death and Photography in America* (1995), the anthropologist Jay Ruby notes that "the

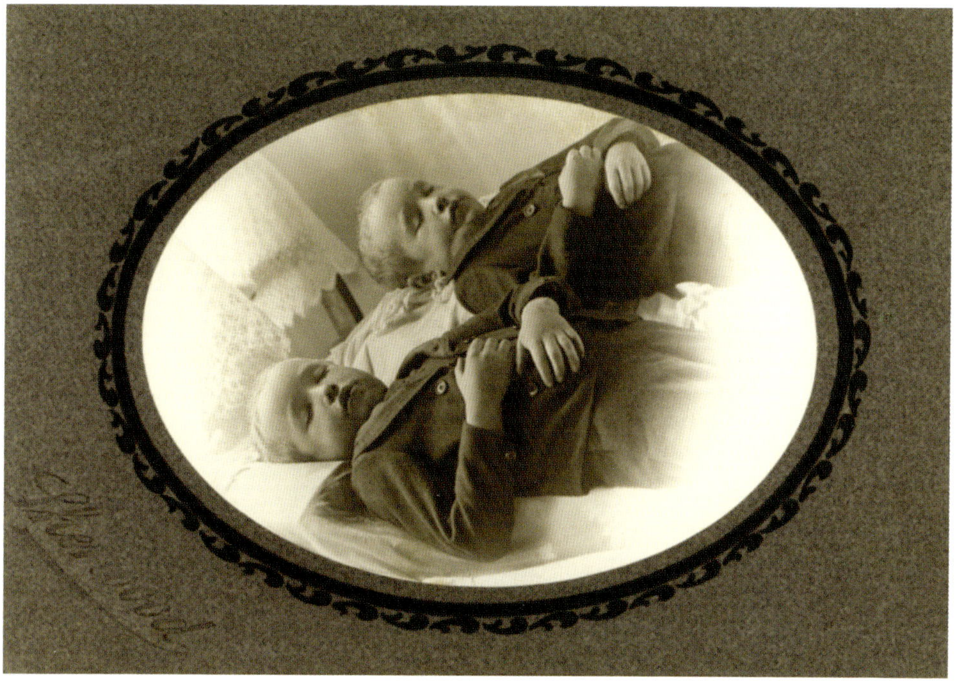

custom of photographing corpses, funerals, and mourners is as old as photography itself."[1] A direct descendant of the "mourning portraits" popular in the eighteenth and early nineteenth centuries—posthumous paintings of the deceased as they looked in life, commissioned by the well-to-do bereaved—the practice of postmortem photography was widespread in nineteenth-century America; "secure the shadow, ere the substance fade" was a popular tagline for photographic studios, exhorting customers to preserve lasting images of the near and dear, even if death had already claimed them. As early as 1846, an ad for the Boston photographers Southworth & Hawes proclaimed,

Image above: Post-mortem photograph. Courtesy of The Thanatos Archive / Thanatos.net.

> We make miniatures of children and adults instantly, and of Deceased Persons either at our rooms or at private residences.

[1] *Jay Ruby,* Secure the Shadow: Death and Photography in America *(Cambridge, MA: The MIT Press, 1995), 50.*

> We take great pains to have Miniatures Of Deceased Persons agreeable and satisfactory, and they are often so natural as to seem, even to Artists, in a deep sleep.[2]

[2] *Ibid.*, 52-3.

Death was a fact of life in the nineteenth century. Childhood mortality took one out of every five children in her first year, two out of every five by their fifth;[3] children were carried off by cholera, dysentery, diphtheria, typhoid, yellow fever, scarlet fever, or measles. "From [baby] carriage to coffin was the fate of over 30 percent of nineteenth-century children," writes Stanley Burns, M.D., in his pioneering study, *Sleeping Beauty: Memorial Photography in America*.[4] Losing all of one's children to an epidemic, in a matter of days, was not uncommon.

[3] *Ibid.*, 179.

[4] *Stanley Burns, M.D.*, Sleeping Beauty: Memorial Photography in America *(Altadena, CA: Twelvetrees Press, 1990), "Caption 57" (unnumbered page).*

In the nineteenth century, especially in rural America, families prepared their own dead for burial by laying the body on a board and washing and dressing it for the wake, traditionally held in the front parlor of the family home. Homes, in Victorian America, "were large to house multiple births and generations," writes the essayist and undertaker Thomas Lynch, in *The Undertaking: Life Studies from the Dismal Trade* (1996). "These were households in which, just as babies were being birthed, grandparents were aging upstairs with chicken soup and doctors' home visits until, alas, they died and were taken downstairs to the same room the babies were christened in to get what was called then, 'laid out.'"[5]

Unlike residents of big cities, people who lived outside urban centers typically had no easy access to a photographer. Among the rural poor, only the momentous occasion of death merited the expense of a portrait; thus, a postmortem photograph was often the only image kinfolk might have to remember a person by, especially in the case of children cut down too soon to have had a studio portrait taken. As evidence for the belief that

[5] *Thomas Lynch,* The Undertaking: Life Studies from the Dismal Trade *(New York: Penguin, 1998),* 35.

"parents were often desperate to have one picture of their dying child," Ruby includes a picture of a baby named Florence May Laser. "An adult hand supports the child," he notes. "[O]n the back of the image someone has written, 'Taken while dying.'"[6]

[6] *Ruby, 179.*

—⁂—

By the first decade of the twentieth century, however, death was disappearing from everyday life, swept aside in the cultural housecleaning called modernism. The Machine Age was revving up, banishing the lugubrious specter of Victorianism (or so it looked, in retrospect). In modernism's revisionist vision of the passing era, the late nineteenth century was the age of the bourgeois paterfamilias, snug and self-satisfied in his sense of entitlement, ruling his domestic castle in a Lilliputian parody of England ruling the waves.

Nothing better served the modern caricature of Victoria's reign as a time of rigor-like social stiffness, suffocating class consciousness, and tight-lipped prudishness than the Victorian conception of stylish decor: rooms stuffed with hulking furniture and bric-a-brac and plunged into a sepulchral gloom by dark colors and heavy drapes. Nothing, that is, except what James Stevens Curl, in his book of the same name, calls "the Victorian celebration of death."

Death, for the Victorians, was the venerated object of a sentimental cult. Unlike sex, it was a subject for polite conversation, prompted, perhaps, by postmortem photographs, which might be prominently displayed in the sitting room. With the rise of the rural cemetery movement in the 1830s, pastoral necropolises such as Mount Auburn in Boston sprang up on the edges of cities, their landscaped greens and imposing tomb houses, obelisks, and cenotaphs affording opportunities, in an era before public parks, for philosophical contemplation, aesthetic uplift, and, not least, outdoor recreation. There was, in fact, a school of mortuary poetry, a branch of which was known as the Mount Auburn school; William Cullen Bryant's "Thanatopsis" (1817), a Transcendentalist hymn to death as the union of the solitary self with the cosmic oneness of nature, was graveyard poetry's greatest hit. †

By the late nineteenth century the genre had degenerated into lugubrious kitsch, so familiar to Victorians that Mark Twain was able to parody it in *Huckleberry Finn* (1884). In the novel, Emmeline Grangerford, a daughter of the Southern gentry, turns out mawkish doggerel inspired by "obituaries and accidents and cases of patient suffering" clipped from the *Presbyterian Observer*—or does, until death stops her pen (a tragedy with a silver lining in Huck's opinion: "I reckoned that with her disposition, she was having a better time in the graveyard").[7] True to form, Emmeline tries her hand at mourning art, too: Huck describes one of her melancholy scenes, a crayon rendering of "a woman in a slim black dress... leaning pensive on a tombstone on her right elbow, ...her other hand hanging down her side holding a white handkerchief and a reticule." There is, of course, the standard-issue weeping willow (a cliché of mourning-picture iconography) and a suitably sachrymose caption, "Shall I Never See Thee More Alas."[8]

Emmeline Grangerford was Twain's sharp-nibbed caricature of the Victorian era's "Sentimental Love Religion," as the literary historian Barton Levi St. Armand calls it, a sensibility that

[7] *Mark Twain,* Huckleberry Finn *in* Mississippi Writings: Tom Sawyer, Life on the Mississippi, Huckleberry Finn, Pudd'nhead Wilson *(New York: Library of America, 1982), 725.*

[8] *Ibid., 724.*

---

†*Proof of the poem's perennial appeal to popular sentiment can be seen in* The Harlem Book of the Dead, *the studio photographer James Van Der Zee's gallery of postmortem images. As late as the World War II era, well over a century after "Thanatopsis" first appeared in print, Van Der Zee is inserting it, through the miracle of double exposure, into his portraits of Harlem residents in their caskets.*

was being elbowed out of the historical limelight, even as *Huckleberry Finn* was rolling off the presses, by a less romantic, more alienated—in a word, more *modern*—attitude toward death.

In America, the Civil War played a pivotal role in the medicalization of death and the professionalization of the funeral. The war sparked improvements in medical science and healthcare protocols, which in turn spurred the spread of hospitals; increasingly, death took place in the operating theater or the patient's room, not the home. As well, the necessity of embalming the dead so they could be shipped home for proper burial had given the fledgling death industry a boost. † On cue, mortuary professionals stepped between Americans and their dead, shrouding death in euphemisms; the undertaker rechristened himself "funeral director," a more anodyne, antiseptic title, and renamed the stark Puritan coffin a "casket," borrowing a term previously used to mean "jewel box." (Nathaniel Hawthorne, true to his Puritan roots, was appalled: "Caskets! a vile modern phrase, which compels a person ... to shrink... from the idea of being buried at all," he groused, in 1863.)[9]

Which isn't to say that the Victorian death cult didn't endure late into the nineteenth century. Dying a "good death" continued to be the done thing, the capstone on a life of Christian virtue and bourgeois propriety. And no good death was better than

[9] *Casket. Dictionary. com.* Online Etymology Dictionary. *Douglas Harper, historian. http://dictionary.reference.com/browse/casket.*

† *For more on this change in cultural attitudes and its effect on the practice of postmortem photography, see Kent Norman Bowser, "An Examination of Nineteenth Century American Post-Mortem Photography, a thesis presented in partial fulfillment of the requirements for the degree master of arts, by Kent Norman Bowser, B.A., B.S., Ohio State University, 1983," archived at http://etd.ohiolink.edu/send-pdf.cgi/Bowser%20Kent%20Norman.pdf?osu1144936478. Another excellent resource on postmortems in general is "Memento Mori: Death And Photography In Nineteenth Century America," an essay by Dan Meinwald included in* Terminals, *an online catalogue for a series of exhibitions that took place at various UC galleries from 1996 through 1999. "Memento Mori" is archived at http://vv.arts.ucla.edu/terminals/meinwald/meinwald.html.*

that of a beautiful child unstained by sin, a cherished icon that harmonized the Victorian romanticization of death with the era's beatification of childhood innocence. The death of Little Eva in *Uncle Tom's Cabin* (1852) was typical of the genre, a histrionic mix of moral instruction and sentimental flummery: her "large clear eyes rolled up and fixed" on a better world than this, she expires with a sign-off from the afterlife, "O, love, — joy, — peace!" Oscar Wilde, the first modern, scandalized his fellow Victorians when he rolled his eyes at the reliably tear-jerking deaths of little angels by remarking, of the beloved heroine of Dickens' *Old Curiosity Shop* (1841), that "one must have a heart of stone to read the death of Little Nell without laughing."

Mourning, in the Victorian world, was a protracted agony, formalized into periods (a premonition of Kübler-Ross' famous stages of grieving?), each of which required its own expensive wardrobe, accessorized with *memento mori* in the form of brooches and lockets containing a lock of the deceased's hair or a photograph. For women of means, widowhood was a two-year death sentence, sartorially speaking. In at least one memorable case, it was a lifestyle: after Prince Albert's death in 1861, Queen Victoria famously retreated into melancholy seclusion for a decade. Commanding that the Prince Consort's things remain untouched, just as he'd left them, and that certain daily routines be maintained, she took the "sentimental love religion" to morbid extremes. "Every night," notes Barton Levi St. Armand, "[Albert's] valet had orders to set out his evening clothes as if he were still going to descend to dinner."[10] It was a taxidermy of everyday life worthy of Miss Havisham.

[10] *Barton Levi St. Armand,* Emily Dickinson and Her Culture: The Soul's Society *(New York: Cambridge University Press, 1984), 66.*

Victoria's veneration of Albert's possessions as memorial relics and her preservation of his quarters as a shrine—a Victorian tendency Twain alludes to in Emmeline Grangerford's disused bedroom, with "all the things fixed in it just the way she liked to have them when she was alive"—are nothing more than a hyperbolic version, fit for a queen, of prevailing mourning practices. In time, the widow of Windsor returned to public life, though she wore mourning costume for the rest of her days. Her widow's weeds set a style that was both a model of grand-opera grief and a fashion trend; punctilious Englishwomen dutifully followed her example on both counts.

All of which has fostered the inextricable myth that postmortem photography came and went with the Victorians, a fiction promoted by Michael Lesy's *Wisconsin Death Trip* (1973). Woven from late-nineteenth century, small-town newspaper accounts of murder, madness, incest, premature burial, diphtheria, smallpox, and suicide (including that of a man who blew his head off with dynamite), Lesy's poetic history of the aptly named Black River Falls mythologizes late-Victorian America as a comic-gothic nightmare of morbidity and depravity. Darkly satirical in the tradition of Sherwood Anderson's *Winesburg, Ohio*, *Wisconsin Death Trip* was an improvisation on the dashed dreams of the '60s in the key of the Victorian Gothic. Intentionally or not, it helped cement the popular perception of the Victorians as death cultists, a vision epitomized by the book's grim period photographs, some of them postmortems. "Some of the most affecting [images] show dead infants in their coffins," the visual-culture critic Rick Poynor observes. "Such photographs were commonplace then, but many viewers, including me, saw them here for the first time."[11]

[11] *Rick Poynor, "Wisconsin Death Trip,"* Design Observer, *April 5, 2005, http://www.designobserver.com/observatory/entry.html?entry=3207.*

Ruby holds Levy, among others, accountable for spreading the misperception that memorial photography was almost exclusively a Victorian phenomenon, a claim he rebuts with peremptory authority: "Sometimes thought to be a bizarre

Victorian custom, photographing corpses has been and continues to be an important, if not recognized, occurrence in American life."[12] Ruby concedes that "after the 1880s the trade journals no longer carry articles about photographing the dead and photographers do not advertise the service,"[13] and that by 1900 advertisements for the service of postmortem portraiture have vanished from newspapers, "a sign of a shift in public sentiment," marking America's passage into the twentieth century, when "death was ignored, forgotten, and denied, at least in public."[14] With our entry into the shiny, happy, death-denying world of machine-age modernism, he implies, postmortem photography went underground.

[12] *Ruby, 1.*

[13] *Ibid., 59.*

[14] *Ibid., 60.*

By the mid-1990s, the time of Ruby's book, the practice was almost exclusively "a middle- and lower-middle-class activity," he writes, "found more frequently among people with a strong ethnic identity, particularly African Americans, Asian Americans, Polish Americans, Russian Americans, and Italian Americans."[15] Case in point: Formal portraits of the deceased, laid out in their Sunday best, were a fixture of the African American "Way of Death" until at least 1944, the most recent of the dated photos in James Van Der Zee's *Harlem Book of the Dead* (1978).[16] Van Der Zee, a commercial photographer who set up shop in Harlem around 1920, took open-casket portraits throughout his career, nearly all of them in funeral parlors, where the subject lay on view in a casket framed by floral displays; in the darkroom, he often added "inserts"—chromos of Jesus or heavenly hosts, inserted through the magic of double exposure, "to take away the gruesomeness of the picture."[17]

[15] *Ibid., 164.*

[16] *"I took some of my first [postmortem] pictures around 1920 or so": James Van Der Zee, quoted in James Van Der Zee, Owen Dodson, Camille Billops,* The Harlem Book of the Dead *(Dobbs Ferry, New York: Morgan & Morgan, 1978), 4.*

[17] *Van Der Zee, ibid.*

Banished from public life, postmortem photography endures behind closed doors, as a private practice. Wary of social taboos, families take covert photos at funerals, mementos intended to help heal what Ruby calls "the social wound of death."[18] (In

[18] *Ruby, 111.*

the flashbulb era, funeral directors often found spent flashbulbs after a wake.)[19] "It is a photographic activity, like the erotica produced in middle-class homes by married couples, that many privately practice but seldom circulate outside the trusted circle of close friends and relatives," Ruby writes.[20]

[19] *Ibid.*, 83.

[20] *Ibid.*, 1.

The analogy is instructive. We've reversed the polarities of the Victorian age, when sex was unmentionable but death was ever present. Despite a *symbolic* realm that is awash in carnage (the zombie apocalypses of videogames, the numbingly numberless victims blown away in Hollywood action movies, nightly news reports of the latest schoolyard shooting or workplace rampage or terrorist bombing, the faraway mirage of casualties in Afghanistan), death at its most irrefutably *literal*—the *intimate* death of someone we know, close enough to clutch at us as consciousness drowns in the oncoming dark, close enough for us to hear the death rattle, watch the light in the eyes wink out—is rarely encountered.

A commenter posting on the website *Metafilter* spoke for many when he described the experience of watching his father die at home in a world where death more typically takes place in hospitals or rest homes, mediated by technology and medical professionals:

> My father died two years ago this December. It was a surprise to all of us and my mother and I were there when it happened. Having the body in the home was okay (it was probably under an hour) and I honestly feel it would have been okay for a while longer. It was dad, you know? He could have been sleeping... I almost felt comfortable with him.
>
> What I did not feel comfortable with was watching the process. I expected a lot of... nothing... at the moment of death. A rattle, a sigh. What I didn't expect was the look of terror in

> the eyes beforehand. I heard once that when drowning, the brain takes even the oxygen under the fingernails. What's the brain thinking about at those moments?
>
> I think we are very isolated from death, and I can't help but think that's a big part of our culture.[21]

—⁂—

In an age where death is regarded as obscene, unapologetically intimate images of death, intended to be stared at without apology, for the viewer's private pleasure, are by definition pornographic. Following that cultural logic, traffickers in such images must be pornographers; likewise, collectors of such images are, naturally, an especially creepy kind of scopophiliac, close cousin to the necrophile. In his discussion of the contemporary perception of postmortem or funeral photography as morbid, Ruby notes that "even the idea of collecting nineteenth century examples of these images upsets some people and causes them to assume the collector has a morbid, unhealthy fascination with death."[22]

[21] *Posted by Brainy at 12:29 AM on October 18, 2006, in the* MetaFilter *discussion topic "I See Dead People,"* MetaFilter.com, *http://www.metafilter.com/55597/I-See-Dead-People#1465992.*

[22] *Ruby, 177.*

The historian of photography Geoffrey Batchen speculates that "the traffic in postmortem photographs probably picked up at roughly the same time that the trade in photographs as collectibles began to accelerate, sometime in the 1970s"—an uptick that coincides with the publication of *Wisconsin Death Trip*. Batchen agrees that books like Levy's and, later, Burns', "probably stimulated the market." Even so, he points out, "there have always been private collectors who specialize in such things. It may seem strange to non-collectors, but it's not nearly as strange as collecting, say, lynching photos, which some people also do."[23]

[23] *Geoffrey Batchen, email to the author, May 23, 2010.*

Jack Mord, an expert on postmortem photography who maintains a collection of such images at his Thanatos Archive website, believes that eBay played a pivotal role in ginning up interest in the genre. "In my 12 years as a member of eBay," he told me, "I have seen the number of postmortem photos for auction there—as well as their prices—skyrocket." Spiking collector interest in postmortem images has given rise, in turn, to niche obsessions, he says—"collectors who tend to collect only a certain type of postmortem image—a mother holding a baby, for example—and are willing to pay plenty for them."

As well, says Paul Frecker, "serious collectors" of "PMs" (postmortems) will pay top dollar for "anything out of the ordinary." A collector and seller of nineteenth-century photography who maintains an extensive archive of postmortem photographs at PaulFrecker.com,[24] he notes that postmortem photographs of children posed to look as if they're asleep are a dime a dozen. Many of the antique postmortems for sale on eBay are paper prints such as cartes de visite and cabinet cards, dating from the latter half of the nineteenth century, when the aesthetic of the day euphemized death as "eternal sleep." Deceased children were often posed with a favorite toy, as if they'd dozed off while playing; deceased adults were posed with open books on their laps.

[24] *Paul Frecker's online "library" of postmortem images can be found at http://www.paulfrecker.com/collections.cfm?pagetype=library&typeID=1&myPage=1.*

At the dawn of the daguerreotype era, by contrast, no attempt was made to conceal the cold, hard fact that the sitter was a cadaver. Its title notwithstanding, *Sleeping Beauty* includes ghastly images from the 1840s—shocking by today's standards—of corpses, neatly attired and ceremonially laid out, but with blood oozing from their noses that no one had bothered to wipe away before the photo was taken. "The terror of death was still taught by some religious sects," writes Burns, "and little attempt was made to beautify the image."[25]

[25] *Burns, "Caption 37" (unnumbered page).*

According to Frecker, "There are umpteen PMs available of children that have been posed to look as if they're asleep.

Image right: "My Tangible Peace". Courtesy of Jenn Stocks.

But a photograph of a dead child with a trickle of dried blood running out of the corner of its mouth would be in a different league altogether, not because it's grotesque but because it's so much more unusual and the photograph has a punctum, a hook that draws you in and establishes a personal relationship with the image and generates a bigger emotional response."

—⁂—

Frecker uses the term *punctum*, Roland Barthes' coinage in *Camera Lucida* for that aspect of an image (often a seemingly incidental detail) that "pierces" the viewer emotionally, charging the photograph with a significance unique to that viewer. In so doing, he directs our attention to the question: what is it about antique postmortem photographs that casts such an uncanny spell on collectors?

For Frecker, such images "resonate in a way that not many other genres do. These are photographs of dead people, yes, but someone loved them and wanted to commemorate their life—to have one last (or perhaps an only) portrait of them before putting them in the earth. One simply doesn't get that level of emotion in a view of Brighton pier. The message of any photographic portrait is 'I was here'; with a PM, that message becomes all the more poignant." In psychoanalytic terms, the image is cathected—charged with emotions so deeply felt they still reverberate in the viewer's mind, a century or more later.

Unsurprisingly, such photographs strike a responsive chord in viewers who've lost a child. "Sadness is definitely part of their appeal," says Mord. "Many postmortem collectors are mothers who've lost children of their own. Their own sadness draws them to these photos, which in some way comfort them."

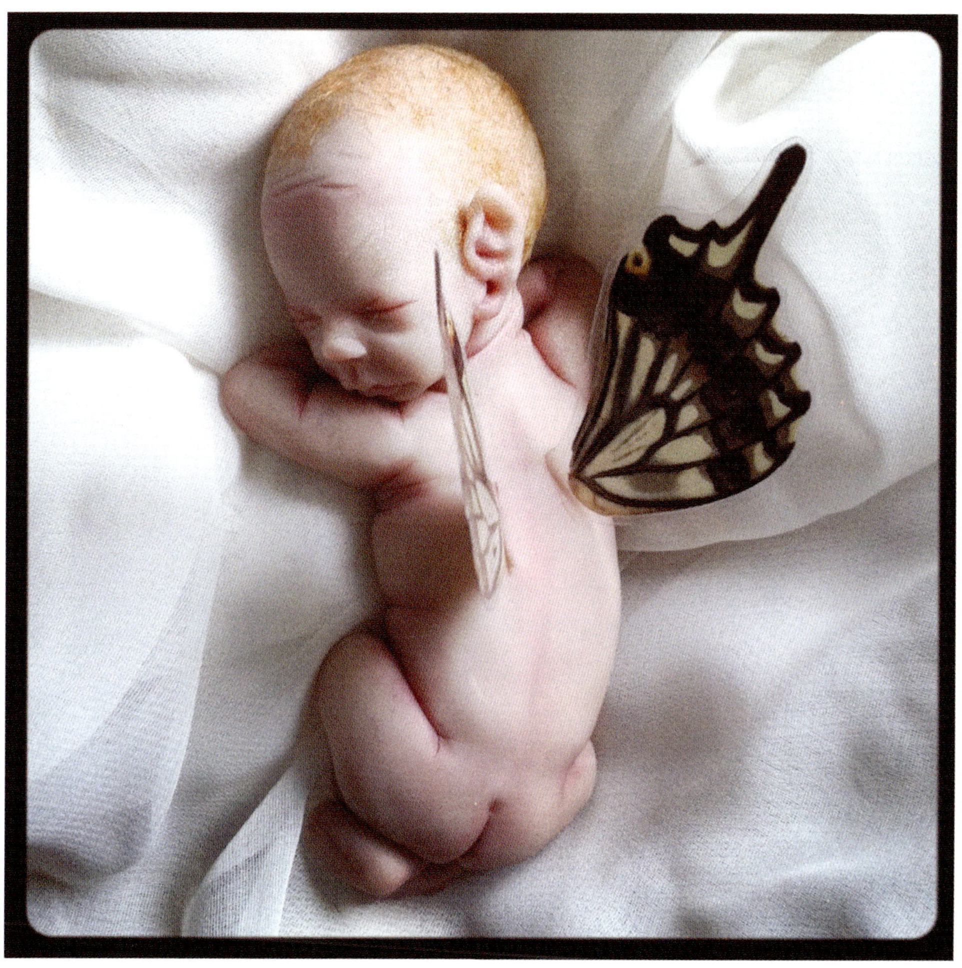

Grieving mothers who take comfort in these images are close kin to the women who find some measure of consolation in the "memorial dolls" sculpted by Jenn Stocks and sold on websites such as Etsy and eBay. Many are commissioned reproductions of babies who died, disconcertingly photorealistic down to the last hair on their little polymer-clay heads. Stocks' creations range from a three-inch "memorial sculpt" of a fetus at twelve weeks,

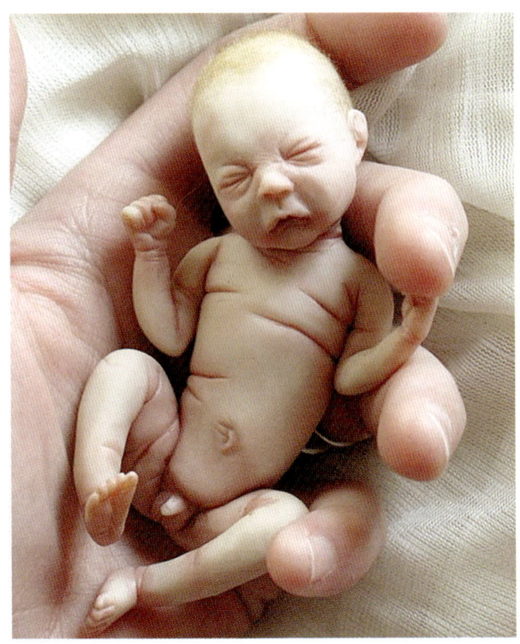

complete with umbilical cord, to tiny fetuses, no bigger than kidney beans, from the earliest stages of gestation, to fanciful "fairy babies" with elfin ears and butterfly wings, to an anencephalic baby apparently modeled on a postmortem photograph.

"I see lots of pictures of dead babies, some beautiful and some horrifying," said Stocks in an email.[26] "Pictures that parents are afraid to share with their close family [members] because they are filled with shame that their baby has died. Many are told to 'just try again,' which is an idiotic statement that negates the experience they're trying to live with." On her website, *My Tangible Peace*, Stocks speaks earnestly of using her talent "to create portrait pieces for families who have lost children in pregnancy, birth, to SIDS, or other illness"—one-of-a-kind simulacra "small enough to be tucked away in a drawer and kept private until an emotional collapse."[27]

[26] All Stocks email quotes taken from email to the author from Jennifer Stocks, April 5, 2013.

[27] Jennifer Stocks, "My Memorial Sculptures," My Tangible Peace website, June 14, 2011, http://www.freewebs.com/mytangiblepeace/apps/blog/show/7391293-my-memorial-sculptures.

Image left: "My Tangible Peace". Courtesy of Jenn Stocks.

Like postmortem photos of dead children, Stocks' dolls flicker irresolvably between pathos and uncanniness, an unsettling ambiguity that seems to divide the minds of many—including the artist herself, who began making memorial dolls after losing her first child to SIDS. "I picked her body up at the medical examiner's office and brought her to the funeral home," she recounted, in an email, "where I was encouraged to take her home and have her service there, surrounded by those who loved us, in an environment that held her memories—her scent, her first steps. Believe it or not, a signed document makes it legal to possess a dead body in Vermont. It was a very powerful experience and I firmly believe that being able to be in control of her body after her death has helped me heal."

An early adherent of the home-funeral movement that, like the home-birth movement pioneered by baby boomers, seeks to wrest intimate care for those we love from rubber-gloved professionals, Stocks has little patience with our neurotic recoil from dying and the dead: "I loathe that our society is so afraid of death. That we fight nature and present our dead as if they are sleeping—cold, chemical-filled sacks of flesh that have been violated with glues, paints, and props, all intended to mask what death does to our bodies."

Regarding the numerous postmortem photographs on eBay, Stocks told me, "What I see in those photographs is love. A mother, wife, friend gently cleaning the body. Putting thought into what [the child's] last dress will be, combing the hair of the deceased, taking pride in how well they're able to present their loved one. Inviting friends and family into their home, the sour smell of death mixing with the meal that is being prepared in the kitchen. It's all part of how it's supposed to be, simple and far from the world that we live in today."

In interviews, however, Stocks sometimes swerves—out of fear she'll be regarded as morbid, she says—into dead-baby-joke territory, referring to her sculptures as "creepy, naked babies" and wisecracking that, because the final stage in her production process involves baking mohair or Tibetan lamb's hair onto their heads, "I always have a baby in the oven."[28] Similarly, comments in an online discussion about her memorial dolls give voice to a wide range of reactions, from shudders of revulsion ("Burn the abominations") to heartsick *tendresse* ("I requested one of these 'creepy' babies in memory of my daughter who passed away at 23 days old. If you think that these dolls are creepy, [you] obviously haven't experienced the death of a child") to profound ambivalence ("This is very morbid. And disturbing. Not unlike the photobooks of the dead. Having had three miscarriages, however, I would have wanted to have had something-anything-like a baby, at least to bury").

[28] *Quoted in Leon Thompson, "A Vermont Artist Finds Healing, and an Income, with Lifelike Infant Sculptures," Seven Days, August 8, 2007, http://www.7dvt.com/2007/vermont-artist-finds-healing-and-income-lifelike-infant-sculptures.*

Likewise, postmortem photographs, especially those of babies and children, inspire radically different reactions, inflected by the viewer's experiences with death. As Mord observes, such images may trigger sympathetic vibrations in mothers who've lost children. But for palely loitering souls who wave their fascination with the macabre as a flag of transgression—code-word: goth, a demographic whose youth makes it more likely than not that its members haven't experienced death firsthand—a postmortem photograph, prominently displayed, is subcultural shorthand for conscientious objection to Middle America, with its Anne Hathaway smile and its power-of-positive-thinking homilies. The writer and illustrator Edward Gorey, the un-witting granddaddy of goth, was fond of postmortem photos.†

—⁂—

Antique postmortem portraits are riveting because they embody *corporeal truth* in an ever more mediated, simulated world, where everyday life is increasingly an out-of-body experience. At a moment when more and more of our interaction with the world around us takes place through tweets, text messages, and Facebook posts, the black-and-white dead of the nineteenth century deliver a visceral jolt. As embodied reality comes to seem like a fading afterimage of our imaginative lives on the other side of the screen, postmortem photos, more corporeal for the dead weight of death, confront us with the inescapable fact of embodiment.

"The postmortem photograph is a relic of a past that has been erased by modernity," says Michael Sappol, author of *A Traffic of Dead Bodies: Anatomy and Embodied Social Identity in Nineteenth-Century America* (2002). "[I]n that lost world, people had more direct and less mediated experiences of shit / sweat / blood / piss / grime / dust / phlegm / pus. And less mediated (less medicated) experiences of death, with a lot more suffering."[29]

[29] *Michael Sappol, email to the author, May 24, 2010.*

Postmortem photos force us to look death in the face, up close and personal. Irony of ironies, the twentieth century—one of, if not *the*, bloodiest in history—bore witness to the medicalization of dying, the professionalization of funeral rituals, and the repression of death in everyday life even as the Nazis applied the logic of Henry Ford's assembly line to genocide

† *"I collect postcard photographs of dead babies," Gorey told interviewer Ed Pinsent. "(Everybody says, 'Don't tell them that.') I got started accidentally. I had a postcard of a baby which looked like it was asleep, but someone said they thought that baby was dead. I said, 'Well, how could it be... I mean, uggh!' Now I discover that there are other pictures [like this], not only babies. You know, when travel was difficult, people had gone out to the frontiers and whatnot, people were losing babies right and left. This is at the turn of the century. They would have a baby all dressed up and photographed—sometimes it's sitting up in a chair, sometimes on a little bed, most often in a coffin, which does give pause.... I have a friend in New York who has a huge collection of postcards. He goes to these postcard shows and sheepishly says, 'Any dead babies?' to the dealers. He tells me, 'I hate it!' I say, 'Well, just keep looking.'" Quoted in Ed Pinsent, "A Gorey Encounter" in* Ascending Peculiarity: Edward Gorey on Edward Gorey, *ed. Karen Wilkin (New York: Harcourt, Inc.: 2001), 195.*

and America brought its genius for push-button solutions to the vaporization of whole cities at Hiroshima and Nagasaki. Death decamped to the hospital, and the ritualized leave-taking of the loved one moved from its traditional domestic theater—the front parlor—to the funeral *parlor,* stage-managed not by the eerily named undertaker but by the more clinical *funeral director.* (This, by the way, is why the front parlor was transformed, by the emphatic decree of a *Ladies' Home Journal* editor in 1910, into a *living* room.)[30]

"There's something fascinating about the juxtaposition of home and death" in postmortem photos, says the cultural critic Mikita Brottman. "Those things just don't go together any more. Home is the realm of shelter magazines and Sunday supplements, and death is the realm of sterile drips, hospital beds, heart monitors, health insurance. To see a corpse in the home is now a jolting juxtaposition."[31]

Our plasma-screen TVs, videogame consoles, and multiplexes are awash in CGI gore, yet few in the so-called first world, where medical advances have made the science-fictional "right to die" movement a reality, have ever looked into eyes of a dead man, trying to meet the gaze that—in the memorable words of the hardboiled novelist Raymond Chandler—you can never quite meet.

Except in a photograph.

[30] *John R. Gillis,* A World of Their Own Making: Myth, Ritual, and the Quest for Family Values *(Cambridge, MA: Harvard University Press, 1997), 212.*

[31] *Mikita Brottman, email to the author, May 25, 2010.*

Postmortem photographs reverberate with uncanniness because their dead are *doubly* dead: done in by injury, illness, age, or another man's hand, then killed again by the camera—trapped by the wink of a shutter in a moment that will last forever. (Not for nothing do they call it "shooting.") Defying time, postmortem people live on, just as those caught on film in the moment of their death will spend eternity dying (as they were in the instant of their immortalization) yet dead (as we know they now are) and, at the same time, undying: Robert Capa's "Falling Soldier" will never stop hanging in midair, splayed out, flailing in the instant the shot hits home; the Vietcong prisoner executed by General Nguyen Ngoc Loan in Eddie Adams' AP photo will flinch for all time from the bullet's point-blank impact, one side of his face scrunched up in that goofy-ghastly way, his hair absurdly mussed.

Of course, the corpses in antique postmortem portraits are no different from the people in *any* old photos in the sense that all photographic subjects are simultaneously dead and undead, and therefore uncanny—phantoms materialized in darkrooms and given ageless immortality as images, images that stare back at us across the gulf of time. Spectrum, spectacle, specter: the common root is instructive. Barthes called photography the flat death[32]; the cultural historian Martin Jay believes that photography, "by violently stopping the flow of time, ... introduced a *memento mori* into visual experience"[33]; Jacques Derrida thought film was "the art of ghosts, a battle of phantoms."[34]

Every photo portrait is a death mask: say "cheese," your frozen grimace baring the skull beneath the skin, anticipating the rictus you'll wear in death. (Inversely, the mortician who fixes a peaceful smile on the loved one's face makes life imitate art, transfiguring mortal remains into a mocking approximation of the "picture face" we all assume, just before the shutter clicks.)

By embalming the moment, photography gives eternal life: that is its paradox. Barthes speaks, in *Camera Lucida*, of "that rather terrible thing which is there in every photograph: the return of the dead." No wonder, then, that he finds photographs

[32] *Roland Barthes,* Camera Lucida: Reflections on Photography, *trans. Richard Howard (New York: Noonday Press, 1981), 92.*

[33] *Martin Jay,* Downcast Eyes: The Denigration of Vision in Twentieth Century French Thought *(Berkeley, CA: University of California Press, 1994), 135.*

[34] *Quoted in* Ghost Dance *(1983), directed by Ken McMullen.*

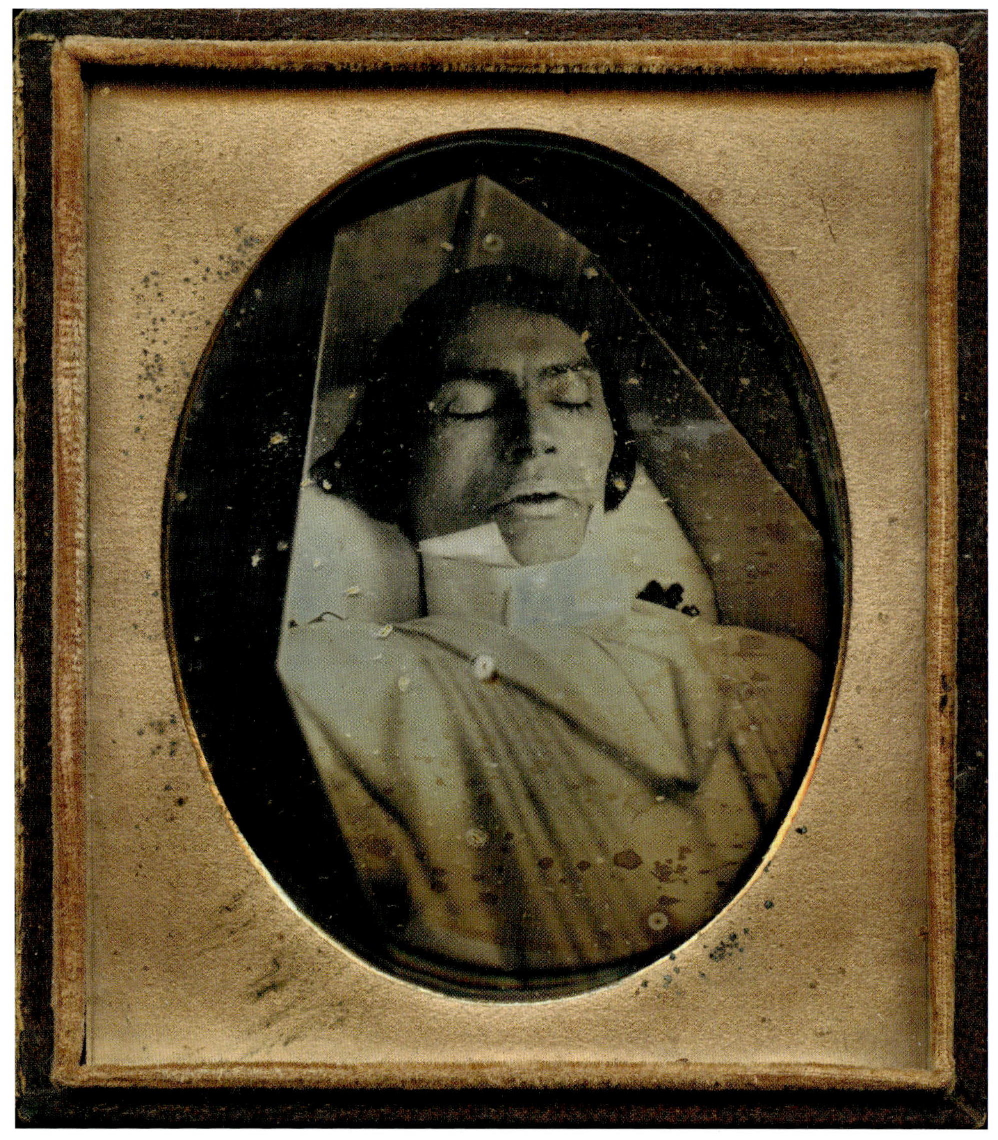

of corpses especially ghoulish: photography, like formaldehyde, fixes life—preserves "the presence of the thing (at a certain past moment)," even if the subject is dead. "If the photograph then becomes horrible," Barthes reasons, "it is because it certifies, so to speak, that the corpse is alive, as *corpse*: it is the living image of a dead thing." Daguerreotypes of Victorians embody these qualities par excellence. Beyond the self-evident uncanniness of photography's counterfeit of reality (in this case a lifelike image of a cadaver long gone to dust); beyond, even, Barthes' revelation that all photography is necromancy, lies the nagging sense that the Victorians, even in portraits taken in life, are always already dead. Their somber garb and lock-jawed expressions don't help, but our perception of the nineteenth century as haunted owes more to the fact that we know it not from moving pictures but from monochrome stills. As the term *nature morte* ("still life") suggests, stills and stiffs are ontological kin. Blotched by the decayed emulsion that always reminds us of blood-spatter patterns, even the most innocuous images seem to whisper of Lizzie Borden and Jack the Ripper. "Life is a movie," wrote Susan Sontag. "Death is a photograph."[35] Pictures of Victorians, even living ones, arrive in our time as postcards from a postmortem world.

[35] *Susan Sontag,* The Benefactor: A Novel *(New York: Picador, 2002), 215.*

[Author's Note: This essay is an extensively expanded version of a piece previously published in the August-November, 2010 issue of the Australian magazine Photofile, *under the headline "Embalmed on eBay," and later reprinted, in revised form, on the website* Boing Boing *on March 25, 2011, as "Ghost Babies." Many thanks to Ashley Crawford, editor of* Photophile, *for commissioning and editing the original version, and to the editors of Boing Boing, for resurrecting it.]*

STUFFED HUMANS

PAT MORRIS

SPECIES FROM ALL THE MAJOR VERTEBRATE GROUPS HAVE BEEN successfully preserved using taxidermy methods, and even some invertebrates (although the octopus does not stuff well). The exception is our own species, about which there is much ambiguity. Many taxidermists tell stories of people asking to have a relative preserved, but it is often unclear whether these were serious requests. Similarly, an undated newspaper article given to me by a friend from the *Ruislip Sunday Journal* headed "I want my late hubby stuffed" appears typical of many such proposals: not fully thought through. It may also reflect the silly season, when journalists experience a shortage of serious news stories. In reality, the preparation of humans by taxidermy involves many special problems and raises a number of specific issues. Such specimens are also extremely scarce, so it seems worth dwelling on the subject here at some length.

Very few humans appear to have been preserved using taxidermy methods, perhaps because anatomical modeling in wax was already well developed long before taxidermy was up to the job. The Romans had used wax to create funeral effigies, and making crucifixion models and other ecclesiastical representations for churches had become commonplace in southern Europe by the 1500s. Highly realistic anatomical modeling in wax was well

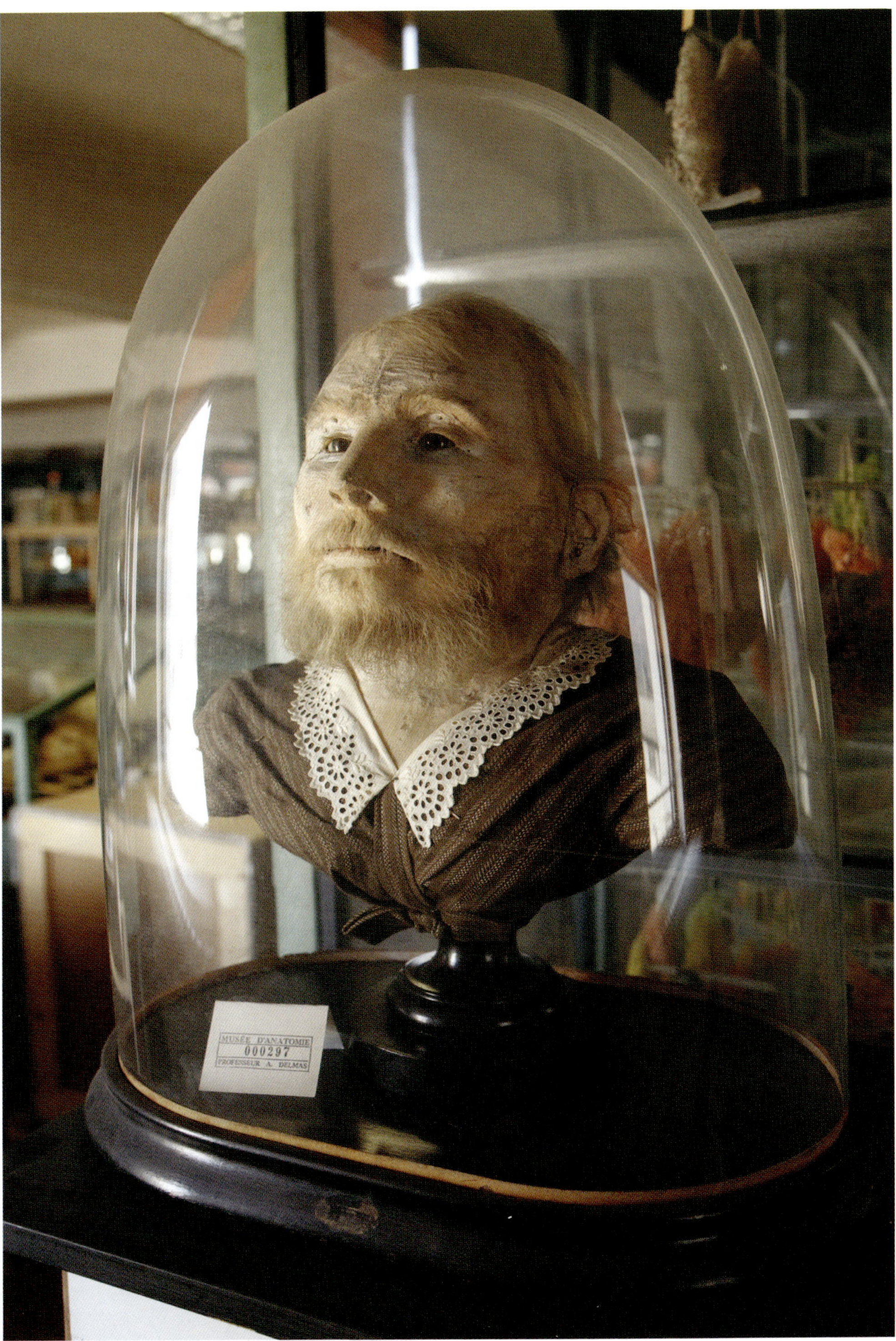
MUSÉE D'ANATOMIE
000297
PROFESSEUR A. DELMAS

Image Previous Page: Femme à barbe (bearded lady under belljar), Musée Orfila, Courtesy Musée Orfila, 45 rue des Saints Pères, Paris 6ème France Courtesy of the Université Paris Descartes, 2010. Photo by Joanna Ebenstein.

established by the mid-eighteenth century in Italy.[1] Techniques for preserving and exhibiting dead humans were needed mainly to serve the requirements of medical training, but the Renaissance also brought fresh interest in the study of the human body as an aspect of art, based on dissection and close observation. In 1740, a collection of anatomical models was begun for the University of Bologna, created by wax modelers and artists, and a wax workshop was later established in Florence specifically to create anatomical models for teaching medical students. High standards were expected, as citizens and sponsors alike were already very familiar with the works of local artists such as Leonardo da Vinci and Michelangelo. The wax models were so good that sets were ordered from as far away as Vienna, and some even ended up in America. Looking at these models today it is hard to realize both that they are not real and that they were created over two centuries ago. Given this high standard of work, so early on, it is likely that humans preserved by the comparatively crude methods of taxidermy would have lacked appeal.

Obsession with human preservation was taken to an extreme by the Dutch anatomist Frederik Ruysch (1638–1731). He not only developed unparalleled skill in anatomical dissection and preservation (using secret ingredients), but also took pride in making his gruesome preparations into works of art. Thus, Ruysch dissected the arm of a child and dressed it "so prettily and naturally" (his own words) in a sleeve and lace cuff sewn by his daughter Rachel, and preserved in alcohol within a glass jar.[2] He also created ornamental tableaux out of human organs. Much of his collection can still be seen in St. Petersburg today. Nevertheless, however startling and skillful, specimens preserved like this in liquid do not constitute taxidermy, being neither stuffed nor (usually) very lifelike.

[1] *Rumy Hilloowala,* The Anatomical Waxes of La Specola *(Florence: Arnaud, 1995).*

[2] *Rosamond Purcell and Stephen J. Gould,* Finders Keepers *(London: Hutchinson Radius, 1992).*

One of H. G. Wells' short stories has an old taxidermist, feet up on the mantelpiece, reminiscing to a young acolyte,

> There never was a man who could stuff like me Bellows, never. I have stuffed elephants and I have stuffed moths and the things have looked all the livelier and better for it. And I have stuffed human beings—chiefly amateur ornithologists. But I stuffed a nigger once. No, there is no law against it. I made him with all his fingers out, and used him as a hat rack, but that fool Homersby got up a quarrel with him late one night and spoilt him. That was before your time. It's hard to get skins or I would have another. Unpleasant? I don't see it. Seems to me taxidermy is a promising third course to burial or cremation. You could keep all your dear ones by you. Bric-a-brac of that sort scattered about the house would be as good as most company, and much less expensive. You might have them fitted up with clockwork to do things.[3]

Today such a tale, albeit tongue in cheek, would be considered in rather bad taste. Yet our contemporary approach to the display of human remains seems ambivalent. A similar confusion exists regarding anthropomorphic taxidermy. Children's story books showing pictures of animals behaving as humans (such as the famous tales of Peter Rabbit by Beatrix Potter) are widely regarded as charming, but attitudes towards real animals set up by a taxidermist to represent humans are highly polarized. Some see them as comical, others as an unacceptable travesty of animal life, denigrating the status and dignity of innocent creatures.[4]

[3] *H.G. Wells, "Story the Fourth: Triumphs of a Taxidermist" in* The Complete Stories of H.G. Wells *(London: A & C Black, 1927).*

[4] *Pat Morris,* Walter Potter and his Museum of Curious Taxidermy *(Ascot: MPM, 2008).*

Exhibiting human remains also provokes widely differing responses. Old postcards show displays of skulls and bones in the crypt of Hythe church (in Kent), obviously set out to catch the eye. Similar displays occur in Malta and in Paris. In southern Italy, catacombs may be visited to inspect the grisly remains of the deceased, set out for all to see. Many museums display ancient mummies, a source of perennial fascination. Little embarrassment or offense is caused, even though they are often entirely naked and despite being the mortal remains of the Egyptian royal family. In Moscow, thousands of tourists would queue daily to view Lenin's embalmed corpse, with no protests (although he needed frequent refurbishment). Embalmed mummies do not constitute taxidermy, nevertheless such things are common and popular museum exhibits. Shrunken heads are viewed with some distaste, but rarely with demands for their removal from display. Around 2000–2005 the anatomist and showman Gunther von Hagens toured Europe with his exhibition of "plastinated" dissections of humans, to wide acclaim and much gruesome comment. His exhibition in London was extended due to its unexpected popularity.

By contrast, human specimens preserved by taxidermy excite strong opinions and defensive reactions from museum curators. When confronted with the notion of stuffed humans, abhorrence is almost universal. This is curious in a way: People seem to have confused and ambivalent attitudes. If humans have to be portrayed in a museum actually doing things or being part of a general exhibit, they are always models, never the real thing. Actual taxidermy mounts are very rare. It is said that Peter the Great did have living exhibits in his collection of natural wonders, including a man called Foma who had only two fingers and toes on each of his hands and feet. His job was to collect money from visitors.[5] When he died he was stuffed and added to the czar's collection of curiosities in St. Petersburg. My recent enquiries as to his continued existence met with no response, so, on a visit to that city, we simply knocked on the door of the Kunstkamera

[5] The Origins of Museums, *eds. Oliver Impey and Arthur Macgregor (Oxford: Clarendon Press, 1985). See also Purcell and Gould,* Finders Keepers *(1992).*

to ask. It appears that Foma fell victim to one of the fires or weedings-out that have whittled down Peter's collection over the centuries and he no longer exists. I have traced only four or five other examples of actual humans preserved for exhibition. Maybe there are more, but museum curators are somewhat secretive, perhaps sensitive to the opprobrium that might result from any public admission that they held such material.

There are legal restrictions on what can be done with dead humans, although this was less of a problem in the nineteenth century, particularly with the bodies of people of non-European origin. There are technical difficulties too. The relatively naked human skin offers no camouflage for even minor defects such as splits or incorrect alignment of the manikin within. We humans are also extremely conscious of the small details in appearance that differentiate individual people and are therefore highly critical of anything which is a less than perfect representation of the living person. For these reasons, stuffed humans are few and the museums in which they reside are not anxious to exhibit them or publicize their existence. Specimens pose a particular problem where they are not Caucasian, leading to accusations of racialism. The Cape Town Museum for example, was heavily criticized for having anthropological displays (not actual preserved humans) in its natural history museum, implying (for those who wished to draw such inferences) that native people were part of the local fauna. Such sensitivities are likely to be inflamed further where actual specimens of humans (particularly black ones) are kept, regardless of the fact that they would have been collected and preserved at a time when different attitudes prevailed. Such was the problem with "El Negro" at Banyoles as recounted below.

In the light of all this, it is perhaps surprising that a number of museums exhibit shrunken heads prepared by Amazonian tribes, particularly the Jivaro people. The preparation of these has been described by a number of travelers and seems to excite little more than morbid curiosity. It appears that the skull was crushed within the skin and the pieces, with attached flesh, were removed through the neck. The lips were sewn up and the skin filled with hot sand and repeatedly rubbed with a hot smooth stone on the outside to remove wrinkles as it dried and shrank. By frequent manipulation, the dried head would end up about the size of an orange and be still more or less recognizable as human. Whether this constitutes "taxidermy" is a moot point. Other forms of dried heads exist in anthropological collections, including those illustrating the elaborate tattoos created by Maori tribesmen in New Zealand. These heads proved popular among collectors and there are stories (perhaps apocryphal) suggesting that some unfortunates were tattooed to order especially for the collectors' market. It is certainly true that removal of preserved Maori bodies from traditional burial sites in dry caves to European museums in the nineteenth century has been a source of political friction.[6]

One famous case of human preservation that lies on the boundary of taxidermy (and well beyond the boundaries of good taste) is the 'mummy' of Julia Pastrana. She was a Mexican Indian who was excessively hairy and had overdeveloped gums. She was exhibited as a lucrative freak during her lifetime, later accompanied by her preserved child. Her manager actually married her, no doubt making international travel easier and also keeping his valuable asset from straying into rival ownership. After her death in 1860, she was embalmed, dressed as a Russian dancer and exhibited in fairgrounds and freak shows around northern Europe by her proprietor/husband and various subsequent owners. The specimen was still extant in 1997 (stored in Oslo) but, not for the first time, under threat

[6] *Michael King,* The Collector *(Auckland: Hodder & Stoughton, 1981).*

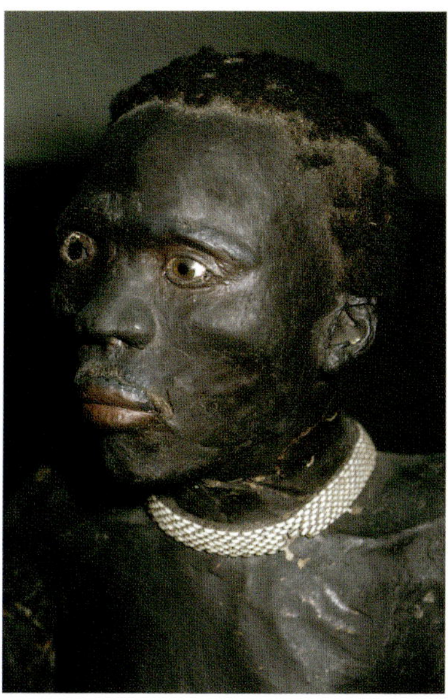

"El Negro". Courtesy of the author.

of destruction or burial.[7] It is astonishing that an embalmed specimen should have survived free standing in the open air without undue shrinkage for over 130 years. Apparently this had been achieved by stuffing the limbs with some sort of filling when the original embalming had been done in Russia in 1860, thus creating an embalmed/taxidermy hybrid.

A famous example of self-preservation is the attempt by Jeremy Bentham, an influential nineteenth-century philosopher, to ensure that his body was used to make a life-like recreation of himself after death. Bentham suggested that when famous people died they should be preserved as "auto icons" as an inspiration to the living and as domestic ornaments. It was normal to have portraits of one's ancestors hanging in the home, so why not the real thing? His pamphlet about the use of human bodies in this way effectively challenged the conventional religious view of going to heaven. Bentham was concerned about the wide-

[7] *Jan Bondeson,* A Cabinet of Medical Curiosities *(London: Tauris, 1997).*

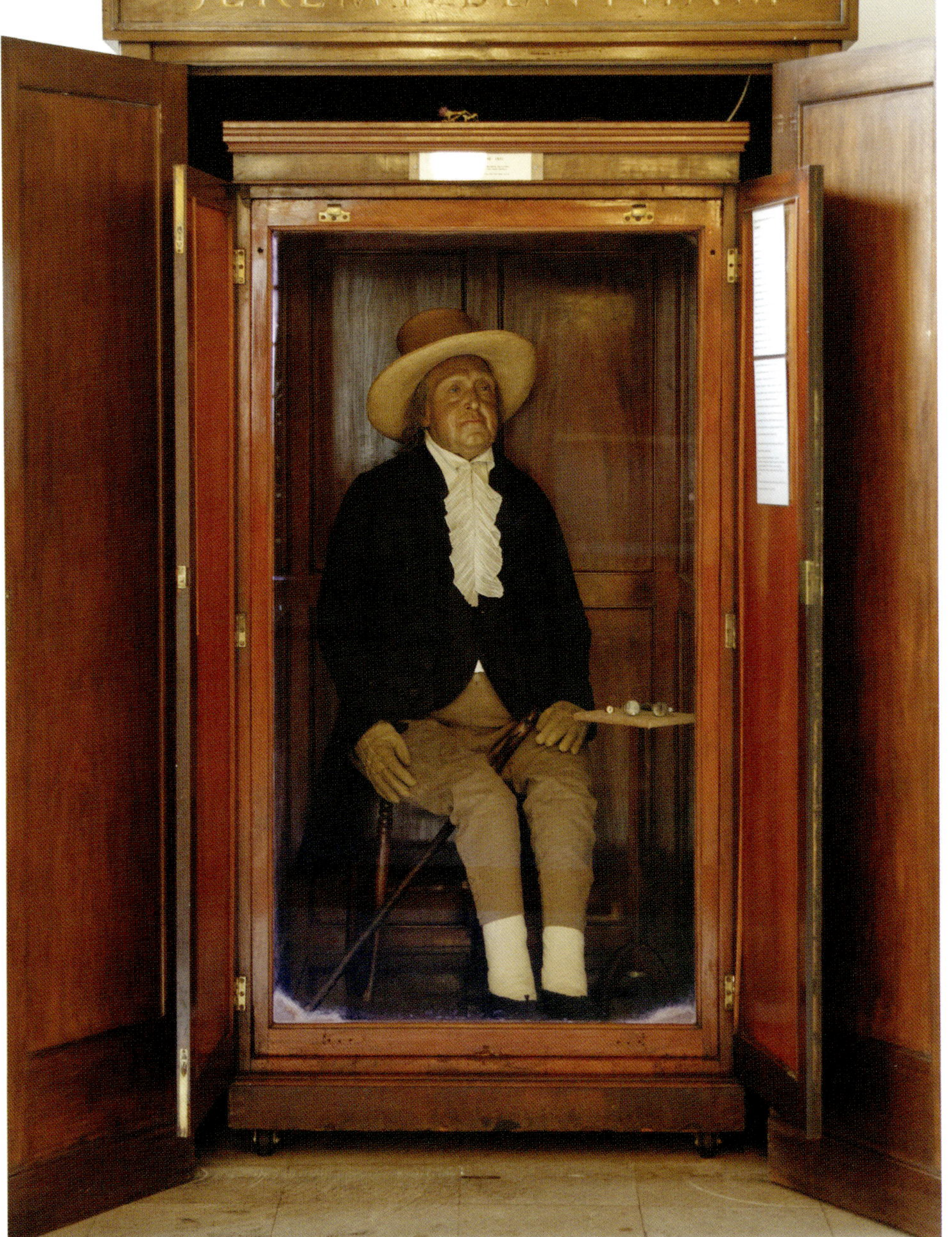
JEREMY BENTHAM

spread fear of being dissected after death (because it would interfere with a serene afterlife) as this reduced the number of bodies available for scientific study. He attempted to set a good example by decreeing in his will that when he died his body should be publicly dissected by an anatomist friend, Woodward Smith, then preserved for display as a memento of himself.

Jeremy Bentham in his case, photo by Joanna Ebenstein. Courtesy of UCL Museums.

For twenty years prior to his death in 1832, Bentham often carried about the glass eyes that would feature in his auto icon. In accordance with his wishes, this consists of the skeleton padded with straw and dressed in his everyday clothes. Bentham suggested that he might be put on display and allowed to attend meetings of liberal-minded persons. Today, Bentham can be seen sitting with his walking stick and spectacles in a large wooden cubicle in the south cloisters of University College London, which he was instrumental in founding. His head was preserved by a form of embalming, but it shrivelled to leave a gaunt and boggle-eyed object that blackened with age. It was replaced by a wax face mask and the original head is kept separately at the College. Bentham's auto icon was reupholstered in 1981 and repairs made to moth damage in the clothing.

There was once a preserved human in the Vienna Museum, a former manservant named Angelo Soliman. He was born in 1721, abducted and sent to North Africa as a slave. At the age of seven he was sold to a noblewoman in Italy at a time when it was fashionable to keep Moors at home as slaves, part of the European fad for exoticism in the eighteenth century. Soliman was baptised and given the name Angelo. He was well cared for, and eventually learned Italian and five other languages, becoming a well-educated man who was widely admired as an outstanding chess player. In 1732, the Prince of Lobkowitz acquired Soliman as a gift, and he later went into service with Prince Joseph of Liechtenstein. Soliman won enough money playing cards to marry in secret, but the marriage was discovered and he was dismissed, then later re-engaged, as a tutor. He became a significant member of a Masonic Lodge, but died of a stroke in November 1796, whilst walking down the road. Soliman was famed for his handsome appearance and fine physique, so the Emperor Joseph II (his good friend) decided to have him preserved for a new museum then under construction. A few hours after Soliman's death, the sculptor Franz Thaller got to work on the body in secret and without the consent of Soliman's daughter, who repeatedly tried to obtain his body. A plaster death mask was made, which is still extant in the Rollet Museum in Baden.

The preserved Soliman was hailed as a fine likeness, although dressed inappropriately in clothes that differed from those he wore in his life as a smart member of an aristocratic household. Instead he wore a feather belt and crown, made from rows of red, white, and blue ostrich feathers. His arms and legs were decorated with beads and he had a braided shell necklace around his neck. This sounds more like an attempt to recreate a "noble savage," rather than a manservant. Subsequently Soliman became the inspiration for books, plays and poems, and even a ballet. He was displayed in Vienna in a fine glass case at least until 1806, but was destroyed by fire in 1848. No drawings or photographs of the preserved specimen appear to exist, only a rather grand painting of him.

Although Jeremy Bentham's auto icon was not really taxidermy, few would take exception to it now, merely regarding it and his ideas as examples of nineteenth-century eccentricity. Rather more controversial was the stuffed "bushman" in the Spanish town of Banyoles. He was part of the collection of Francisco Darder (1851–1918), a noted scientist in Barcelona who operated a biological supply house, selling anatomical preparations, models, glass eyes and sundry scientific equipment. He also indulged in taxidermy, no doubt assisted by being director of Barcelona Zoo. His taxidermy included a rat writing a letter and a squirrel holding an ashtray, as well as ordinary work of generally poor quality. His specimens also included two mummies, a shrunken head and two flayed skins of humans (one black and one white) prepared by students in Barcelona from unclaimed bodies. Darder gave his entire collection to Banyoles in 1916 in gratitude for the kindness and assistance he had received from the local people during his researches on fish production in a nearby lake. The collection, housed in its own museum, included a full mount of a human known locally as "El Negro," who made his first appearance in British newspapers in May 1992.

Darder's collection catalogue, printed in 1888, says that this man came from the French taxidermist Edouard Verreaux, who had attended a native funeral searching for specimens. Together with his brother, Verreaux returned at midnight after the mourners had departed and dug up the body. It was then shipped home to Paris. This tale may have been embroidered somewhat in order to sell the specimen to Darder, or the latter may have sensationalized it to create greater interest in the specimen and his collection. Either way, El Negro was prepared by Verreaux, in 1830, and brought to an exhibition in Barcelona, where Darder purchased him in 1880. He was said to be a bushman and his glass case was labelled "Boixima del Kalahari."

It appears that a campaign to remove El Negro from display and give him a proper burial was started in 1991 by a resident of Taragona who spread misleading and racially based information to African countries and the USA. This aroused international concern and a threat by the International Olympics Committee and some African countries to boycott the Olympic Games in Barcelona, parts of which were due to be held at Banyoles.

However, the mayor and townspeople refused to be intimidated and insisted that El Negro had been on display for 75 years with nobody objecting. T-shirts and lapel badges went on sale locally in support of the museum and its "bushman." Subsequently, the town council unanimously passed a resolution stating that the Darder Collection was an important social and historical record of attitudes at the turn of the century; it should remain intact and not be selectively dismantled in response to twentieth-century ideas. The resolution also pointed out that many museums displayed Egyptian mummies and other human remains without arousing protest.

In view of the historic interest of this specimen, I arranged to visit Banyoles in April 1997, then read a newspaper story claiming that agreement had been reached to repatriate El Negro to Senegal (why Senegal was not apparent). Fortunately, although removed from public display, he was still in the museum and I was allowed to inspect him closely. El Negro had originally been skinned through a mid-dorsal incision from the end of the coccyx to the crown of the head. The stitching was covered over with papier-mâché and almost invisible except among the hair of the head. Preparation was otherwise exactly as normal for medium-sized antelopes in the nineteenth century. The limbs had been turned inside out and skinned to the tips of the toes and fingers, with the bones of feet and hands left inside. The skull was intact, but the main parts of the skeleton and ribs had been removed. The whole was supported on iron rods, linking the limbs and head to a central wooden board. Two rods supported the head, others (one to each limb) were bent to lie alongside the limb bones and were probably tied to them with string, although this was not visible in x-rays. The bones and rods were then probably wrapped in tow before the skin was pulled back over them. The stuffing was soft and there was no modeling compound under the skin. Traces of a trimmed moustache on the upper lip suggest this was a man of at least 20 years old.

The skin had the texture of stiff paper. It had not been tanned, but may have been preserved in a salt and alum bath after removal from the body (this was the normal way of saving skins for mounting later). In places the colored (painted) epidermis had flaked off. The scrotum (hidden by a relatively modern piece of lion skin) was filled with modeling compound to retain its shape and around the face large masses of what appeared to be clay had been applied to the skull, allowing the skin to be modeled, retain a smooth texture, and create prominent cheeks. The same techniques were used by nineteenth-century taxidermists to reproduce the facial details of big game trophies. The lips, nose (and perhaps ears) were also modeled with a soft compound inside, which was transparent to x-rays and may have been papier mâché. This would suggest a two-stage process for making the head: First build up the features on the skull, using clay, and embed the glass eyes in the orbits (again in clay), then the skin, with papier mâché inside the lips and nose, would have been placed over the skull, and the facial details modeled from outside. The modeling around the eyes was quite detailed and the facial skin only a little distorted.

For years, the people and the Museum of Banyoles repeatedly refused to give up El Negro, but under pressure from the Spanish government and the Organization for African Unity, they were finally forced to relent. In October 2000, it was reported that El Negro had been taken to Botswana to lay in state before being buried with full military honors. The ceremony was attended by local dignitaries, including the Foreign Minister, who declared "we are prepared to forgive but we cannot forget, lest the same acts are repeated in future generations."

There are said to be other preserved humans of different types in Paris, perhaps also set up by Verreaux. Apparently they served to teach trainee soldiers how to recognize the enemy in his various forms. I have been unable to confirm the potentially apocryphal tale or a story in the *Sunday Times* (9 March 1997). This reported that a Captain Wills had exacted nineteenth-century retribution on some raiding Aborigines at his farm in Australia and shot them. He had one stuffed and sent it back to his old school, Rugby, where it was shown hanged in a mahogany case until the school sold it at a London auction in 1878. If this tale is true, where is it now?

There is, however, a full, mounted human specimen in Italy. He was called "Steve," and was one of two slaves that belonged to Napoleon's sister, Pauline Bourgèse, wife of the Governor of Turin in the early nineteenth century. When he died, in 1813, a taxidermist from Bologna was called in to prepare the skeleton and set up the skin on a wooden manikin. Steve was on display in 1830 in the museum of a scientific academy, in a glass case labelled "*Homo africanus*," a reminder that there were formerly considered to be several different species of humans. Later, when his taxonomic and social affinities were reappraised, Steve was transferred to the local anatomy museum. For many years he stood in a corridor, passed each day by students attending lectures. I saw him in March 2000 in a basement open to the outside air, where he had been standing for about thirty years among various debris, without a glass case, and was thickly covered in dust. He was dressed in a skirt made from macaw feathers and wore a small straw boater hat. At one time he may have had a spear and a shield in his hands, but these were no longer present. He was about 1.8 meters tall, with relatively straight hair and may have originated in the West Indies rather than come directly from Africa (where there are no macaws

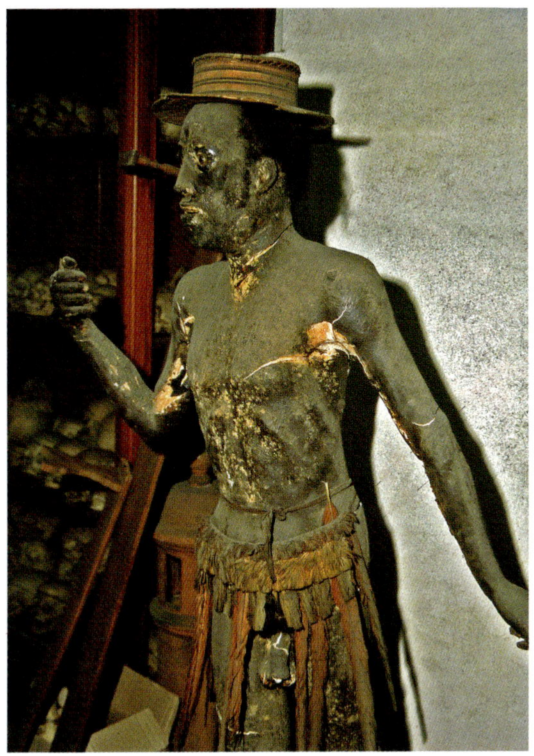

"Steve". Courtesy of the author.

for the skirt). Steve is also a likely name to have acquired in the West Indies. Moreover, Napoleon had family connections in Martinique.

The skin had been removed by a mid-dorsal incision, with further cuts along the insides of the arms and legs. The arm incisions went to the armpits and then across the scapula region to the dorsal incision. These were skillfully stitched up, with the threads largely hidden. The wooden manikin was carved to depict ribs and pectoral muscles quite accurately. The skin was probably glued direct to the carved wood to prevent it "drumming," but had split in a few places and the epidermis had peeled back on parts of the legs. The head was of wood (the skull being elsewhere with the skeleton), with glass eyes inserted. The mouth was slightly open, revealing carved wooden teeth, and the lips were filled with clay (or a similar material) to allow a natural horizontal shape to be preserved (unlike dried heads where the lips tend to shrink to form a near circular hole, exposing the incisors, but covering the canine teeth). Some clay appeared to have been used in modeling the face, genitals, toes and fingers. Steve's future seems uncertain as the whole building in which he stood was in a similar state of neglect.

Among the thousands of heads mounted by Rowland Ward Ltd., the leading London taxidermist, there is a human one that may still exist. It was sent to London by J. S. Jameson, the zoologist on Henry Morton Stanley's Emin Pasha Expedition to central Africa. Apparently, some local men had stolen guns from the expedition's Base Camp in 1888 and refused to return them. A punitive raid was launched on their village across the river and Jameson reported that "A number of natives were shot, but I cannot tell how many as most of them sank in the water; however, they captured one man and brought back one head with them, which Ward and I sketched. Afterwards I skinned and preserved it and shall try to get it home with me."[8] The Ward referred to was Rowland Ward's nephew Herbert.

[8] *James S. Jameson,* The Story of the Rear Column *(London: Porter, 1890).*

Jameson died before reaching London again, but his specimens arrived safely and were exhibited in the Rowland Ward showroom, where the *Times* (29 November 1888) reported them in generally admiring tones, but described a headdress made from a human scalp as "repulsive" without mentioning the mounted head. In fact it had been prepared in Ward's studio and became the property of Jameson's widow. She later complained about the smell it exuded on damp days and also the "atrocious comments" directed at her late husband in the Press. In fact the head appears to have been soon forgotten as even more lurid tales emerged of the expedition's behavior in connection with cannibalism. This was so severely censured in the press that Stanley himself was moved to deny all responsibility and Herbert Ward also claimed it had nothing to do with him. Others stepped in to publish their own accounts of what had gone on, including Assad Farran (published in the *Echo* and other newspapers in November 1890). He claimed to have known the African personally and to have shaken hands with him on many occasions. A reporter confronted Rowland Ward, a friend of Jameson, asking directly whether or not he had mounted the head of an African native. Ward replied "My relations with the family of the late Mr. Jameson are such that I must decline to make any statement regarding the matter. You will therefore kindly excuse me. I cannot talk upon the subject." He also refrained from mentioning it in his autobiography, while describing many other famous specimens his firm had prepared. This was in spite of the care with which he had preserved dozens of the relevant contemporary newspaper articles in his personal scrapbooks that he used when writing his autobiography. In 1923, the head was presented to a museum, but it was another twenty-one years before it was formally accessioned into the collection.

This particular piece of taxidermy seems to have been associated with controversy and embarrassment on such an epic scale that details of its preparation seem rather mundane. Using x-rays in 1982 revealed that it had been skinned by an incision at the back of the scalp, as one might with a small antelope, and the skin pared down until it was very thin. The skull was removed in the field and cleaned, probably by maceration. Back in the London workshop, this was anchored to a baseboard by two large nails and then used as a framework on which to build up clay or plaster to replace facial muscles, exactly as would be the procedure for mounting a small game head trophy. However,

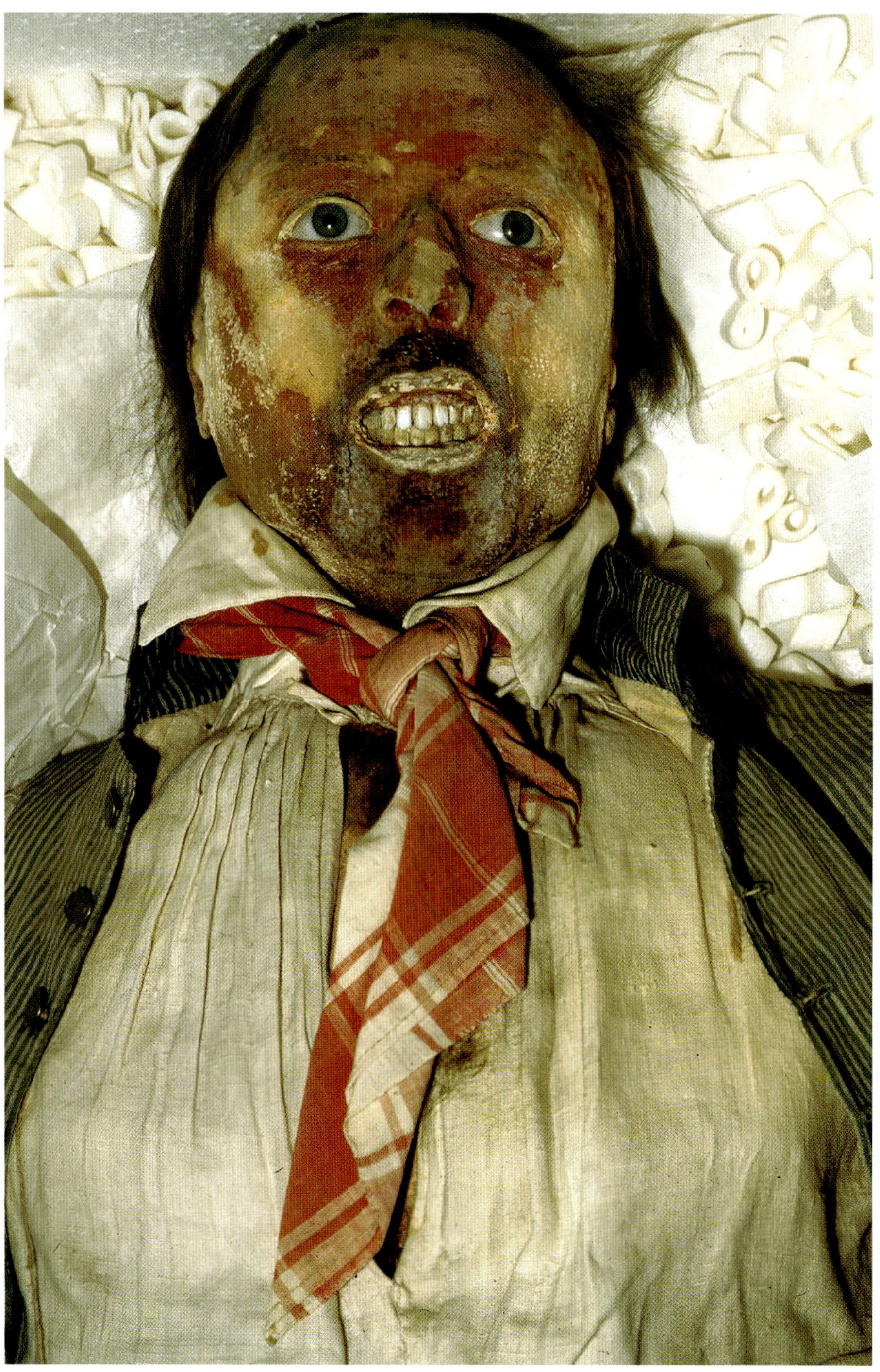

an excess of clay was added at the front, making the face rather prognathous in profile. Perhaps this was an accidental fault, or maybe this is what a London taxidermist imagined an African native should look like? Packing out the face in this way resulted in the ears being drawn forward by about two centimeters. They were not lined with clay or other material. Eyelashes and eyebrows were still present although rather sparse. The glass eyes were of the highest quality, but the skin was faded in places, although it had been suitably touched up with paint. The smell that had troubled Mrs Jameson was not evident.

Image left: Montbrison Man. Courtesy of the author.

The Museé d'Allard at Montbrison, France, has a stuffed man prepared about 1825 by the French taxidermist, Dupont. Apparently he had been a prisoner at the local jail, where the governor allowed trusted inmates to go and work in the local town during the day. Oral tradition has it that he fell off the roof of the museum where he was working and was added to the collection inside as nobody knew how to contact relatives to arrange for a funeral. He looks as though he may have been Caucasian, with straight hair and narrow nose. Although the skin now appears dark, this may be an artifact. He stands, wearing a worker's shirt and vest, with his open mouth revealing regular dentition. Good-quality glass eyes had been used, but the skin has been affected by time, being cracked and with small red and yellow spots. He is not normally on display, but in November 2000, he was borrowed for an exhibition in the Natural History Museum at Neuchâtel. Here, visiting children apparently seemed less bothered by him than the adults, perhaps because the latter could imagine the processes involved in taxidermy. However, the exhibition was acclaimed by visitors and excited almost no adverse comment. A local newspaper reporter clearly had little idea what to say about it and wrote only a very bland account of the displays.

Perhaps the public reaction to the exhibition of human taxidermy will always vary according to its context. What might be acceptable in London, New York, or even Neuchâtel, might cause deep offense in some other cities. Perhaps, like other forms of taxidermy, it depends upon how the items are shown. Portrayed as a novel and "edgy" form of art, human material might be regarded as exciting, a fresh departure from the staid and unimaginative past. Shown as illustrating the different races of man, an entirely logical approach in years gone by, human taxidermy would today create uproar. Perhaps we humans are still not quite ready to resolve our own contradictions.

AT THE [HUMAN] ZOO

A Sampling of Ethnographic Exhibitions in the Modern World

ELIZABETH L. BRADLEY

Nor is there any mercy in Hagenbeck's layout with trenches and without bars.... The more that civilization preserves and transplants unspoiled nature, the more implacably the latter is controlled.
—Adorno, *Minima Moralia*

THE LOUISIANA PURCHASE EXPOSITION WAS A SMASH HIT. THE 1904 World's Fair seemingly had something for everyone: exhibition halls and an "anthropology reservation," hair-raising rides and sideshows, foods from the future (the debut of cotton candy), and even an anthem—"Meet Me in St. Louis," of course. But the Fair would have succeeded without these signal attractions, for the simple reason that it was the site of the 1904 Olympic Games, the first such competition to take place in the United States. The Americans, perhaps by virtue of the fact that they outnumbered foreign athletes by six to one, took home the most gold medals of any country. There was, however, one Olympic tournament at which the Americans did not triumph, because they were not invited to take part: "Anthropology Days." This two-day competition, also known colloquially as the "Special Olympics" (not to be confused with the contemporary events for disabled athletes), pitted the Fair's

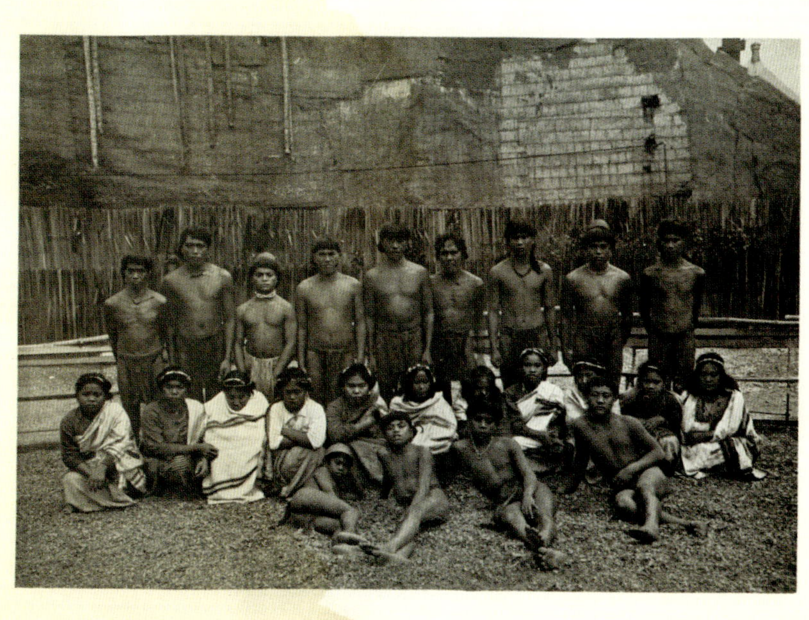

IGORROTES FROM THE PHILIPPINES, LUNA PARK

An Igorrote village occupies twelve acres at the northeast end of the Luna Park enclosure. Here fifty-one head-hunting and dog-eating savages from the Bontac Province, Island of Luzon, have incorporated all the wild features of their distant mountain homes. Among them are two war chiefs and a witch doctor. Their chief occupation, to which they give the larger part of their time, is building their native style of houses.

"anthropology reservation" residents against one another in a crude series of Olympic-style events, for which these conscripted athletes received no preparation, instruction, or recompense. It was not a tournament so much as a large-scale experiment: the chance to illustrate the theories of scientific racism with living, breathing "exotics" from around the globe. To this end, "Patagonian giants" from Argentina and "hairy Ainu" from Japan were assigned to archery; members of the Mohawk and Seneca tribes were instructed to do battle on the lacrosse field (and, oddly, at tug-of-war); aboriginal Filipinos the Igorots and the Moros raced each other; and every "ethnographic" group, from the Congolese pygmies to the Patagonians, was handed a shot put.

Image above: "Igorrotes from The Philippines, Luna Park," from Luna Park Souvenir and Programme Book, 1905. *Courtesy of the Coney Island Museum.*

The result of all this choreography was, not surprisingly, a dismal fiasco. Participants were panicked by the (unfamiliar) starting gun and baffled by the finish line. They had never seen or trained with track-and-field equipment (high jump, anyone?). They resented being asked to do for free what they did for pay in their Fair enclosures, and to be calipered and questioned by staff anthropologists for their pains. And they all found the shot put to be a clumsy, pointless joke.

"Anthropology Days" was an embarrassment by the standards of the day, as well as by our own—but not for the reasons that the contemporary reader might expect. The organizers of the Fair were not embarrassed by the bigotry of the spectacle they had created. They were, instead, critical of the performance of the hastily assembled teams. The official report of the Fair admitted that the "Anthropology Days" were the "only disappointing feature of the season... destroying the common belief that the greatest natural athletes were to be found among the uncivilized tribes in various parts of the world."[1] The Fair's chief anthropologist even tried again, holding a second set of ethnographic games a few months later with mostly Native American athletes who had been coached in their sports. This time, "Anthropology Days" was a success, with thirty thousand Americans watching "primitives" at play. "In no place but America would one have dared to place such events on a program," Baron Pierre de Coubertin, the founder of the Olympic Games, would later write of the "Anthropology Days," adding, "but, to Americans, everything is permissible."[2]

But de Coubertin's "permissible" Americans were only indulging in one of the oldest of European spectator sports: the human zoo. Although the court dwarf has been replaced by the reality show, the human impulse to put others on display is remarkably durable. In the early Renaissance, exhibitions of

[1] *Susan Brownell,* The 1904 Anthropology Days and Olympic Games: Sport, Race, and American Imperialism *(Nebraska: University of Nebraska Press, 2008), 206.*

[2] *Ibid., 150.*

people were largely private and exclusive arrangements: the explorer Hernán Cortés claimed that the fifteenth-century Aztec ruler Moctezuma had a collection of human "freaks" in his royal menagerie, while Cardinal Ippolito de' Medici, the illegitimate grandson of Lorenzo the Magnificent, reportedly kept a collection of African, Native American, Tatar, and North African Arab slaves on view at his Florentine palace. But by the early nineteenth century, these titillating *tableaux vivants* were designed for the widest possible public, promising audience members an existential encounter with living marvels (generally of a different, exoticized race) in exchange for a modest fee.

The most famous of these displayed persons in Europe at the time was the South African slave Sarah "Saartjie" Baartman, known as the "Hottentot Venus." Baartman was a Khoisan (which the Victorians called "Hottentot") woman with pronounced buttocks and elongated labia. Her curvy, lightly clad figure was a subject of scandal in London and Paris, where she was exhibited under coercive conditions from 1810 until her death five years later. Americans made celebrities out of other marginalized people, such as the African American slave Joice Heth, who was advertised as the 160-year-old nursemaid of George Washington, or the conjoined Chinese-Thai twins Chang and Eng Bunker, advertised as "the most wonderful and extraordinary of all human curiosities." Unlike Baartman, the Bunker brothers, who were genuinely conjoined, were free agents (who sometimes worked for P.T. Barnum) and naturalized American citizens. Joice Heth, on the other hand, was neither emancipated nor the real thing: she was Barnum's earliest blockbuster hoax, the spiritual ancestor of the Feejee Mermaid and other "gaffed" artifacts in his extensive collection. Heth might have made the reputation of her young promoter, but she died a slave.

—※—

The exhibition of "curious" and foreign people might have stayed in the sideshow but for European imperialism. The late nineteenth and early twentieth century saw a mad dash to claim as much of Africa, Latin America, the Indies and Central Asia for Europe as possible, a claim that often, in some form or other, included the people who already lived there. The first entrepreneur to successfully import native peoples to Europe for purposes of entertainment (rather than slavery) was a German zookeeper named Karl Hagenbeck (1844–1913). Hagenbeck began his career in 1864 as a menagerie-maker, purchasing and brokering the sale of live exotic animals from big-game hunters based in Africa. Some of these imported specimens were for his own zoological gardens, the Tierpark Hagenbeck in Hamburg, while others were bound for zoos and circuses throughout Europe and the United States, including Barnum's (Hagenbeck was his exclusive animal dealer for more than thirty years).

Hagenbeck began to import people in 1874, when, as he notes in his memoir, "the supply of wild beasts had begun to exceed the demand, and the profit on my business somewhat decreased." At the suggestion of a colleague, he decided to add a little human interest to his living dioramas, and put in an order that his next shipment of Lapland (Finnish) reindeer be "accompanied by their native masters," the Sami people. Hagenbeck was not looking to discover the next Chang and Eng, but rather their opposite: "finely moulded... unspoiled children of Nature" whose features and traits conformed to the physical type of their ethnicity, thus upholding the imperial racial theories of the day. The visiting Sami delighted the German public, who quickly developed an appetite for *Völkerschauen*, or human zoos. These ethnographic displays were radically different from a solo sideshow performance: instead of a single ambassador from the realm of the exotic or freakish, the Tierpark Hagenbeck offered visitors the chance to experience extended families and tribes from other continents, dropped down in the middle of their city as if from outer space. And indeed, the animal dealer was looking for a Martian effect: "strangeness," or *Fremdheit*, was one of his criteria for human display.

Such assemblies functioned as a kind of glib primer in ethnology for average Anglo-Saxons, by creating a series of artificially reconstructed worlds for them to inspect and analyze. The Sami were followed by a group of Inuits from Greenland and a tribe of Sudanese "wild men" and their dromedaries, among many others. Most of these invitations to native groups were made through their colonial governments (such as the Danish governors of Greenland, home to the Inuit) or through missionary groups who could attest to the legitimacy of Hagenbeck's project. His agents were also not above appealing to patriotic sentiment in the effort to recruit native ambassadors to the task of edifying the West about their faraway homeland.[3]

[3] *Carl Hagenbeck,* Beasts and Men *(Longmans, Green, 1911), 15-16, 20.*

The truth, however, was that the *naturmenschen* had not been brought to Europe to "enlighten" white visitors about their homeland. They were there to perform, and the enclosure of the zoological garden that served as their stage only made their quotidian rituals seem more alien and their ancestral costumes more outlandish. With or without the papier-mâché icebergs (brought in for the Inuits), Hagenbeck's ethnographic exhibitions were living snow globes, pantomiming a pretense of ordinary freedom from the other side of a deep trench (Hagenbeck's innovation to deter animal escape without unsightly fences). They must, in other words, be actors, capable of convincing the spectator of their "naturalness" and their exoticism, despite the blatant fakery of their surroundings. Such an assignment was paradoxical by definition: Hagenbeck's performers had to have deep reserves of sophistication in order to demonstrate the most believable simplicity. This intersection—of so-called innocence and performance—would prove to be a hallmark of the human zoo.

Although Hagenbeck's ethnographic tableaux were lucrative, they were not the cornerstone of his business; that was animals. (And this remains true at the Tierpark Hagenbeck, now Hamburg's foremost zoo and aquarium, which is advertised with the tagline "*Hamburgs tierisches original*," literally, "Hamburg's beastly original". But Hamburg's original humans proliferated beyond Hagenbeck's park with lightning speed; within five years of the Sami visit, no patriotic exposition or world's fair was complete without a living exhibition. The cities that hosted these exhibitions are today among the most cosmopolitan in the world, but at the turn of the twentieth century, the very idea of a nonwhite, non-Western person could inspire an intoxicating mixture of excitement and anxiety.

Prior to the 1878 Paris Exposition and the Amsterdam International Colonial Exhibition in 1883, Victorian fairs had, of necessity, confined themselves to illustrating ethnography in wax or plaster. The Sydenham Crystal Palace had shocked mid 19th century London with thirteen life-sized dioramas of the "races of man," illustrating the theories of scientific polygenism, which holds that the different races shared no com-mon human ancestry.[4] By comparison, the colonial displays in Paris (1878 and 1889) and Amsterdam offered the chance for a close encounter with an actual Caribe or Creole from Surinam, Javanese gamelan players in a model "kampong" (hamlet), or Senegalese living in a patchwork assemblage of picturesque housing culled from all over their home country. These *villages negres*, based

[4] *Edward Ziter,* The Orient on the Victorian Stage *(Cambridge: Cambridge UP, 2003), 124.*

on Hagenbeck's pioneering work, were a revelation; instead of a wax replica behind glass or one exotic body on a stage, here were whole tribes and families, talking, cooking dinner, making tools, goofing off, in *plein air* and, in some cases, at arm's reach.

The effect, however, was hardly humanizing. Millions of pairs of eyes gazed upon these aboriginal visitors, most of whom were darker than their European hosts, required to wear their most "traditional" or ceremonial garb (however inappropriate to the occasion), and to live in makeshift approximations of their native dwellings. To heighten the sense of objectification, many of the transplanted natives accepted donations from the public, or required them as a condition of their cooperation while on view. But there was no summit, no exchange, no conversation to be had, and without the benefit of firsthand facts or context, how could European spectators hope to connect with their otherworldly guests? Under these circumstances, it is little wonder that the colonial displays of Paris and Amsterdam made orientalists out of spectators and fetishes out of the spectated. How else could Europeans understand this display of difference, except through the lens of empire? Without a cultural interpreter of their own, the native performers were easily reduced to Hagenbeckian typologies, and transformed, by Western tourists, into a living panorama of the "races of man." It was an arrangement of semiconsensual captivity that is hard to make sense of at the present day: analogs such as historic site interpreters (such as Colonial Williamsburg), exploit the distant past rather than the Victorians' bloody imperial present.

Despite their lavishness, the European expositions were ultimately just a dress rehearsal for the main—American—event: the Columbian Exposition of 1893, held in Chicago. While the stated reason for the Exposition was the 400th anniversary of Christopher Columbus' discovery of the "New World," the

Fair really gave Americans the chance to show their erstwhile colonizers—and themselves—how very far they had come. The Exposition served as an all-encompassing illustration of the United States' superior commerce and culture, the better to prove conclusively that the young nation had earned its place among the capitals of the "Old World." It was an exhaustive goal, but by all accounts the "White City" of the Fair more than delivered: its monumental Beaux Arts campus was stuffed to the rafters with arts, innovations, and entertainments. Among the offerings in this last category were some "new worlds" fit for twentieth-century eyes: more ethnographic exhibitions than had ever before been seen in one place.

Exposition organizers had mapped two paths for those seeking an encounter with "primitive" people on the streets of the White City. The first revolved around the Anthropological Building, which housed a vast array of archaeological and ethnological artifacts curated by anthropologist Frederic W. Putnam of Harvard University with the assistance of a young colleague, Franz Boas. In addition to their careful selection of objects, many of which were on loan from the Smithsonian Institution, the Anthropological Building housed a bewildering number of didactic and patriotic exhibits, not to mention old-fashioned *Wunderkammern*. These included (to mention just a small sample) model health, hygiene, medical and correctional displays from Europe and the United States; a "Physical Anthropological" chart comparing the physical measurements of fifty thousand North American schoolchildren and twenty thousand Native Americans; and the entire contents of Ward's Natural Science Establishment, a private museum in Rochester, New York. In Ward's Establishment, the Exposition Directory extolled, "one sees all forms of animal life from the sponges to man, all admirably classified and arranged."[5]

But the "animal life" inside the Anthropological Building was largely static and two-dimensional: living exhibitions could be found just outside, in the form of a campground village of "the native people of America." The other ethnographic path a visitor could take was decidedly less scholarly: a route through the Midway Plaisance, the Exposition's headquarters for commercial programming, under the management of theater entrepreneur Sol Bloom. Bloom, in concert with Putnam, Boas, and recruiters such as Hagenbeck himself, transformed the Midway into a kind of polyglot paradise. It was home to "Javanese, Egyptian, Moorish, Dutch, Japanese, Malay, Austrian, German, Irish, Dahomian, Algerian, Tunisian and Arabian pavilions, booths, villages, streets, and settlements," all of which were plunked down amid the more traditional "midway"-style amusements of the Fair, which included cycloramas, a natatorium, a "captive" (tethered) hot air balloon, wild animal shows (also courtesy of Hagenbeck), and the first Ferris wheel. Pedestrians walking through the Midway faced a bewildering array of foreign-seeming options: camel rides, exotic pastries, snake charming, or "Russian style" high tea at the supposed home of the Shah of Ispahan.

This was vaudeville ethnography, with no attempt at colonial spin or scientific inquiry. "The scene, as one views it," a contemporary reviewer wrote, "is one of striking curiosity... [A]fter returning from a day spent in investigations of its wonders, one feels indeed that he has returned from a trip around the world."[6] In contrast to the decorous hierarchies of the Anthropology Building, the Midway Plaisance had a democratic, even anarchic spirit, which gave visitors the chance to get impossibly close—by Edwardian standards—to native performers, and to each other.

It was a distinctly urban atmosphere, polyglot and crowded: more like Chicago (or Cairo) proper than the gracious and

[5] The Official Directory of the World's Columbian Exposition, May 1st to October 30, 1893 *(W. B. Conkey Company, 1893), 1092.*

[6] *Trumbull White and William Igleheart,* World's Columbian Exposition, Chicago, 1893: A Complete History of the Enterprise: A Full Description of the Buildings and Exhibits in All Departments: and a Short Account of Previous Expositions *(Historical Publishing Company, 1893), 595.*

tidy avenues of the campus it abutted. And it was mesmerizing. Little wonder, then, that the signature spectacle of the Columbian Exposition was found not in the White City's crystalline palaces but inside the Midway's "Streets of Cairo" attraction: the *danse du ventre*, or belly dance. In addition to proximity to their flesh, the crush of the Midway gave spectators unusual access to the most private facts of performers' lives, too, as in the case of Nancy Helene Columbia Palmer, the Inuit baby born out of wedlock in the "Eskimo Village" concession, just before the Exposition opened. The serendipitous arrival of baby Nancy, a photogenic "mite in seal skins," who was christened by the Exposition's patroness, Mrs. Potter Palmer, was better than any publicity stunt.[7] Columbia's family would ultimately break with the Eskimo Village and open their own establishment outside the fairgrounds, but it didn't matter: the winsome infant was already the mascot of the Midway.

[7] *Jim wick,* Inuit Entertainers in the United States: From the Chicago World's Fair through the Birth of Hollywood *(Infinity Publishing, 2006), 34.*

While the Columbian Exposition did not have an explicit *village negre,* as Paris had done, the ethnic enclosures created by the displays of both Frederic Putnam and Sol Bloom had the same segregating and diminishing effect. Frederick Douglass, who made his headquarters in the Haitian Building, pointed out that the Dahomian natives were the only Africans represented at the Fair, and organized a Colored People's Day at the Exposition in protest. The white director of a model Indian school complained bitterly when his students were forced to share space with Buffalo Bill's Wild West Show, as if educated Native Americans were just another set of curious artifacts, to be inspected alongside the teepees and tomahawks. Despite all this, the Exposition was a tremendous success, and its ethnographic displays both on and off the Midway helped to attract nearly twenty-six million visitors in the space of five months. Americans, with their talent for scaling up, had only managed to make the human zoo bigger.

—⁂—

If Chicago introduced America to the high- and low-culture potential of *Völkerschauen*, then the St. Louis Fair took that potential to its most profound extremes. The Louisiana Purchase Exposition of 1904 was no rival to the Exposition in grandeur, size or scale, but it was the first American exhibition that actively sought to elevate and professionalize the field of anthropology through both static and living exhibits. It succeeded, however, only in blurring the lines between science and spectacle beyond all recognition. The anthropologist in charge of the ethnographic exhibitions in St. Louis was William McGee, director of the Smithsonian Institution, and a firm believer in physical anthropology, or what we might today describe as a kind of racial Darwinism that has since been thoroughly discredited as bigotry and pseudoscience. McGee was not shy about his agenda. "The aim of the [St. Louis Fair] Department of Anthropology," he declared, " ...will be to represent human progress from the dark prime to the highest enlightenment, from savagery to civic organization, from egoism to altruism."[8]

[8] *Brownell, 200.*

The impact of McGee's philosophy on the tone and events of the Fair cannot be overestimated. Like Chicago, the St. Louis Exposition showcased a range of "exotic" persons that was typologically consistent with Western evolutionary ideology, and ranged from African pygmies (small) to Argentinian Patagonians (tall). Even the Native Americans recruited through the Office of Indian Affairs met the criteria: from Dakotas (tall) to Pueblos (small). Anthropologists and armchair anthropometrists were delighted at the variety, and the possibility for research that it represented. "Never before in the lives of living anthropologists had so varied a collection of

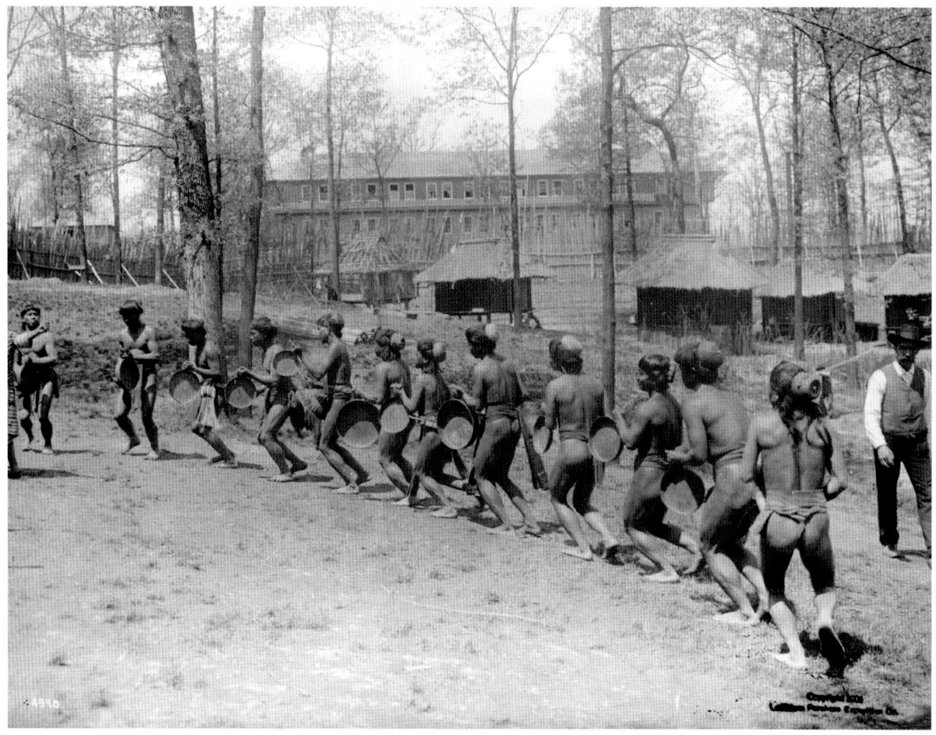

primitive races been brought together, fresh from their wild and savage haunts," rhapsodized the *New York Times.*[9]

[9] The New York Times, *May 7, 1905.*

St. Louis also offered visitors a number of "official" ethnographic villages to visit, the most popular of which was the government-sponsored Philippine Reservation. It is difficult, at the present day, to see the Reservation as anything other than a pure political statement. The Philippine-American War had ended just two years before, sealing the fate of Filipinos as an annex of the United States, and the Reservation embodied this annexation at the Fair: it was a literal (as well as metaphorical) containment of Filipino identity. 1,100 performers worked on (and in most cases resided full time on) the Philippine Reservation alone, and included representatives from all the tribal populations and native peoples of the Philippines: Tagalogs, Visayans, Muslims, Tinguianes, Pampangans, Kalingas, Mangyans, Negritos, and Bagobos. Fairgoers found the Bontoc, Suyoc, and Tinguian tribes particularly appealing, largely because they were marketed to the public as "Igorrote" [sic] headhunters and dog-eaters. The practice of eating dog meat garnered the tribesmen a large amount of disgusted press and drew them even larger crowds.

Image left: Igorot men from the Philippines wearing loincloths and carrying hand drums, dance in a semi-circle; huts and a building in background at the Louisiana Purchase Exposition; November 13, 1904. Library of Congress.

Some of the other performers, as well as tourists, were intrigued by the Igorots at St. Louis—particularly the Native Americans who had been recruited to feature in their own ethnographic encampments on "Indian Hill," or to attend the Fair's model Indian school. Interestingly, it proved difficult for the St. Louis organizers to find Native Americans willing to live in traditional housing, wear buckskin and demonstrate artisanal crafts —by 1904, many were too accustomed to Anglo culture to volunteer for the privations of a previous way of life, while others were already professional showmen, courtesy of Buffalo Bill's Wild West Show and its many rivals. In one instance, Fair organizers discovered that many of the Oglala (Sioux) Indians they had hired performed their tribal dances wearing wigs made from their own hair, since they preferred short, Western hairstyles for every day. It was a substitution that had been deemed sufficiently authentic by Oglala elders, but not by St. Louis ethnographers.

With or without his hair, there was at least one warrior of unimpeachable authenticity among the Native American performers at St. Louis—Geronimo, the famous Apache raider and (by 1904) American prisoner of war. Guidebooks to the Fair played up Geronimo's reputation, calling him "the red devil... [who] made every white settler tremble with fear, as his extreme cruelty was dreaded... bloodthirsty.... Long years of captivity have broken his spirit and he is docile because he has met his masters.... Geronimo will be practically free at the world's fair, but still a prisoner of war."[10] Because Geronimo refused to wear anything but Western attire while at the Fair, the media spun that too, suggesting that Apache garb had been forbidden because it made the chief violent and ungovernable. Geronimo himself understood the Fair as a moneymaking opportunity; he sold feathers and autographs (making more than two thousand dollars over the course of six months), rode the Ferris wheel with journalists, and made appearances at the daily Wild West shows—at once the Fair's unofficial mayor and its official prisoner. Geronimo did not take part in the infamous "Anthropology Days," the nadir of the St. Louis Fair, but the athletes who did may be seen as fellow test subjects, if not as fellow captives. This series of lesser Olympic Games was meant to prove, once and for all, which ethnic types were the best at which feats of athletic prowess, while at the same time providing anthropometric data about the different participating races. The resulting chaos dashed the hopes of evolutionary scientists, in part because their quest for timeless authenticity was thwarted by a very twentieth-century professionalism. Like Geronimo, and like Chang and Eng before him, many performers simply refused to participate in the unpaid competition—why would they volunteer their signature talents, when the same audience would gladly pay to see them? Final score: Ethnographic subjects, 1, Ethnographers, 0.

[10] *Nancy J. Parezo and Don D. Fowler,* Anthropology Goes to the Fair: The 1904 Louisiana Purchase Exposition *(Nebraska: University of Nebraska Press, 2009), 112.*

Among the most famous ethnographic subjects at the St. Louis Fair was Ota Benga, a Mbuti pygmy who had been recruited during a talent scouting expedition to the Belgian Congo. A hostage of the Congo Free State army, Ota Benga was "redeemed" by the missionary Samuel Verner in exchange for a pound of salt and some cloth, making him the first—but perhaps not the only—performer to technically be "owned" by the St. Louis World's Fair, much as the Hottentot Venus had been owned by her promoters, almost a hundred years before. Ota Benga, along with four Batwa pygmies, was displayed at the Fair as an "emblematic savage," representative of a "primeval dwarfish race," and thus, if not the missing link, then the poster child for scientific racism.[11]

Ota Benga's story did not end with the Fair, however: in 1906 he was hired by the Bronx Zoo to live in the Zoo's Monkey House, where he was to be "exhibited each afternoon in September," according to the Zoo's signage. This most literal of human zoos came to a speedy end after the Colored Baptist Minister's Conference of New York City mounted a vociferous public objection to "making an exhibition" of the Mbuti man " to corroborate the [Darwinian] theory of evolution." Interestingly, Ota Benga's original chaperone, Samuel Verner, vehemently refuted these allegations, arguing for the "humanitarian" nature of his recruitment. Ota Benga is *not* meant to stand in for the "missing link," he insisted to the *New York Times*, adding "the zoological and the psychological gap between the pygmies and the apes constitutes a cataclysm."[12] It was a surprising admission in 1906, and an early sign that anthropology was beginning to discard, or at least modify, its race theories. Progress did not come fast enough for Ota Benga, however; he committed suicide ten years later, unable to integrate into American society or to return home to the Congo.

[11] *Supplement to* Scientific American *71 (March 4, 1911): 137.*

[12] The New York Times, *September 11, 1906.*

The spontaneous, well-publicized outrage over the treatment of Ota Benga, coming on the heels of the embarrassment of "Anthropology Days" did not put an end to the display of aboriginal peoples in the twentieth century, but it served as a catalyst for gradual change, particularly in the United States.

This philosophical shift made sense in the new century: the field of anthropology had begun to veer away from race theory (leaving that to the nascent pseudoscience of eugenics) and American manifest destiny had been reduced to a few, final colonial land-grabs (such as the U.S. Virgin Islands). In addition, as immigration restrictions tightened between the World Wars, it grew more difficult to bring foreign performers into the United States—a sign of institutionalized racism, rather than increased civil rights, but the outcome for "exotic" natives was the same. But it was publicity, not policy, that was ultimately responsible for the demise of this particular kind of human trafficking. By making human zoos silly, the media rendered them moot.

One example of this kind of deflation can be found in the reporting surrounding Filipino ethnic villages at Coney Island's Luna Park and Dreamland, where press releases abandoned scientific rhetoric in favor of comedy. To this end, when the "Igorotte" performers of Luna Park decamped for a rival park because they had been refused the opportunity to cook dog in their village, the headline teased "Clams and Crabs a la Bowery All Right For A Time, But They Prefer To Do Their Own Cooking," and when the Orphans' Automobile Day Committee brought two thousand motherless children to Coney Island, the encounter between "Pete McGuire, orphan, age 10" and "Wila, the pride of the Igorrote Village," read like a *People* magazine cover story rather than a physiometric investigation:

> The first glances over, Wila took a poke at Pete with a pink sun shade which he held in his hand, and which constituted his wearing apparel. Then he muttered a few words of that language which is understood in the Philippines. Pete looked reflective and replied, 'Gee, I should think you'd be cold.'[13]

[13] The New York Times, *August 10, 1906 and June 12, 1909.*

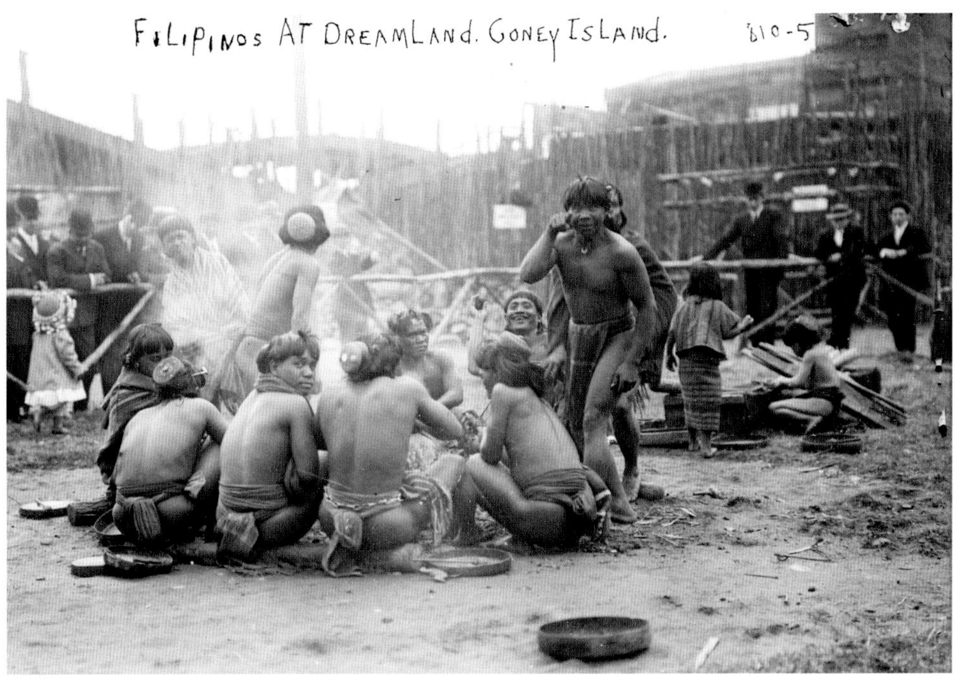

Filipinos in loin cloths sitting in circle together at Dreamland, Coney Island, N.Y., 1907. Library of Congress.

Even the ten-year-old spectator sees through the pantomimed ferocity of these urbane exotics, with their sunshades and boardwalk menus. Six years later, a silent film entitled *Josie's Coney Island Nightmare* takes the spoof of the ethnic village to its logical extreme, recreating an Igorot enclosure for a satire on gullible Coney Island tourists fearful of the spear-shaking natives and their cannibalistic dinner plans. Not long after that, the surviving Coney Island parks abandoned expensive, large-scale ethnographic displays altogether. They were replaced by the kind of living *wunderkammer* made popular by Barnum more than fifty years before: the ten-in-one sideshow.

Some of the performers in these programs, such as the Dreamland Circus Sideshow, were veterans of the ethnic villages. One of these was "Chief Amok," a Filipino actor whose

1924 pitch card advertised him as a "Bantos Head Hunter" [sic], and offered to tell "The Story of Myself and My People." It would be eleven more years before the Philippines was granted Commonwealth status, but the addition of a Bontoc person—and a Bontoc narrative—to the Dreamland bannerline can be seen as a liberation, of the Coney Island kind: the freedom to profit from your own curiousness, your unlooked for *Fremdheit* in the global human zoo.

PART III

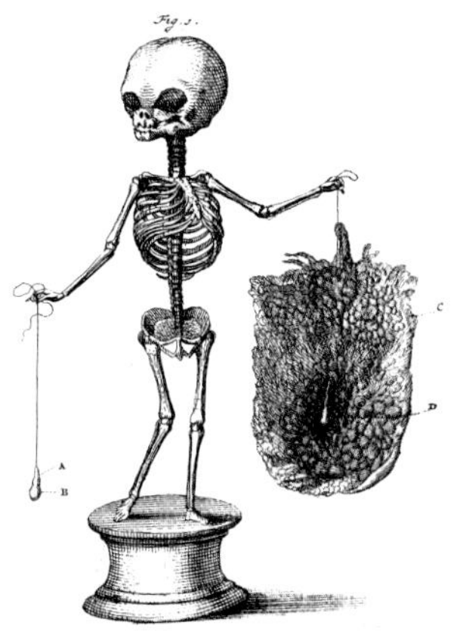

THE WITHERING CROWD

EVAN MICHELSON

DEATH HAS TRADITIONALLY BEEN THE FIRST STEP IN THE PROCESS of decay but in Palermo, Italy, a combination of casual mummification and formal attire has imposed an unusual kind of stasis. Here the bodies of the dead are put on display and the result is a singular, eerie, beautiful, grimly whimsical gathering to which no one else will ever be invited. I recently visited this place as a clear-eyed researcher, an obsessed pilgrim and a curious chronicler; I did not expect to mourn.

This journey was of particular importance to me; I have been preoccupied with the historical preservation and display of the human corpus for as long as I can remember. As a child I had family stationed in Europe, where I was a frequent visitor to many of the great churches and cathedrals of Christendom—always diving into crypts and traipsing though cemeteries and graveyards, a dedicated lurker in any place that is quiet, old, and intended for solemn remembrance. I believe it was in Italy, in some poorly-lit side chapel, that I encountered my first sacred reliquaries, and those bits of human skin, bone, hair and teeth that make up a first-degree relic. I was instantly and fatally smitten by the tiny, exquisitely cut and polished rock crystal portholes, the gleaming silver and golden vessels which contained those incongruously humble, brownish-grey, dry bones.

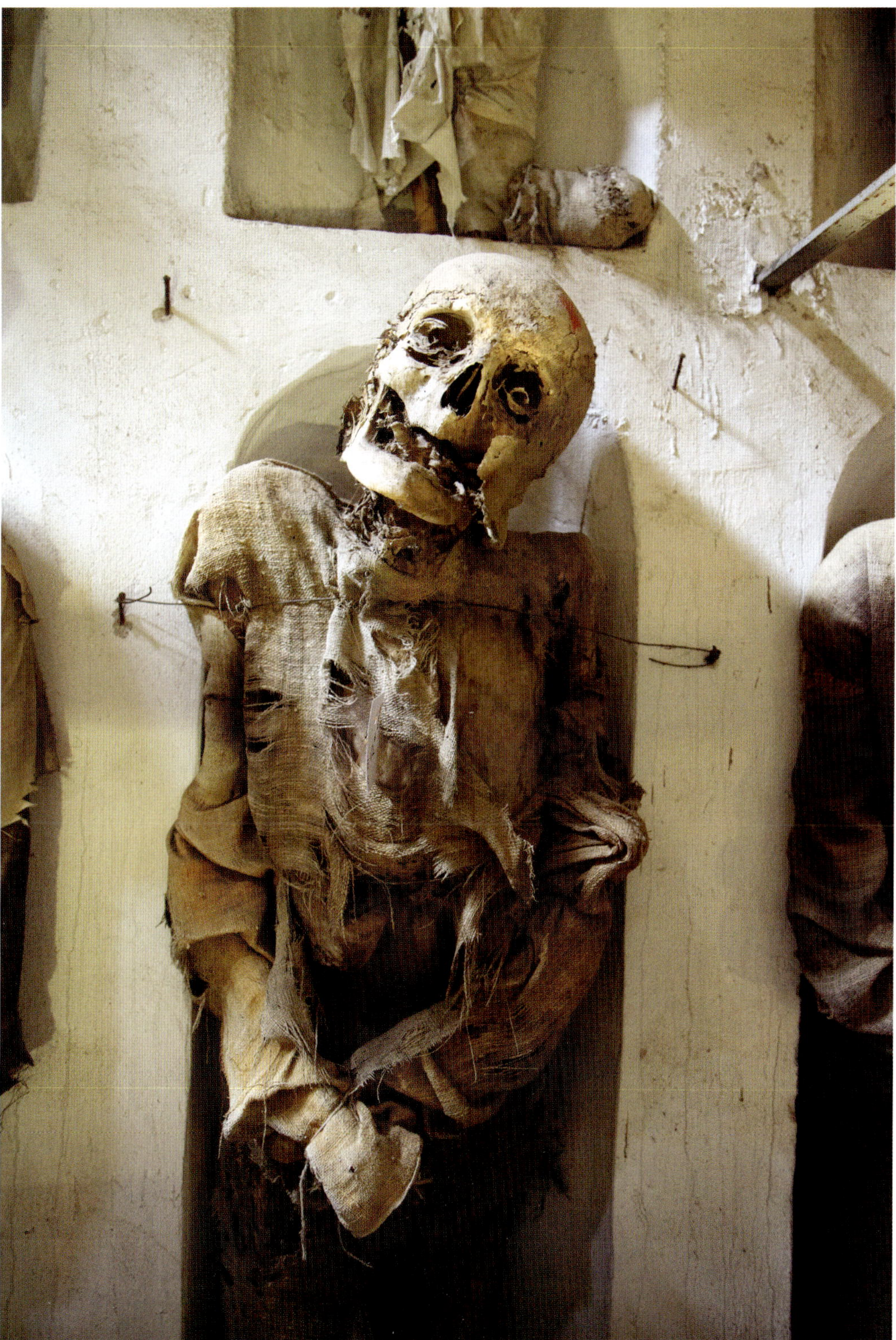

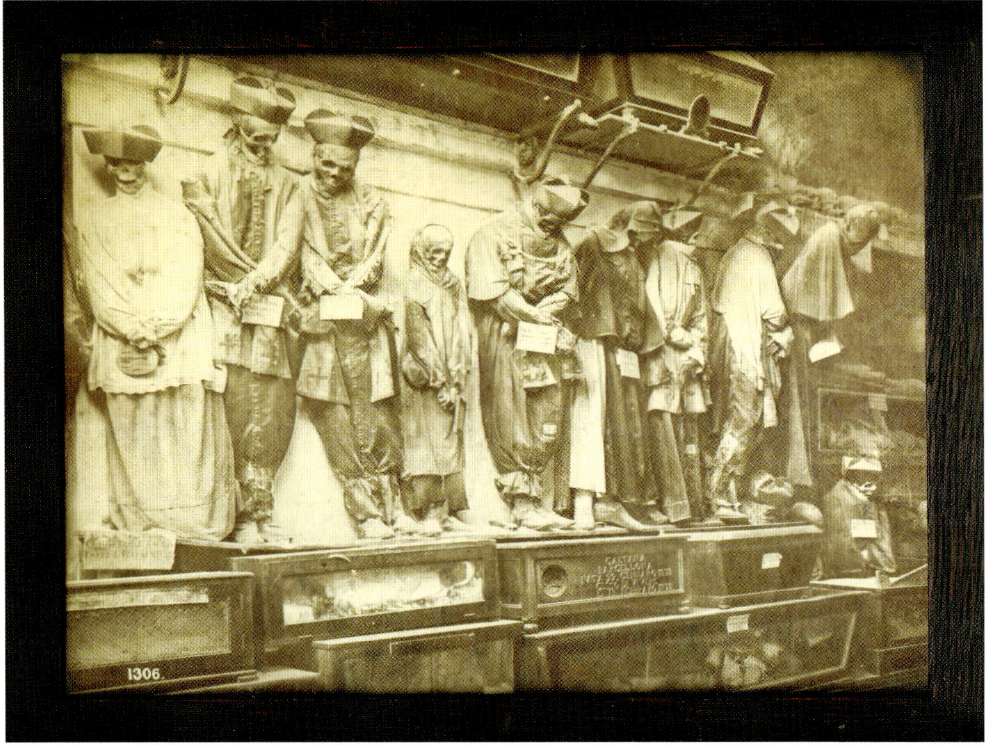

The course of my life would return to this aesthetic again and again. Indeed, I have been an antiques dealer for a few decades now, and I regularly buy, sell, collect and swoon over preserved remains (both human and animal) under glass; eventually the time came to write a book on the subject, and I finally found an opportunity to visit the ultimate gathering of the dead: the famed Capuchin catacombs of Palermo.

The Palermo catacombs have been a tourist attraction since at least the nineteenth century. Over the course of my career I have collected a few of these tokens of morbid tourism: some framed, early photos, stereoviews, and tiny souvenir postcards that fit into the palm of your hand. My mental image of the catacombs had always been of the place as it exists in these old photographs, where the beautifully dressed bodies are lined up behind piles of messily stacked, ornate wooden coffins, skulls sprinkled whimsically (and somewhat haphazardly) about. In my mind's eye the catacombs were frozen in time, the living visitors consisting of ladies in fine linen dresses and gentlemen in frock coats carefully picking their way through the crowded maze of sloughing bodies while holding delicate lace handkerchiefs and quoting the latest poetic stanzas on the passing of the body and the immortality of the soul. The catacombs have always been, to me, a sepia-tinged, nineteenth-century place of informal intimacy and dust: a place of eternal stasis.

Image left: Photograph of Capuchin Catacombs, circa 1900; collection of the author.

Of course, such is not at all the case. When I finally made it to Palermo (after so many years of dreamy anticipation) I was both surprised and taken aback by the modern lighting and the tasteful, raised-glass floor. There are now protective barriers and fences up in front of the bodies, and those teetering stacks of ornate, rotting coffins have long since been sensibly packed away. Although a certain amount of dust is unavoidable, the place seemed so very clean. Here, at my primary (and perhaps overly anticipated) place of deathly pilgrimage I felt an initial flutter of disappointment, my dramatic notions of time travel and dank exploration shot down by some very reasonable modern precautions. Such is often the case when we encounter people, places or things with which we've become infatuated from afar—reality can seldom hold a flaming torch to the vivid chambers of the imagination.

And yet, and yet—it was when I started inspecting the mummies, so beautifully dressed and hung (rather unceremoniously) by wire on hooks on the whitewashed walls that time began to slow down a bit, then slowly reverse; I found myself entering another world—*their* world. I was able to pick out familiar corpses: There were the very unseeing, grimacing faces that I had been staring at in antique photos for so many years, and they were still wearing their familiar clothes—the melancholy gentlemen in their sturdy woolen suits (with their still neatly folded pocket squares), the screaming clerics in their rough muslins, the grinning ladies in their fine linens and delicate, ruffled silks. It didn't take long before I began to feel more at home, and the true power of the place started to seep in.

The history of the catacombs is fairly straightforward: The Capuchin friars first came to Sicily in the early sixteenth century, where they settled in the outskirts of Palermo, amidst the beautiful hillsides of Sicily. Here the friars buried their dead near the Church of Santa Maria della Pace in a then-customary mass pit (burial inside a church then being forbidden by the order). In the course of a late-century exhumation of one of these mass burials it was discovered that a great majority of the corpses had been naturally mummified. The friars considered this a sign of divine intervention and they moved the miraculous mummies indoors, to take their place in a specially constructed room behind the main altar. What was seen as miraculous was (at least in this case) entirely natural: this region of Sicily lies in the shadow of Mount Etna, and the soil in the area is rich in tuff (compressed volcanic rock), a very porous substance that soaks up moisture like a sponge. The volcanic soil is a perfect vehicle of desiccation, which explains why so many of the deceased friars came out of the ground looking very much like they did going in.

At some point the Capuchin brothers decided to aid the natural process by mummifying the bodies themselves using a very simple process of evisceration, drying and chemical exposure. The friars built special preparation cells (some still visible along the catacomb corridors) where the bodies of the

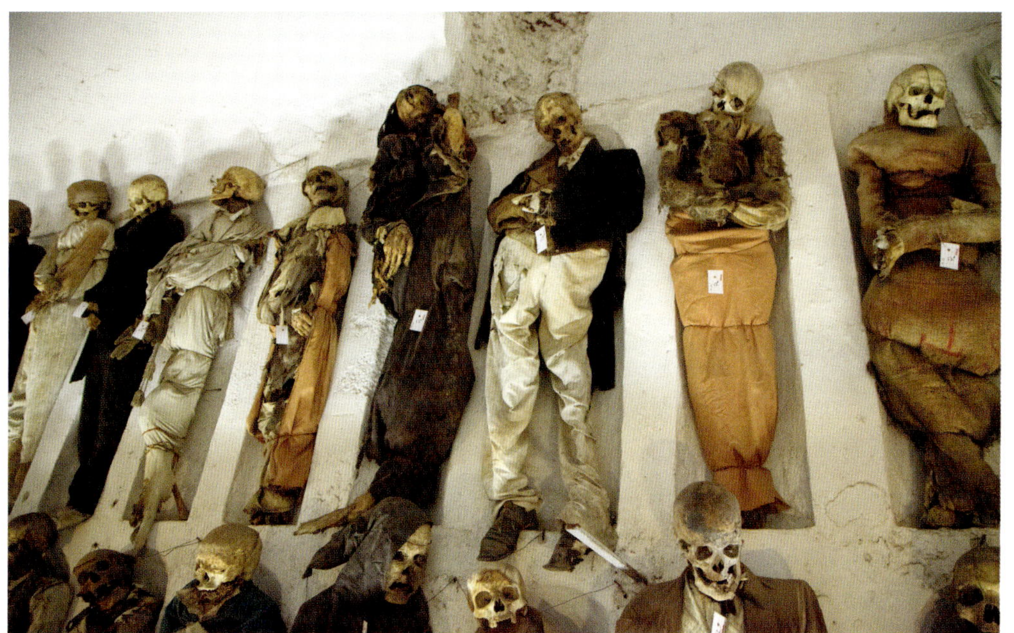

This photo and all following in this essay were taken by Joanna Ebenstein, and are included here courtesy of the Order of the Capuchin Friars, Palermo.

deceased were opened and the inner organs removed; the corpses were then left on a drainage surface and sealed in for a period of roughly one year. At the end of that time the cells were opened and many of the dried-out bodies were then dipped in vinegar before being put on display for all eternity. On occasion a body was treated with lime (as was often the case during a plague outbreak or other instance of mass infection), and some of the best-preserved, nineteenth-century mummies show evidence of lime preservation. Yet other bodies were injected with mercury and arsenic, popular nineteenth-century preservatives (and highly toxic poisons). If a body had not mummified after one year in the sealed room, the friars would remove the rotted soft tissues and replace them with straw or some other stuffing, and so it is that many of the bodies on display resemble large dolls or taxidermy mounts (indeed, one of

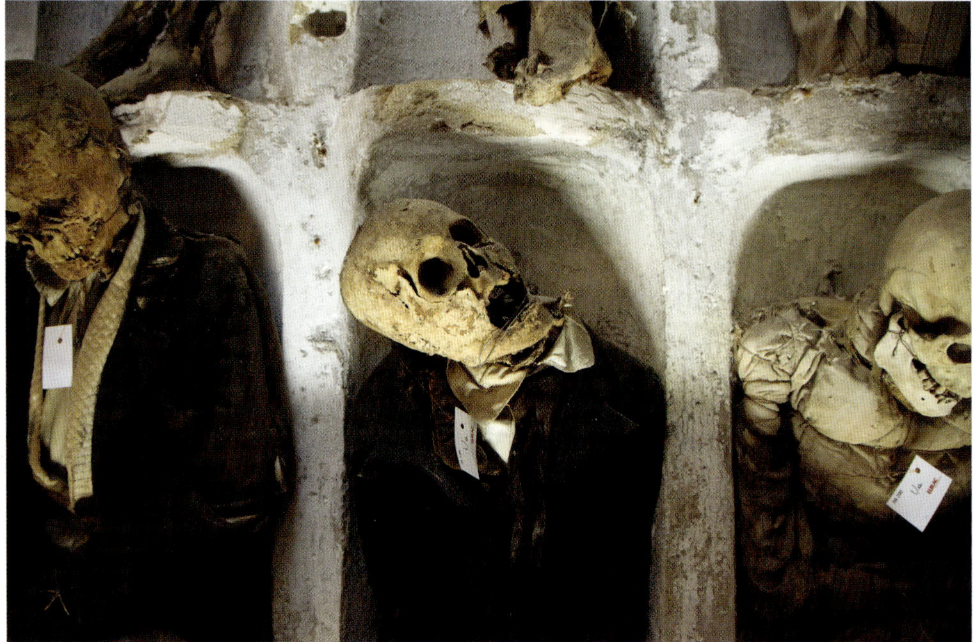

the Palermo preparers was a taxidermist). The ultimate result of these various methods of mummification are bodies in wildly differing states of preservation.

By the turn of the seventeenth century so many friars had died and been preserved that more room was needed, and underground corridors and chapels were created to house all the mummies; this is when the Palermo catacombs that we know today really began to take shape. Eventually wealthy patrons (apparently impressed with the spectacle) requested that their remains be preserved and displayed alongside the ever-growing ranks of dead friars and by the late eighteenth century the catacombs and the surrounding cemetery had become a popular place of burial and preservation. The wealthiest patrons were interred underneath marble and majolica slabs in the floor, but other socially elevated citizens chose to be mummified and displayed in the underground corridors and chapels; the rest of the populace had to make do with anonymous burial in mass graves. So it was that the Capuchin catacombs of Palermo became a surreal, underground city of the well-dressed dead, a place where high society continued the social parade and announced its privileges, even after all earthly life had ceased.

By the mid-nineteenth century modern sanitary awareness signaled the end of the friar's mummification process, and by the beginning of the twentieth century relatively few bodies were interred. The miraculously preserved little Rosalia Lombardo (skillfully injected with paraffin) was given a special dispensation and placed in the catacombs in 1920. She is the most perfectly preserved body laid to rest there, and she was the very last.

In death we all look very much alike: the greater the decay, the less individual we are. This rather obvious fact was never more viscerally evident to me than when I encountered the Palermo mummies wearing their eternal Sunday best (right down to the fine shoes, slippers and elegant, leather gloves). The effect of all this sartorial splendor is grimly fascinating and strangely intimate. These bodies, as they slowly slough their withered skins, make a mockery of such social niceties as kid gloves and cravats; the effect is the very essence of the uncanny. These splendidly dressed corpses walk that unsettling line between living and dead, animate and inanimate, real and unreal. They display undeniably distinct personalities, their post-mortem body language a grotesque parody of life. Long after the muscles stiffen, the skin continues to shrink, harden and slough away, giving rise to hideous and comical expressions that

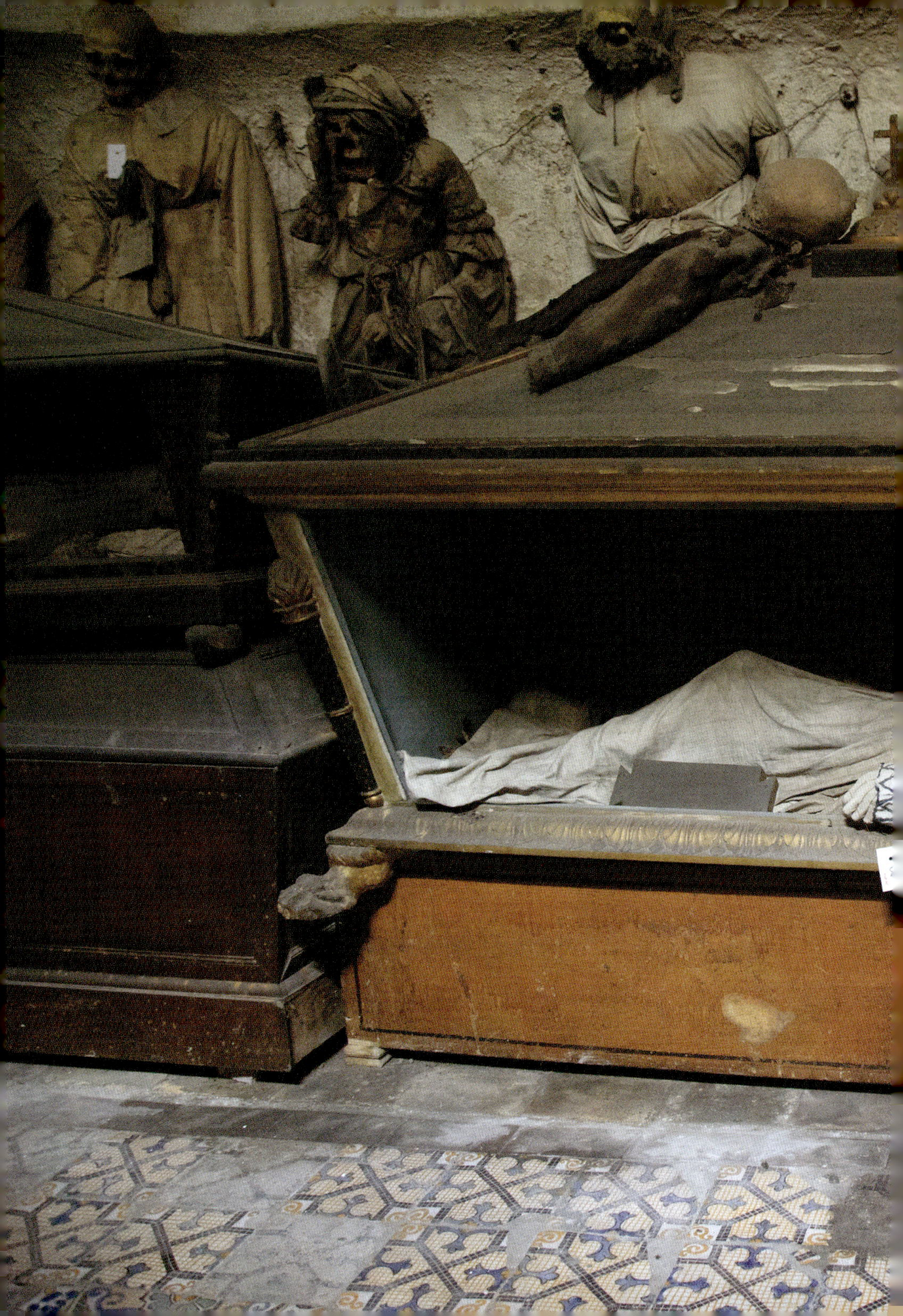

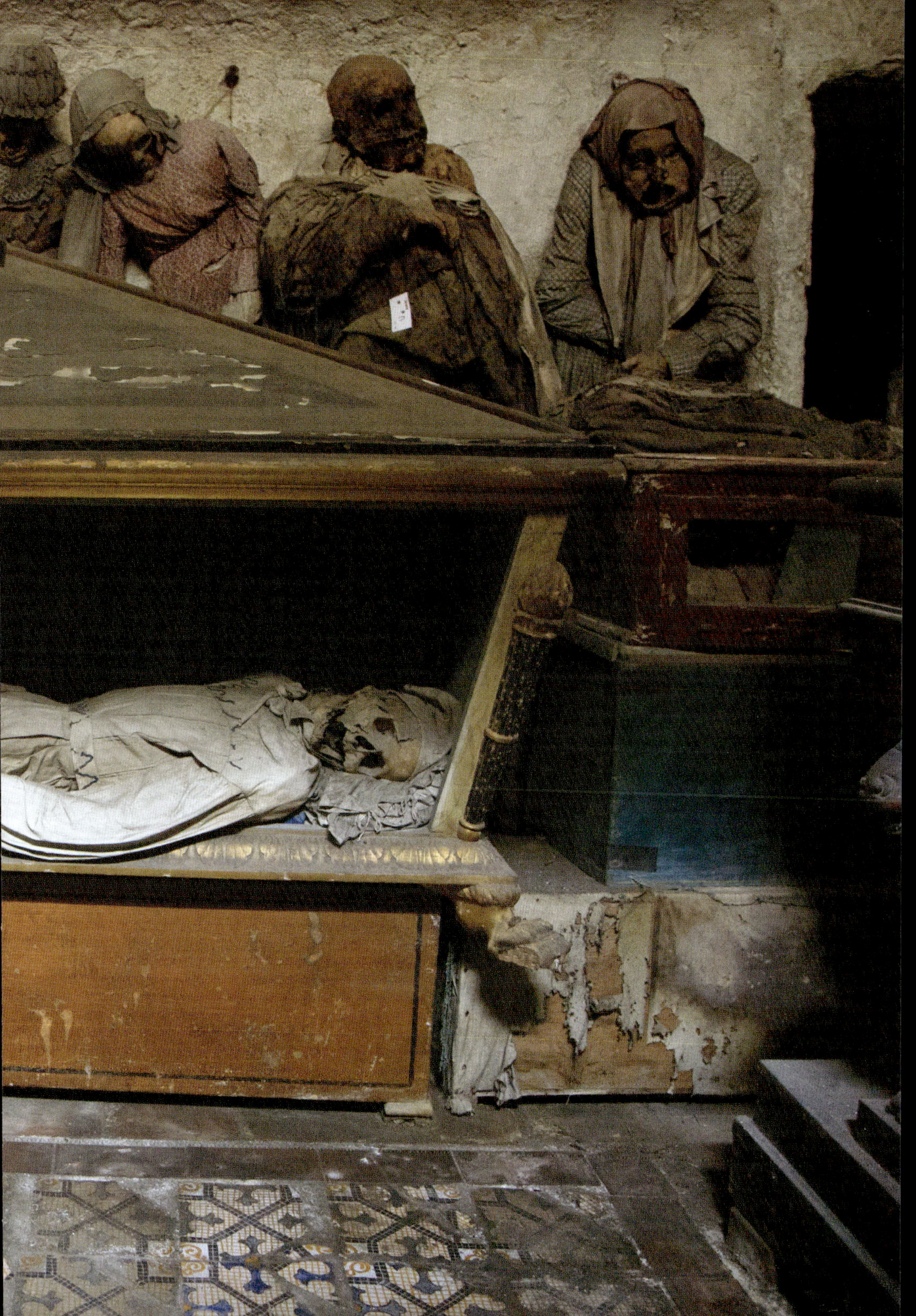

mirror the entire range of living emotion. Everywhere in this underground complex one encounters expressions of pain, fear, laughter, agony, surprise, resignation and sadness. The hanging bodies, obeying the call of gravity, slump and lean in intimate ways, and strangers in life are locked into decades of apparent conversation, whispering into one another's ear or lending a comforting shoulder.

The friars would occasionally redistribute the bodies, organizing them into categories according to profession, age, sex or class. There are what appear to be family groups, but most of the identifying records were destroyed in a fire long ago, and the true relation between the various slumping corpses is largely a mystery. Some of the bodies are placed together in chapels, the most eerie and devastating of which is undoubtedly the children's room; I had never seen old images of this particular cell, and it came as something of a surprise. Here the corpses of young children are hung very much like the adults outside, and the little slumping bodies in their niches highly resemble skeletonized dolls, the delicate cotton bonnets resting on bare skulls. Perhaps it is the fact that young children are so often in frenetic motion that the stasis in this room felt even more unnatural than the stately quiet of the corridors of the adult dead. The newborn babies, mummified and naked as they came into the world lie woodenly in their cradles in a brutal display of the madness of a parent's grief. One little boy in a particularly jaunty hat stands at attention in his Sunday best, inviting uneasy smiles as he welcomes decades of curious strangers. In this room, more than anywhere else, the grieving is still palpable, and the existential emptiness gapes wide.

It was in a disused work area at the back of one of the corridors that I fell utterly into the spell of the place. This room was set aside as a restoration area, a place where the bodies could

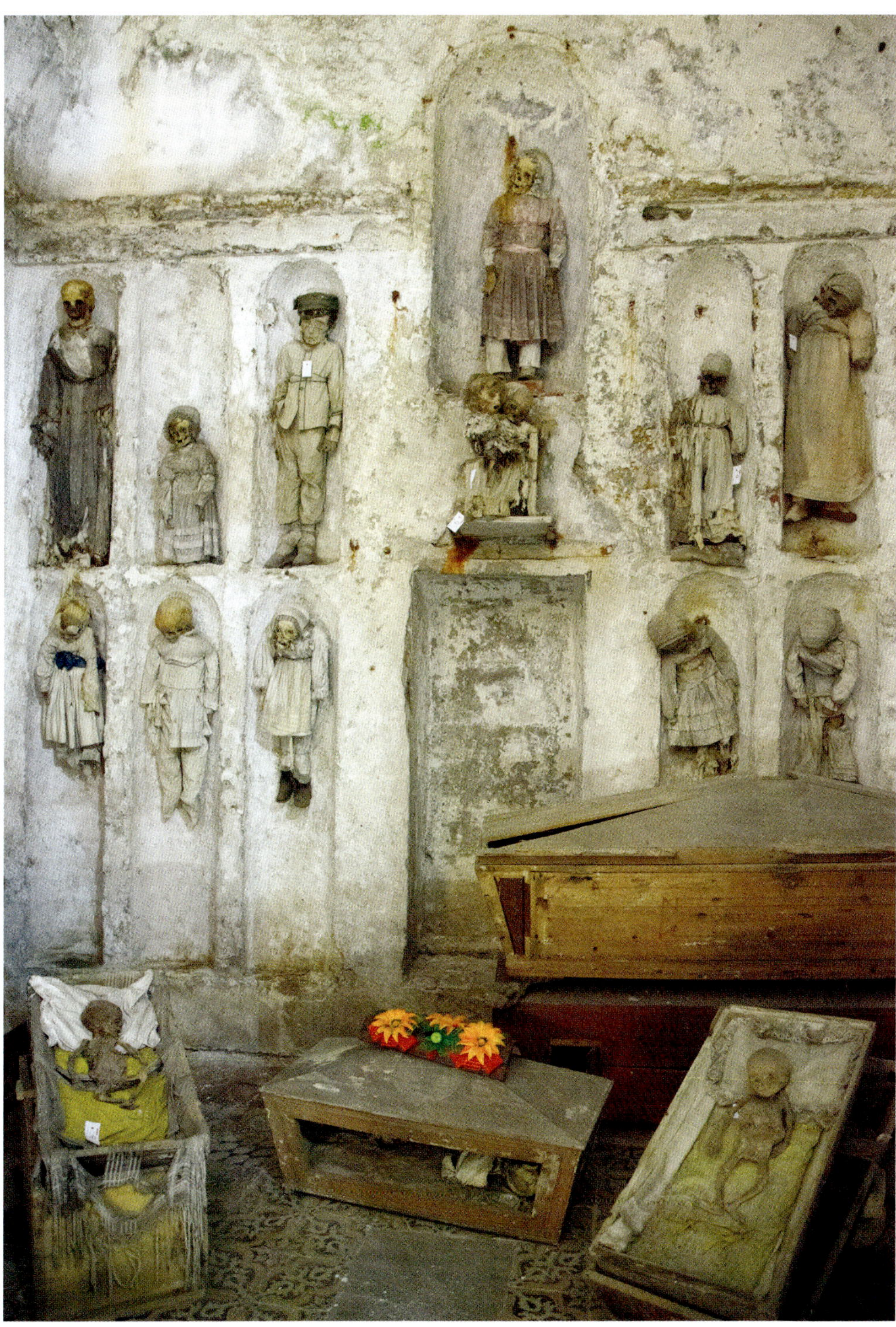

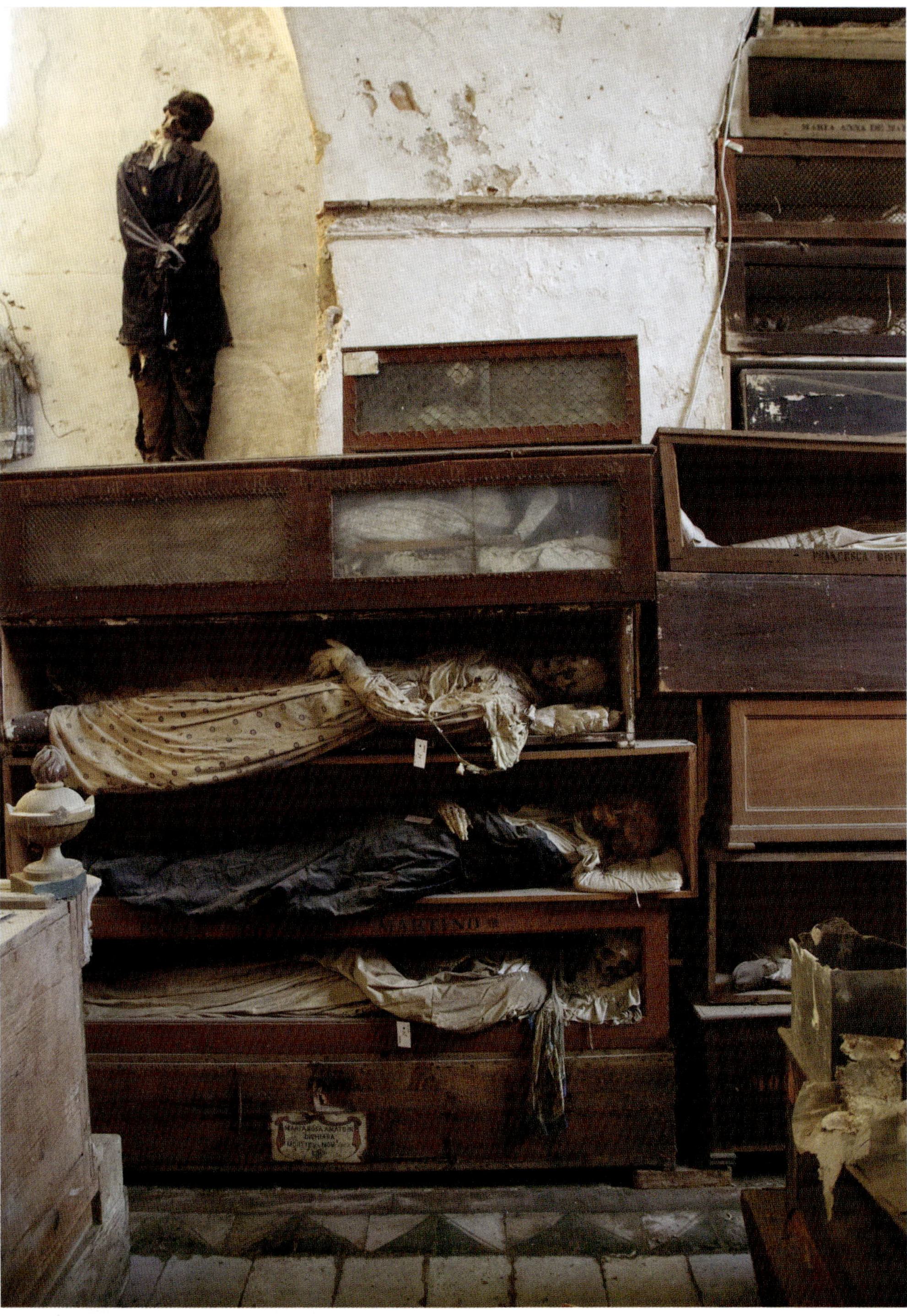

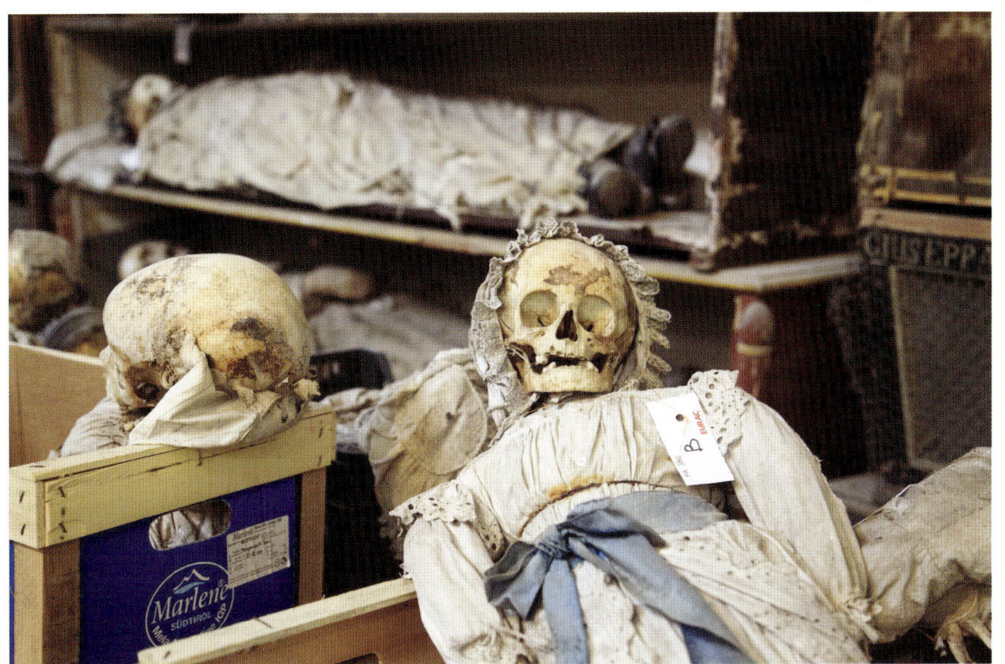

be maintained and restored to counter decades of damage from pollution, flooding, fires and the bombings of World War II. It was in this room that the catacombs finally looked and felt like those old sepia images hanging on my wall: Here were the stacks of ornate little coffins; there were no modern barriers of any kind. The mummies of small children were lying in boxes and plastic crates, waiting patiently for caregivers; in this state they looked even more like dolls—genuine examples of human taxidermy. Many of the bodies are stuffed with straw and cotton batting, which is now leaking and protruding out of various cracks and orifices. The babies' heads are mounted separately on wooden rods that run up through the small stuffed bodies, looking very much like the specimens of stuffed Victorian birds that I spend so much time restoring back home. I so wanted to put a few of them back together, but I touched nothing.

It was perfectly quiet, and I was alone, and I began to really take in the tiny, telling details: the fading of the fabrics, the settling of the skin on bone, the mothing of wool, the worming of dried flesh, the shattering of silk. One woman in particular caught my attention: She was lying on a lower shelf, and her dress (a dusty blue fabric with a yellowing machine-lace overlay) looked to date from about the 1870s. I was struck by the pattern of the lace—it was so like a dress that I had brought with me for the trip. I began to wonder who picked out this particular outfit; did this woman know she was dying, and choose to be laid out in this dress forever? Was the choice made by a grieving husband or fiancée? Her parents? Did she die slowly of a wasting disease? Perhaps it was sudden, or the result of an accident or even foul play. As I leaned closer still, I had a sudden, intense sensation of her *presence.* Unlike graveyards with their stone monuments or columbiums with their plaques and flowers, the dead here speak for themselves. Unlike ossuaries, where the bones are anonymous and speak to a more abstract notion of eternity, these skeletons and mummies are as specific as can be. I found myself involuntarily speaking to her: "What a lovely dress you're wearing," I said, and I felt an entirely unexpected stinging of tears.

It occurred to me suddenly that all of these people were laid to rest here when the place was still active. The other denizens would have been far fresher, and their clothing would not have been the fascinating stuff of museums but common, everyday wear. Anyone choosing to be displayed here could see that the process was highly imperfect, that one's body would continue to age in unexpected (and sometimes alarming) ways, and yet the choice was still made to join this somewhat ghastly spectacle. In the nearly 150 years since the woman in blue was interred here, Western attitudes towards death have changed utterly; something like this simply could not happen again. These catacombs are in part a holdover from earlier, pagan

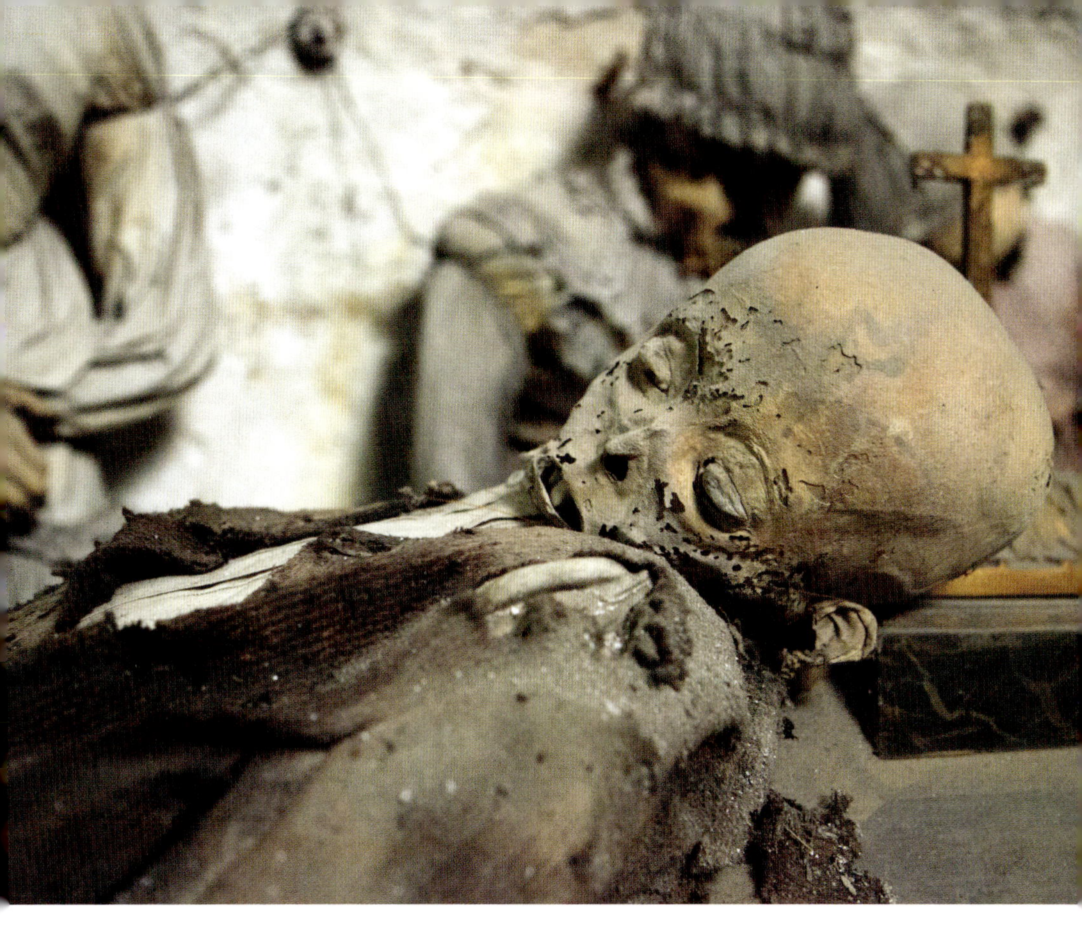

times, when ancestor worship required the talismanic presence of the actual ancestor. They are also a crowning example of a certain kind of Christian materiality that sees preservation and the cessation of decay as evidence of God's grace. All these mummies are secular incorruptibles who have been lifted from the earthly corruption of sin and set into a more celestial sphere beyond mortality. These bodies reside here in a state of highly improbable grace (bought and paid for in life), to be the stuff of dreams and nightmares for as long as their mortal remains can cohere. They are a paean to the uniquely human desire to transcend nature, move beyond the boundaries of our physical world, and become one with the angels.

LOOK NOT UPON THEM!

Maternity & the Monstrous Imagination

STEPHEN T. ASMA

"I HAVE TODAY COME ACROSS A VERY REMARKABLE CASE OF animal monstrosity with the particulars of which you will I think be interested." So begins a curious 1865 letter to Charles Darwin from George Maw, a Shropshire tile-maker and amateur botanist. Maw relates a recent pig birth at the local inn, in which a sow gave birth to ten normal piglets, and one deformed creature resembling a little elephant. The monstrous offspring possessed a distinct trunk-like proboscis and the ears and mouth of an elephant. The creature was born alive but the mother smothered it, and the local pharmacist pickled it in a jar of spirits.

Maw's letter to Darwin asks advice. Does Mr. Darwin think it is interesting enough for scientific analysis? Should Mr. Maw purchase the monstrosity and bring it to the Hunterian Collection in the Royal College of Surgeons in London? Maw has investigated the case thoroughly and eagerly shares a tentative theory about the genesis of the elephant pig. A day or two after the sow was impregnated, he explains, a traveling menagerie passed through town and one of the elephants tried to attack the sow. She was

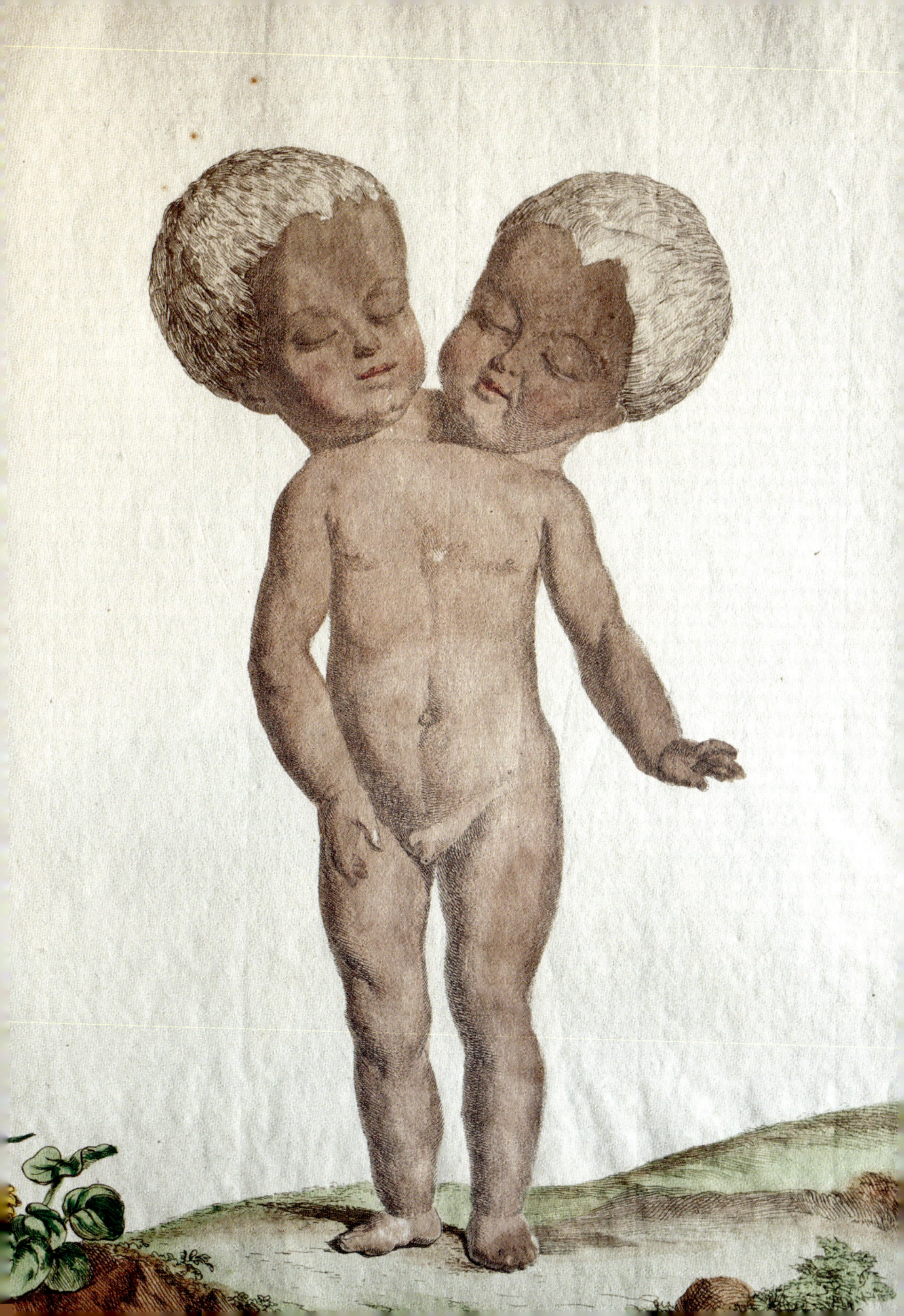

[1] It's unclear whether Joseph actually believed this or whether it was constructed as part of his promotional biographical material.

terror stricken by the experience, and Maw suggests that this trauma had a distorting effect upon the embryonic pig gestating within her. The frightening impression of the aggressive elephant traveled through the perceptual faculty of the sow and imprinted an isomorphic disfiguration upon the forming matter in utero.

The theory of monstrous maternal impression was widespread in the nineteenth century. It was often employed to account for organic distortions in human, as well as animal, embryology. One is reminded of Joseph Merrick, the "Elephant Man," who claimed that his own unfortunate condition was the result of his pregnant mother being frightened by a dangerous elephant in 1859. In his autobiographical pamphlet, Merrick says, "I first saw the light on the 5th of August, 1860, I was born in Lee Street, Wharf Street, Leicester. The deformity which I am now exhibiting was caused by my mother being frightened by an elephant; my mother was going along the street when a procession of animals were passing by, there was a terrible crush of people to see them, and unfortunately she was pushed under the elephant's feet, which frightened her very much; this occurring during a time of pregnancy."[1]

Image previous page: Jacques Louis Moreau (1771-1826), Description des principales monstruosités dans l'homme et dans les animaux précédée d'un discours sur la physiologie et la classification des monstres ... avec figures coloriées par N.F. Regnault... *Paris: Fournier, 1808. Courtesy of the New York Academy of Medicine Library.*

Intentional Monsters

Monstrous births have always been theorized and contextualized in moral terms, from the prodigies of ancient Greece and Rome to the theology of parental sin in the Medieval period. Christianity tended to see monstrous births as punishments, and if the afflicted lived to adulthood they were further theorized. Do conjoined twins, for example, have two souls or one soul? The seventeenth-century magazine *Athenian Mercury* considered the famous Italian conjoined brothers, Lazarus and Baptista. Theologians wondered if both brothers had rationality (reason was evidence of soul) but they also wondered whether the *bodies* of these extraordinary creatures would be resurrected at the Day of Judgment.

Lazarus toured all over Europe in the 1630s and '40s, exhibiting himself for money. His parasitic brother Baptista, consisting of a head, torso and leg, emerged from Lazarus' chest and hung upside down. Baptista showed negligible signs of consciousness, and no speech, but did respond reflexively to pain. According to the *Athenian Mercury* (1691), Lazarus would probably go to the beatific eternity alone—without his more deformed brother. The magazine suggested that since Baptista did not demonstrate rationality, Lazarus would surely "rise without him at the Day of Judgment, for there will be no monsters at the Resurrection."[2] And if Baptista should turn out to have a very rudimentary, passive mind, then he will be raised up with children and imbeciles, but housed in a new, perfected body.

Less well known is a monsterology tradition from St. Augustine to Michel de Montaigne that conceptualized deformed babies as "wonders" of nature. Instead of being a punishment or even contrary to nature, the monster is a *token* of a mysterious *type*. The creature probably has its own species somewhere in the grand plan of the deity, and we are privileged to witness such a unique ambassador. As Montaigne says, "Those that we call monsters are not so to God, who sees in the immensity of His work the infinite forms that He has comprehended therein; and it is to be believed that this figure which astonishes us has relation to some other figure of the same kind unknown to man. From His wisdom nothing but good, common, and regular proceeds, but we do not discern the disposition and relation."[3]

Whether they are divine punishments or divine wonders, they are heaven sent. In other words, both these negative and

[2] *The story of Lazarus and Baptista, and this quote from the* Mercury, *are nicely discussed in Stephen Pender's "No Monsters at the Resurrection" in* Monster Theory: Reading Culture, *edited by Jeffrey Jerome Cohen (University of Minnesota, 1996).*

[3] *Michel de Montaigne, "Of a monstrous child," trans. Charles Cotton, in* Quotidiana, *ed. Patrick Madden (2010).*

positive traditions see monsters as "intentional" freaks. Their alternative morphologies are a kind of message, sent from a divine agent. They mean something. Now contrast these traditions with what I'll call the "accidental" tradition.

Accidental Monsters

Accidental monsters are not secret codes that need to be deciphered. Their causal story may be obscure, but they are not designed for some transcendental communication. The monster, in this tradition, is a glitch or malfunction of natural laws. Giants and multi-limbed creatures, for example, may be the result of too much matter in the reproduction process, or, in the case of dwarfs, midgets, and missing limbs, there may be too little of the needed gestational matter. Blended parts too may be a concoction problem rather than an intentional sign.

Darwin's elephant-pig and the Elephant Man's putative origin are species of this accidental tradition. These monsters of maternal impression are a subset of the naturalistic teratology that brought embryology under a more scientific umbrella. The idea that monsters can be caused by unpleasant impressions is considered highly superstitious today, but it was once a partner in the naturalization of the more metaphysical tradition.

Russian Czar Peter the Great (1672–1725) celebrated the monstrous and freakish in his early museum collections, and in some of his official proclamations he prohibited the killing of deformed children and requested that local officials send the "marvels" to his St. Petersburg museum. Peter was himself a marvel, at 6 feet 7 inches, and may have purchased a French giant named Bourgeois to become his constant companion (his personal servant) because Bourgeois made Peter look "normal" by comparison.

Obsessed with breeding giants and dwarfs, Peter looked more deeply into the science of teratology, the proximate mechanisms of deformation and variation. In one of his proclamations, he states:

> Ignoramuses think that such monsters are born from the action of the devil which is, however, impossible for there is only one creator of all creation, and that is God. And the Evil One has no power over any living creatures. For monsters are the result of internal damage, of fear and the thoughts of the mother during her pregnancy, of which fact there are many examples. For example, when the mother is frightened, hurt or injured in any way the child will be influenced.[4]

A hundred years before Peter's psychologizing of monster embryology, the French surgeon and scholar Ambroise Paré (1510–1590) also emphasized the role of the mother's imagination in teratology. Paré started "rescuing" monsters from the melodramatic arena of spiritual and moral meaning, but failed to affect a complete revolution in monsterology, toggling between highly superstitious and scientific. He certainly paved the way for future medical scientists to study birth anomalies. Paré's book *On Monsters and Marvels* (1573) took a relatively empirical approach to monsters, preferring the collection and dissection of oddities rather than the pursuit of hearsay natural history.

[4] *This 1718* ukaz *is included in Anthony Anemone's excellent article "The Monsters of Peter the Great" in* Slavic and East European Journal *44, no. 4 (2000): 583-602.*

Working slowly toward a general and naturalistic procreation theory, he sought to explain a variety of pathology cases. And this can be seen, for example, in his treatment of hybrid monsters. Creatures that appear to be half animal and half human are not the result of supernatural causation. They are not omens or signs sent to us as coded messages. They are more mundane than that. Paré includes many woodcut images of hybrid monsters: a figure of a child/dog fusion, a goat with a man's face, a pig with a man's face and hands, and more. These sad monsters are no mystery, he explains. They are the results of "sodomites and atheists" who have sex with animals. These impure humans "join together and break out of their bounds—unnaturally—with animals, and from this are born several hideous monsters that bring great shame to those who look at them or speak of them. Yet, the dishonesty lies in the deed and not in words; and it is, when it is done, a very unfortunate and abominable thing, and a great horror for a man or a woman to mix with or copulate with brute animals; and as a result, some are born half-men and half-animals."[5]

[5] *See Chapter 20, Ambroise Paré,* On Monsters and Marvels, *trans. Janis L. Pallister (Chicago: University of Chicago Press, 1982).*

"Monsters," Paré explains, "are things that appear outside the course of Nature... such as a child who is born with one arm, another who will have two heads, and additional members over and above the ordinary."[6] Notice that, despite terminology, Paré is not disagreeing with the much earlier theological naturalism laid down by writers like Isidore of Seville, for he is only expressing that monsters deviate from the norm. Well beyond the abnormalities of monsters, however, are the "marvels" or "prodigies" according to Paré. "Marvels are things which happen that are completely against Nature as when a woman will give birth to a serpent, or to a dog...." In other words, even the barriers of taxonomic kinds are violated or transgressed in the case of true prodigies.

Lastly, he distinguishes monsters and marvels from "maimed persons." "Maimed persons include the blind, the one-eyed, the humpbacked, those who limp or [those] having six-digits on the hand or the feet... or any other thing that is against Nature." Notice the strangeness of this category, which seemingly contains both congenital defects and accidental wounds. Paré's logic here cannot be entirely appreciated, because he only mentions the maimed briefly and focuses instead on monsters and marvels.

His list of the *causes* of monsters demonstrates his cusp status—at once progressive and enlightened, but also backward and uncritical. "There are several things," he says, "that cause monsters":

The first is the glory of God.
The second, his wrath.
The third, too great a quantity of seed.†
The fourth, too little a quantity.
The fifth, the imagination.
The sixth, the narrowness or smallness of the womb.
The seventh, the indecent posture of the mother, as when, being pregnant, she has sat too long with her legs crossed, or pressed against her womb.
The eighth, through a fall, or blows struck against the womb of the mother, being with child.
The ninth, through hereditary or accidental illness.
The tenth, through rotten or corrupt seed.
The twelfth, through the artifice of wicked spital beggars.‡
The thirteenth, through Demons and Devils.[7]

A typical example of a monster born from too much seed is the two-headed girl of Bavaria. Paré describes a sad story, and offers a woodcut of a girl whose body was "perfect and well-

[7] *See Paré, Chapter 1.*

† *He offers an illustrated tour of conjoined twins, parasitic anomalies, and hermaphrodites, all of which are explained by the presence of too much seed at the time of generation. "On the generating of monsters," Paré explains, "Hippocrates says that if there is too great an abundance of matter, multiple births will occur, or else a monstrous child having superfluous and useless parts, such as two heads, four arms, four legs, six digits on the hands and feet, or other things." This view, which was continued by Aristotle, is upheld by Paré as superior to those who think that the womb is a multichambered vessel. Some theorists believed that the womb, being composed of many cells or cavities, has the ability to gestate.*

‡ *Here we see an interesting aspect of Paré's notion of causality. In most of the other list items, he is trying to isolate some actual mechanical process that causes monstrosity. But "cause" twelve reveals that he is also considering the appearance of monstrosity, even when no monster is present—in other words, how are certain deceptions regarding monsters foisted upon us? It is noteworthy that Paré feels no need to separate out this epistemic consideration from the other metaphysical considerations on the list. The case he refers to is one where a beggar led many citizens of Angers, France, to believe that he had a monstrous rotting arm, when in fact he had only stolen the decaying arm of an executed man and tricked the public by sewing it into his jacket sleeve.*

proportioned" save the fact that she had two heads. She lived for over twenty-five years, "which is not natural for monsters, who ordinarily live scarcely any length of time at all because they grow displeased and melancholy at seeing themselves so repugnant to everyone, so that their life is brief." This rare moment of recognition—acknowledgement of the inner psychology and subjectivity of the monster—is abandoned quickly and the pariah status is underscored in the rest of Paré's story. "This girl," he continues, "went begging from door to door for her livelihood, and people gladly gave to her on account of the novelty of such a strange and such a new spectacle. Nevertheless, she was at last driven out of the Duchy of Bavaria because she could spoil the fruit of the pregnant women by the apprehension and ideas which might remain in their imaginative faculty, over the form of this so monstrous a creature. It is not good that monsters should live among us."

The Impressionable Woman

For our purposes here, we are most interested in the fifth item on his list, the imagination.[8] Paré follows his ancient predecessors (i.e., Hippocrates, Aristotle, and Empedocles) in upholding a theory about the role of the mother's imagination at the moment of conception and in early gestation. If a woman in coitus is exposed to some frightening, or disturbing, or just strong imagery (either through the senses or memory), then her offspring may be impressed upon by the offending image. Paré accepts the reality of a physiological process—one that begins as a disturbing sense impression, and ends with a distorted fetus. He offers a few cases to illustrate his point, some of which seem quite credible to him, while others strain this credulity.

[8] *See Paré, Chapter 9, for a discussion of the role of the imagination.*

Undermining his own embryonic empiricism, Paré cites the authorities of old. He tells of Queen Persina, the Queen of Ethiopia, who together with her black King Hidustes mysteriously produced a white baby "because of the appearance of the beautiful Andromeda that she summoned up in her imagination, for she had a painting of her before her eyes during embraces from which she became pregnant." Likewise we are told of another girl who was born as furry as a bear. Her unfortunate state was a result of her mother "having looked too intensely at the image of Saint John [the Baptist] dressed in skins, along with his [own] body hair and beard, which picture was attached to the foot of her bed while she was conceiving." The potential convenience of this particular explanation is nowhere more evident than in his retelling of a story from Hippocrates. Hippocrates, it seems, saved a young woman from the accusation of adultery, "because she had given birth to a child as black as a Moor, her husband and she both having white skin; which woman was absolved upon Hippocrates' persuasion that it was [caused by] the portrait of a Moor, similar to the child, which was customarily attached to her bed." [9]

A more contemporary example is offered in Paré's story of a baby born, in sixteenth-century France, with the face of a frog. When asked what the cause of this monster might be, the father of the child explained that his wife had been ill with a fever and had taken the curative advice of her friend. The friend offered a folk cure, saying that the wife should carry around a frog in her hand until the frog died—at which point she would be cured of the fever. "That night she went to bed with her husband, still having said frog in her hand; her husband and she embraced and she conceived; and by the power of her imagination, this monster had thus been produced."

From these cases, Paré, the medical man, offers some advice. It is important, he says, that women "should not be forced to look at or imagine monstrous things" at the time of conception

[9] *Presumably Paré is using "Moor" in a generic sense here, meaning someone of African descent.*

or during the early formation of the child (which takes thirty to thirty-five days for males and forty to forty-two days for females). But once the formation of the child is complete, no images or imaginings will have a detrimental effect upon the offspring.

Paré is drawing upon an ancient tradition that started in Aristotle's *Generation of Animals* and found full force in the writings of Albertus Magnus (ca. 1193–1280).[10] This tradition explains conception and development as the impression of male "substantial form" (contained in semen) onto the menstrual blood or matter (contributed by the mother). This is in keeping with Aristotelian and later Scholastic metaphysics of hylomorphism. Forms become instantiated in matter, and this makes one animal different from another (our species definitions are meant to capture these different substantial forms). But the mind itself is, according to Aristotle, the "form of forms." The mind receives the forms of the natural world, not the matter (there's no room in my mind for the material world). My mind takes in a form of a hippopotamus (and manipulates it as a representation), not the hippo itself. The imagination is the receiver and manipulator of these forms and it must be pliant enough to receive the impression, but durable enough to hold the forms. From Aristotle to Albertus Magnus, it was thought that the imagination of women was more susceptible to unhealthy impression because the female mind was more moist. Excessive moisture made the imaginative faculty easily corrupted with frightening external images and inner ideations. This impressionability put the fetus at risk of malformation. Inner humidity "explained" certain kinds of monstrosity, but also the fickleness of females, who get impressed easily but lose focus because the mental substrate cannot hold the information properly.

[10] *See an excellent discussion of this tradition in Katherine Park's "Impressed Images: Reproducing Wonders" in* Picturing Art, *eds. Caroline A. Jones and Peter Galison, (Routledge, 1998).*

These sorts of causal explanations may seem ridiculous to us, but they represent a naturalistic turn in the sense that they opened up possible research avenues. There may not have been a discoverable physiological *mechanism* that transmits disturbing sense impressions to the conceptus, but at least Paré didn't just throw up his hands and say "the devil did it." Invoking the imagination also indicates some sense of psychological effect; psychology can lead to very concrete manifestations (e.g., a deeply troubled woman can result in a miscarriage). In this respect, Paré seems to foreshadow psychosomatic theories that flourished during Freud's generation and beyond.

Of course, Paré was not a secular humanist, and devilish demons were quite real for him. He did not take an ironic or literary response to the demonic. "Satan's actions," he says, "are supernatural and incomprehensible, surpassing the human mind, [it] not being able to explain them, any more than [it can] the magnet which attracts iron and makes the needle turn." But he goes on to say that we should not fall into a general skepticism about the "principles and reasons of natural things." Here we find an inconspicuous boundary marker in Paré's thinking. The natural monsters are appropriate subjects for medical study, but the supernatural monsters exist in a domain that cannot be penetrated by science. The proper response to this latter domain is prayer and piety, not scientific exploration. This important concession to the Church, reiterated by most scientists of the subsequent century, helped to create an autonomous domain for previously forbidden explorations of nature.

French philosopher Nicolas Malebranche (1638–1715) continued the exploration into monstrous imagination, trying to bridge the dualist divide of mind and matter. The bond between mother and unborn child is the strongest that exists for humans,

> And although their soul be separated from their mother's, their body is not at all detached from hers, and we should

> therefore conclude that they have the same sensations and passions, i.e., that exactly the same thoughts are excited in their souls upon the occasion of the motions produced in her body. Thus, children see what their mothers see, hear the same cries, receive the same impressions from objects, and are aroused by the same passions.[11]

Malebranche illustrates the point with a recent specimen that "all of Paris has been able to see as well as me, since it was preserved for a considerable time in alcohol." A woman had been looking too intensely at a portrait of St. Pius, and gave birth to a baby that resembled perfectly the face of the saint. The baby had the face of an old man, and even his forehead was shrunken due to the foreshortened angle of the portrait.

[11] *Nicolas Malebranche,* The Search After Truth *in Cambridge Texts in the History of Philosophy, eds. Thomas M. Lennon and Paul J. Olscamp (Cambridge, 1997). See especially Book Two, Part One, Chapter Seven. Thanks to my colleague Dr. Katharine Hamerton for suggesting the Malebranche text.*

When a mother desires a pear too much, according to Malebranche, the pear shape (object of desire) will actually re-form in the extremely soft flesh of the embryo—distorting the body. The mother is spared this transformation because her body is no longer as soft and impressionable. Women are more impressionable than men, but less than babies.

The mysterious mechanism that links mother-mind to baby-body is not as troubling for Malebranche because of his unique metaphysics of occasionalism. For Malebranche, bodies and minds don't really act upon each other. Technically, events don't need to cross some Cartesian divide from soul to body, because all such causal connection is an illusion. Changes in the body and changes in the mind are divinely coordinated parallel events (without direct causal communication). This idiosyncratic "solution" failed to inspire subsequent teratologists, however, and more naturalistic or mechanical explanations continued to mount.

From Aristotle, through Ambriose Paré, to Peter the Great, the monstrous imagination played an important role in the naturalized tradition of pathological ontogenesis. Things began to change, however, in the first few decades of the nineteenth century. But breaking with such historical inertia was difficult. Mary Shelley's friend, professor William Lawrence (1783–1867), was an early scientific martyr in the demystification of monster gestation.[12]

[12] William Lawrence eventually overcame the rocky start of his early scientific career. After denouncing his own early work, his career trajectory resumed its upward climb. Being ahead of his time, the next generation, including both Darwin and Wallace, finally acknowledged Lawrence's foresight in many areas.

Shelley apparently added the moralizing, anti-materialist tone to *Frankenstein* (1818) in later editions because she feared the same condemnation that her friend William Lawrence received. He had been suspended from the Royal College of Surgeons because of the radical materialism contained in his controversial book, *Lectures on Physiology, Zoology and the Natural History of Man* (1819). Fearing that her own book might be withdrawn, Mary Shelley tempered her original 1818 edition. †

Lawrence, however, paid a great service to embryology and laid to rest many popular misconceptions about monsters. Regarding the theory that a mother's imagination can corrupt the fetus, he asks what sort of mechanical process could operate from the mother's imagination down to the womb, where it would then have to destroy the normally developing head and reconstruct a new monkey head, or frog head, or whatever. Furthermore, he states, we have extensive evidence that women can suffer serious disorders (e.g., diseases, amputations, etc.), with no ill effect on the fetus, so frights and imaginings seem far too weak for fetal reconstruction. ‡

---

† *Marilyn Butler, "Frankenstein and Radical Science" in the Modern Criticism section of Norton's Critical Edition of* Frankenstein, *eds. J. Paul Hunter (W.W. Norton & Company, 1996). Butler points out that the earliest versions of Shelley's Dr. Frankenstein show him as a scientific bumbler who knows "too little science rather than too much." The earliest versions of the story are not indictments of science itself.*

‡ *Next, Lawrence counters the theory that severe monsters are caused by blunt or acute traumas to the mother's gravid abdomen. For one thing, Lawrence argued, a majority of cases of unfortunate offspring are born to women who suffered no such violence. Furthermore, if the heads were caved in or broken in half, then we should discover some excess matter in utero and some bruising or signs of trauma. "[H]ow does it happen," he asks, "that the head should be*

Preformation, Epigenesis and Pangenesis

Throughout the eighteenth and nineteenth centuries, before the discovery of the microscopic human egg, biologists argued over the true gestational mechanisms.[13] Preformationists and epigeneticists offered alternative explanations for how embryos grew into babies. The mystery was how an undifferentiated blob could become a fully articulated body, when no shaping forces are observed. Some vitalists suggested an occult invisible force that molded the intrauterine matter into a recognizable form. But the preformationists (from Nicolaas Hartsoeker to Charles Bonnet) suggested that a tiny homunculus existed (in the semen or menstrual blood) and conception triggered mere *growth*, not development. Little potential people were nested within us, and, in turn, their descendants were contained like Russian dolls within them. Embryonic organisms were fully formed, miniature versions of their adult selves.

[13] Karl von Baer discovered the mammalian egg in 1826, but the first human egg was not properly described until the 1920s.

Epigeneticists, on the other hand, accepted the reality of development: homogenous material substrate, in the uterus, becomes more complex and heterogeneously structured over several months of gestation. From Johann Friedrich Blumenbach to Caspar Friedrich Wolff, epigeneticists argued that matter and form change qualitatively (not just quantitatively) in utero. In a time before genetics, preformationists had a certain advantage when trying to explain hereditary *continuity* and *species integrity* over generations, but epigeneticists had the upper hand when explaining *variation* over generations. Peter the Great was interested in this debate and seems to have engaged in some "monster breeding" as an attempt to figure out the underlying logic of

---

destroyed in all cases just so far as the orbits?" These and other such arguments refine Lawrence's belief that internal fusions might arise in utero, causing monsters like conjoined twins or parasite/autosite twins, but sudden external force does not appear to create monsters.

trait mixing. He arranged extremely short and tall people to procreate, and other permutations of anomalous traits to gain some understanding of heredity.

The whole issue of heredity was confused before Mendel's laws and twentieth-century molecular genetics, but by Darwin's time it was clear that procreation needed the predictability of preformed heredity patterns and the flexibility of parental trait mixing. To that end, Darwin tentatively offered a "pangenesis" theory (1868), suggesting that gemmules (hereditary particles) contain micro-patterns of our body parts, and these migrate from parents' bodies down to the parents' sex cells and then get transmitted to a substrate during conception. This creates a true composite of mother and father that includes the unique physiological characteristics of each.

Mutations and monsters offered an interesting, special case in the heredity debate. Preformationists held that the disfigurements of terata (monsters) were somehow contained in the germ itself, and only grew large through nutritive gestation. Darwin's friend (and later enemy) Richard Owen held a version of this view. Epigeneticists, on the other hand, argued that monsters could arise midway through the developmental process, due to external interference—too much heat or cold, for example. A perfectly normal germ could be corrupted in the course of epigenetic development, but there were law-like regularities to these teratologies, too. This view was forwarded by the French naturalists Étienne Geoffroy Saint-Hilaire (1772–1844) and his son Isidore Geoffroy (1805–1861). The younger Geoffroy, in particular, made monsters his life's work, penning the highly influential *Histoire générale et particulière des anomalies de l'organisation chez l'homme et les animaux* (1832).

When George Maw wrote his 1865 letter about the elephant-pig monster, Darwin's response came quickly—and it provides us with insight into late nineteenth-century embryology. Together with Richard Owen, Darwin had toured the many monsters of the Hunterian collection, but he was convinced, after reading the Geoffroys, that monsters were epigenetic glitches.† They were not "messages" or signs from the beyond, and they were not preformed in the germ. They were caused by environment. This environmental epigenetic view of monsters left open the question: did the mother's imagination absorb and translate some shock to the piglet (perhaps via pangenesis), or did common mechanical causes distort the fetus because of environmental flux? The answer is in the rarity or regularity of such occurrences. In his response to George Maw, Darwin doesn't rule out the imagination thesis entirely, but he refers to Isidore Geoffroy's work. Darwin writes, "The monstrosity of a proboscis-like prolongation of the snout occurs much more frequently as stated by Isidore Geoffroy than with any other animal; and therefore I presume is not rare." A pig trunk is, in fact, a common aberration and correlates with developmental patterns of craniofacial formation. Like the case where the prosencephalon fails to properly divide the orbits into two cavities and Cyclops anomalies occur, the pig trunk is a common teratology. Darwin says that he "must believe that the coincidence of the visit of the elephant and the birth of the monster was a simple accident."[14]

[14] *Darwin Correspondence Project. Dated June 4, 1865.*

Increasingly, monsters came to be seen as the result of pliable epigenetic causes, but the pliability was not like the radical folk version—maternal imagination cannot rearrange embryonic matter. Heredity theories like Darwin's pangenesis were toppled

† *In the 1830s, Darwin considered the possibility that monstrous birth might be a launching pad mechanism (a drastic variation) for the birth of new species. He abandoned this idea around 1838 in favor of natural selection and micro-mutations. Stephen Asma, "Darwin's Mutants" in* On Monsters: An Unnatural History of Our Worst Fears *(Oxford University Press, 2009).*

by the rise of molecular genetics, DNA, and the central dogma of biology—all of which coalesced into the neo-Darwinian synthesis. Genetics restored some of the preformationist thinking—in the sense that some terata are the result of "germ" mutations rather than environmental forces. And once we understood the directional path of genotype to phenotype, we had even less reason to believe that a mysterious communication system connects a mother's mind to her baby's body.

[15] *See Chapter One in Ronan O'Rahilly and Fabiola Muller,* Human Embryology and Teratology, *3rd ed. (Wiley-Liss, 2001).*

Teratology Today

Modern genetics helped us understand that some deformations are code glitches.[15] But surprising data in the 1940s and 1950s swung the pendulum back toward the external environment as a major cause of terata. A rubella epidemic in Australia was found, in the early 1940s, to be the major cause of a spike in congenital cataract. And the popular sedative thalidomide, used by pregnant women in the 1950s, was shown to cause major limb defects (hands arising directly from shoulders is a common result). These rather dramatic cases, mixed with new wisdom about the "environmental" influences of maternal diet and radiation exposure, resulted in a more pluralistic view of abnormality causation.[16]

[16] *K. S. Parthasarathy, "Heath Effects at Hiroshima, Nagasaki" in* The Hindu, *September 6, 2001.*

Contrary to popular mythology, there was not, according to the Radiation Effects Research Foundation (RERF), an increase in morphological birth defects among the children of Hiroshima and Nagasaki survivors—an outcome that one might expect based on the morphological mutations in mice and fruit flies due to radiation exposure. But there was indeed an increase in the mental retardation of children who were exposed to the explosions during weeks eight to fifteen of their development (neuronal propagation and cell migration in the cortex is most vigorous during weeks eight to fifteen), while incidences of mental retardation were at normal rates for children who were in earlier or later stages of development during the explosions.[17]

In the last fifty years we have accrued evidence that alcohol, lead, nicotine, thalidomide, X-rays, cocaine, dioxin ("agent orange"), and lithium, among other substances, all act as teratogens.[18] In addition, we understand that vitamin deficiency (and excess) can have teratogenic effects, and that most of these causal stories have to be contextualized in terms of *when* the fetus is exposed to the teratogens—timing is important. In addition to the "timing" issue of the Hiroshima exposures, we have significant data showing that temporal "windows" of vulnerability exist in embryogenesis. A critical exposure period in the thalidomide cases, for example, appears to be between post-ovulatory days twenty-one and thirty-six, when it seems that the drug blocks the formation of new blood vessels.

Our current scientific understanding of teratology is still in its infancy. Roughly speaking, we know that twenty-five percent of anomalous births are attributable to known genetic and chromosomal factors (e.g., fragile X syndrome, Huntington's disease, Down syndrome, cystic fibrosis, etc.), while ten percent are attributable to environmental factors (e.g., chemical teratogens, virus infections, radiation, etc.), leaving sixty-five percent to unknown causes. We now know that most malformed fetuses, ninety percent, are spontaneously aborted before birth (compared with only eighteen percent of phenotypically normal conceptuses). Those anomalous humans who survive to birth are calculated to be between two and seven percent of total human births.[17]

[17] Dioxin, or "agent orange," increases cases of limb deficiency and the incidence of conjoined twins.

[18] See Chapter Nine in Ronan O'Rahilly and Fabiola Muller, Human Embryology and Teratology, 3rd ed. *(Wiley-Liss, 2001).*

Folk Wisdom and the Maternal Environment

The folk belief in "imagination distortion" has persisted throughout the twentieth century. When my Chinese wife was pregnant with our son, I was regularly told (by my in-laws and other Chinese relatives) that I should keep my wife calm and away from disturbing imagery. This advice was offered by highly educated, urban professional Chinese, not uneducated rural villagers.[†]

In southern India pregnant women are cautioned against looking upon temple decorations of lion figures or disturbing deities. "If she does," ethnographer Edgar Thurston says, "the tradition is that she will give birth to a monster." And in a telling example that completes the circle of monster-to-collection-to-monster, Thurston writes, "some Hindus in Madras believe that it would be unlucky for a newly-married couple to visit the museum, as their offspring would be deformed as the result of the mother having gazed on the skeletons and stuffed animals."[19]

[19] *See Edgar Thurston's 1912* Omens and Superstitions of Southern India.

More recently, the *Ethnicity and Disability Fact Book*, updated regularly by the Multicultural Disability Advocacy Association of New South Wales, reminds us that many people around the world still believe that disabilities can be "caught" like a contagion by encountering other disabled people or frightening events. "The idea that disabilities can be caught is quite common across the world. This results mostly in actions to protect pregnant women from seeing, hearing or touching people with disability or even their technical aids." In addition, disabilities are frequently blamed on "perception negligence" of the mother. "In the Philippines," the *Fact Book* explains, "a woman gave birth to a baby who was unable to move his limbs. Her explanation of her son's disability was that she had worked in

† *The Chinese have a long tradition of monsters being produced by disturbing maternal perceptions and imaginings. For an interesting discussion of the relevant Qin Dynasty texts, see Chapter Two in Frank Dikotter, "Torments of Imagination" in* Imperfect Conceptions: Medical Knowledge, Birth Defects, and Eugenics in China *(Columbia University Press, 1998).*

view of a statue of a national hero during her pregnancy and must have caught the 'stiffness of the limbs'."[20]

[20] *Excerpts of the recent Fact Book can be found at the Multicultural Disability Advocacy Association website: http://www.mdaa.org.au*

In Ghana, women must not look at blood, or monkeys, or disturbing carvings. In Jamaica, mothers are advised against seeing a human or animal corpse. The same is advised by North American Indians, and Nigerian mothers are advised to make sure that no ugly people walk behind them. Sami mothers in Lapland are to avoid conversations about deformity as well as witnessing reindeer calving.[21]

[21] *This list was compiled at the website* Pregnancy and Childbirth Around the World.

All this superstition is easy to dismiss and we're tempted to write off the maternal impression thesis as retrograde magical thinking. But as usual, these folkways contain deeper truths. We will not, I suspect, find any mechanism that translates bad thoughts or disturbing perceptions into monstrous babies, but we now accept the more general mechanisms by which maternal stress negatively impact offspring.

Stressed mothers release high levels of cortisol and adrenaline into their systems. Ordinarily these hormones are useful for fight-or-flight adaptive responses to threats, but if their levels stay too high for too long, they can damage the mother's body and brain, and compromise the health of the child. Acute stress (like seeing something very disturbing) or chronic stress (like living in an unsafe environment) can bring unhealthy hormone levels into the baby's system. These changes can alter brain development and corrupt blood flow in the fetus, reducing oxygen levels and negatively impacting organ integrity. Moreover, a stressed mother tends to eat and sleep poorly and these are not optimal behaviors for the baby's health.

High stress in the mother can lead to shortened gestation and increased chance of miscarriage or premature birth. Stress during pregnancy also has measurable impact on the postpartum infant, the subsequent childhood stage, and eventually even the adult stage of the offspring. Problems with temperament, attention, emotional sensibility, intelligence, motor function, and mental illness have all been correlated with maternal stress.

Perhaps a little superstition about maternal imagination and monsters helped generations of mothers and babies stay healthier. As we enter a new kind of epigenetic paradigm, we may have even more reason to celebrate the paranoid preventions of prenatal monsterology. "Epigenetic" formerly meant embryological development from simple to complex structure (as opposed to preformation), but the term has a new meaning these days. "Epigenetic" has been resurrected by biologists recently to refer to the newly discovered layer of molecular triggers and switches that ride on top of our genetic code.

The new epigenetics is rendering the old distinction between nature and nurture obsolete. It is also revealing how the mother's prenatal uterine environment can "communicate" features of the outside world to the baby's epigenome (switching system) and set new default traits that may last for multiple generations. For example, recent data from the *Hongerwinter*, or Dutch famine of 1944, show an epigenetic switch for obesity. Longitudinal studies of the Dutch population have demonstrated that if a fetus was in its second or third trimester during the period in which the Nazis diverted food from the Netherlands to Germany, the fetus "learned" that the environment was extremely poor in nutritional resources and adapted in utero by calibrating its physiology to aggressively conserve incoming fat, sugar and other nutritional necessities. The fetuses that were developing in this hostile uterine environment of the "Hunger Winter" automatically reprogrammed to store every bit of incoming calories. The result, many years later, was a high degree of obesity in the adults who were epigenetically changed during their fetal experiences. Lab testing on rodents has isolated the actual

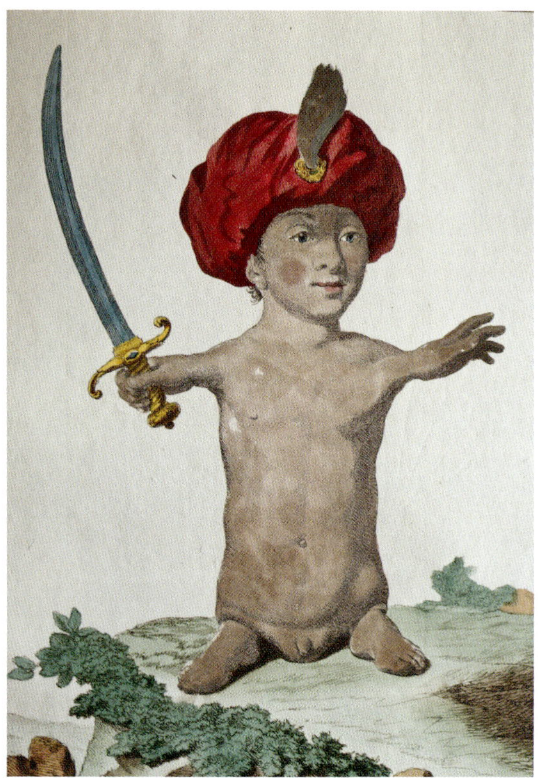

Image above: Jacques Louis Moreau (1771-1826). Description des principales monstruosités dans l'homme et dans les animaux précédée d'un discours sur la physiologie et la classification des monstres ... avec figures coloriées par N.F. Regnault... *Paris: Fournier, 1808. Courtesy of the New York Academy of Medicine Library.*

epigenetic switch for fat storage that can be turned on or off. [22] The point of this, for our purposes, is that maternal experience can have shaping influences (beyond genetics) on the gestating offspring—both short-term and long-term influences. The developing fetus is unrolling a genetic program, but it is also a very plastic and impressionable system—open to real time changes in the mother's experience.

None of this is meant to suggest that maternal imagination can distort embryos and fetuses in the traditional manner.

Science has not confirmed earlier magical thinking, and it won't. But it's interesting that we're more culturally sensitive than ever to the importance of "womb safety"—not only avoiding disturbances but also playing Mozart and Bach to the gravid belly. We're reminded that chemistry emerged slowly out of alchemy, and evolution theory arose out of natural theology. Maternal monsterology reveals a complex dialogue between folk obstetrics, teratology and medical embryology.

We've come a long way in understanding disability. For starters, we are all monsters. We are all deviations. Variation is the true norm. We must recognize that many women and differently-abled children were needlessly demonized and blamed in previous eras—and such tragedies are not past tense in parts of the developing world. Scientific progress, in this story at least, humanized us. To appreciate how far we've come, see Marc Quinn's wonderfully controversial sculpture, *Alison Lapper Pregnant* (2005), displayed on the Fourth Plinth of Trafalgar Square. A gigantic version was recreated and featured in the 2012 opening ceremony of the Paralympic Games in London. It shows a naked and very pregnant Alison Lapper, who was born with phocomelia (defined in Stedman's Medical Dictionary as a defective development of arms, legs or both, so that the hands and feet are attached close to the body, resembling the flippers of a seal). It portrays Lapper, a friend of the sculptor, as dignified—majestic almost, in tons of white marble—not to mention healthy and sexual. It's an arresting image.

Of course, we have a long way to go before the old stigmas of disability disappear altogether. Maybe they never will. Still, the imagination is a powerful faculty—however its mysterious mechanisms work—and if the imagination can make monsters, then maybe it can unmake them too.

[22] *David Crews, "Epigenetics and Its Implications for Behavioral Neuroendocrinology" in* Frontiers in Neuroendocrinology *29 (2008): 344-57 and Nessa Carey,* The Epigenetics Revolution: How Modern Biology Is Rewriting Our Understanding of Genetics, Disease, and Inheritance *(Columbia University Press, 2012).*

DEMONIC CHILDREN & THEIR CURIOUS ABSENCE IN THE EUROPEAN WITCH TRIALS

CAITLIN DOUGHTY

Son of a Demon

It is the year 1308 and Guichard, the Bishop of Troyes, has been arrested and imprisoned by the French court. The charges against him include sodomy, extortion, practicing harmful magic, and making a pact with the devil to murder the queen by inserting pins into a model of her body.[1] At Guichard's trial the next year, the first accusation against him is that he is the son of a male demon (an incubus), a charge confirmed by twenty-seven witnesses. The witnesses testify that Guichard's mother had been sterile for seven years before he was born and that his father refused to look at his child because he was, "the incubus' son."[2] Guichard is convicted, and will stay in prison for five years before being released in 1314.

Guichard was not alone in finding himself accused of practicing harmful magic; the details of his trial would be repeated again and again over the next three hundred years during the height of the witch trials. What makes Guichard's case so unique is the one accu-

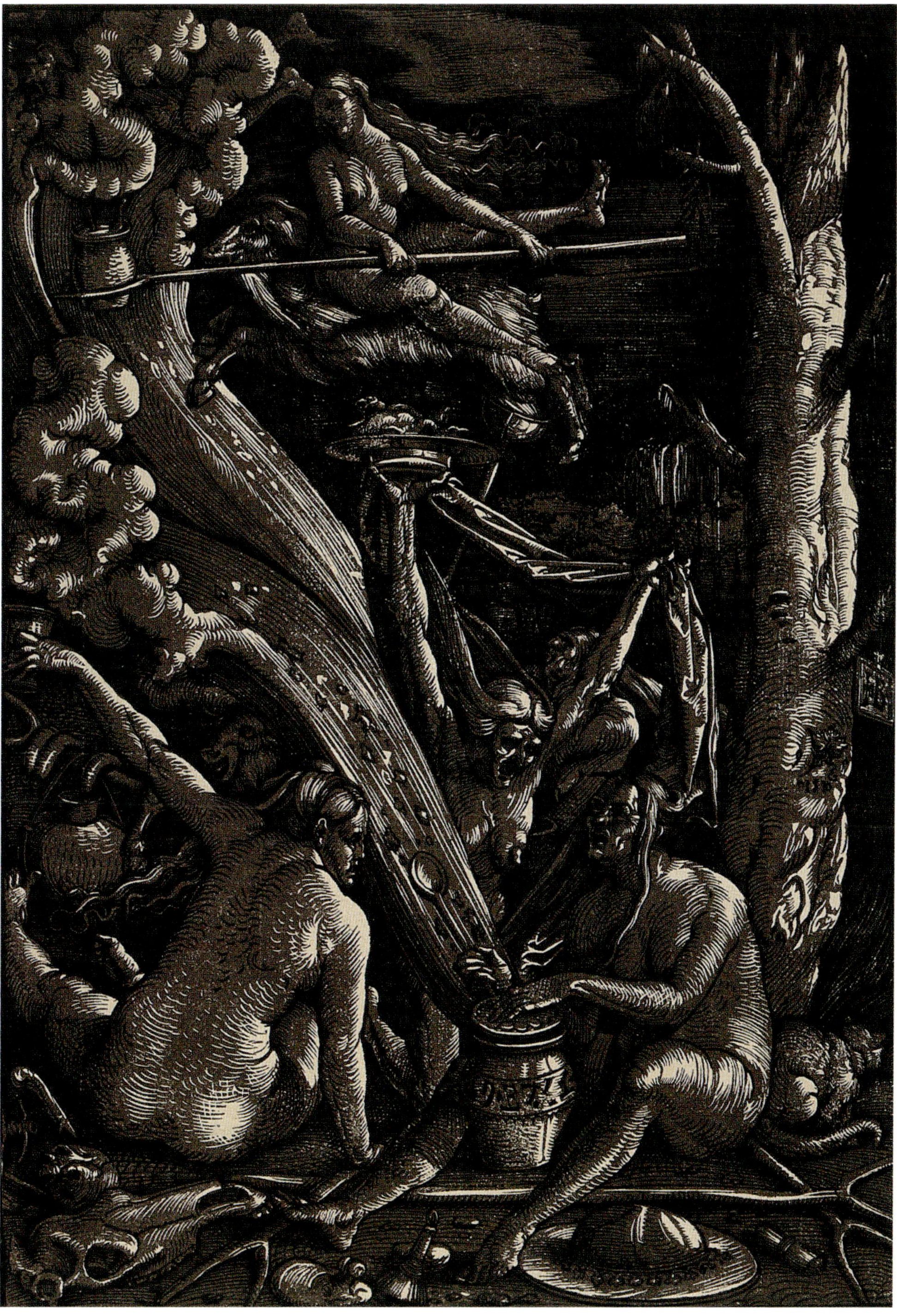

sation that Guichard could call his own—a demonic bloodline, the label "son of an incubus." Charges of harmful magic and sexual relations with incubi (a male sexual demon) and succubi (a female sexual demon) would be repeated *ad nauseum* in the trials of accused witches, but the charge that a baby was born of this unholy union with demonic forces would be *very* rare indeed.

The Late Medieval Witch Trials

There was a time in Europe's history when it was believed—by lawmakers, the church, and the people alike—that a conspiracy of witches lurked, secretly, within society. Historically, the definition of a witch in the late Middle Ages ranged from a healer to a evil outsider, but at the outset of the fifteenth century a new definition emerged: a witch was a human (usually a woman) who had made a sexual pact with the devil.[3] Since virtually all women were illiterate and unable to sign their names, sex was considered the alternative to an official signature on a document. The sexual pact allowed the woman to be the bearer of all manner of bad magic: killing crops, killing farm animals, killing infants, causing impotence in men, and causing droughts or inclement weather.

Manuals for rooting out witchcraft began to appear in increasing numbers after the decade of the 1430s, and roving inquisitors like German Dominican monk Heinrich Kramer, author of the *Malleus Maleficarum* or "Hammer of the Witches," went from town to town to help bring those in league with Satan to justice. In 1484, Pope Innocent VIII removed all limits on torture when it came to witchcraft, meaning inquisitors like Kramer were able to engage in sexual and physical torture to force the accused women to admit their fornication with the devil. If the women admitted their crimes, which they often

Image previous page: A naked witch flies to the sabbath mounted on a goat, while her companions continue to prepare their drugs. Photomechanical reproduction of a chiaroscuro woodcut by H. Baldung Grien, 1514. Courtesy of the Wellcome Library, London.

[1] *Robert E. Lerner,* The Heresy of the Free Spirit in the Later Middle Ages *(Berkeley: The University of California Press, 1972), 45.*

[2] *Norman Cohn,* Europe's Inner Demons *(New York: The Random House Group, 1975), 190.*

[3] *Lyndal Roper,* Witch Craze: Terror and Fantasy in Baroque Germany *(New Haven: Yale University Press, 2004), 153.*

did under severe torture, their immortal souls were saved, but their bodies burned at the stake.

The Demonic Babies of Early Christianity

The very possibility of demonic children comes from no less a source than the Bible. In Genesis 6, after men and women were created and began to multiply on earth, the "sons of God" took a fancy to the daughters born of these new human couples.[4] In the Middle Ages, these "sons of God" were usually interpreted not as mortal men, but as fallen angels, the same fallen angels that became the demons of hell. The passage goes on to say that not only did the fallen sons of God marry the daughters of men, but that the pairing gave rise to giant children, the Nephilim, the first human/demon hybrid.[5]

The possibility of literal interbreeding between demons and mortal women was not dismissed by the early church fathers, either. Augustine, considered by scholars in the Middle Ages to be the most authorative of the early church theologians,[6] argued in his *De Civitate Dei* for the existence of demons, which included all the gods of the Greek and Roman pantheon. Augustine also believed that humans had copulated and produced offspring with both the half-god Pan and the mythical sylvans,[7] which would both be used as prototype ideas of incubi and their demonic spawn.

The transition into the Middle Ages saw no shortage of demonic babies. Folklore and didactic literature gave the devil an entire family, including a grandmother, seven daughters representing the seven cardinal vices,[8] and wives who were once mortal women. There are also tales of the devil's sons—monstrous, giant children produced when the devil impregnated Jewish or otherwise "sinful" women. In the tenth century the monk Adso of Montier-en-Der wrote a treatise on

[4] *Gen. 6:4 (King James Version).*

[5] *Gen. 6:4. There are other references to giants in the Bible, including Og the King of Bashan and Goliath of Gath.*

[6] *Augustine is cited frequently in the work of Aquinas.*

[7] *St. Augustine of Hippo,* The City of God, *trans. Henry Bettenson (London: Penguin Books, 1984), sections 15, 23.*

[8] *The vices being pride, greed, lust, envy, gluttony, wrath, and sloth. Jeffery Burton Russell,* Lucifer: The Devil in the Middle Ages *(Ithaca: Cornell University Press, 1984), 77.*

the birth of the Antichrist, a man conceived and born in sin from copulation between the devil and a yet to be determined Jewish woman.

So the question becomes: if there were strong examples of demonic babies in the Bible and folklore, why wasn't a trial like Guichard's the rule instead of the very rare exception? In short—where were the demon babies?

The Transition to Demonic Artificial Insemination

The first possible answer to the disappearance of demonically inspired children may lie in simple sexual mechanics. *De Secretis Mulierum* [The Secrets of Women], written in the late thirteenth century, was a commentary on the intersection between women and science. It defined a man's nature as hot and dry. In contrast, it defined a woman's nature as cold and damp, causing her to desire intercourse at an alarming rate to create heat.† In order to counteract the effects of a woman's frigid womb, the semen of a man must be extremely warm.

Unfortunately, the devil's penis and semen were extremely cold. The confessions of accused witches undergoing torture described the devil's semen as not only as cold as his penis,[9] but "yellow, corrupt, and fetid."[10] Alternatively, Barbara Dameter, an accused witch who believed the devil was her husband until she realized she kept having intercourse with him when he was scheduled to be away, testified that the devil's penis was cold and hard, but there was no ejaculation or semen of any kind.[11] If the combination of hot and cold is a physical requirement for the conception of children, how could the frigidly cold devil create

[9] *Robert Muchembled,* A History of the Devil: From the Middle Ages to Present *(Cambridge: Polity Press, 2000), 66.*

[10] *Russell, 250.*

[11] *Roper, 94.*

† *In fact, "coitus is beneficial for women because they lose their superfluous cold and receive heat." Women's Secrets: A Translation of Pseudo-Albertus Magnus' De Secretis Mulierum with Commentaries, trans. Helen Rodnite Lemay (Albany: State University of New York Press, 1992), 70.*

the semen heat necessary to impregnate a human woman?

The answer provided by the great church theologian Thomas Aquinas was surprisingly simple. The devil did not need to create his own semen if there were still mortal men available to create it for him. In his *Summa Theologica*, Aquinas put forth that demons, using air and vapor, are able to create the body of a succubus (female demon) and steal semen during intercourse with a human male. The demon then transgenders itself into an incubus (again, a male demon) and deposits the semen into a human woman. Thus, the "child so begotten would not have the Devil for its father, but the man whose semen had been used,"[12] eliminating the possibility that a child would be born that was literally the offspring of Satan.

However, that did not mean that such a child would come into the world unscathed. Heinrich Kramer, mentioned above as the author of the infamous witch hunter's manual, 1484's *Malleus Maleficarum*, took Aquinas' theory of demonic parentage a step further by adding witchcraft to the equation. When Aquinas was writing in the late thirteenth century, he did not equate his theory of incubi and succubi with maleficium and witchcraft. Aquinas stated only that sex with a demon was mechanically possible, not that it would give those who had demonic sex special powers or a relationship with the devil.[13]

It was Kramer's contention that until the year 1400, demonic sex was involuntary. That is: incubi had been raping women against their will. It was only in 1400, approximately 84 years before the *Malleus* was written, that women stopped resisting demonic advances and gave in to their "insatiable wombs" and carnal desires to copulate with the devil willingly.[14] Kramer kept the mechanics of Aquinas' original theory, but added that although the devil could easily act invisibly to impregnate

[12] *St. Thomas Aquinas,* Summa Theologiae*, vol. 9,* Angels*, ed. Kenelm Foster (Cambridge: Blackfriars/ McGraw-Hill/ Eyre and Spottiswoode, 1968), 43.*

[13] *Cohn, 174.*

[14] *"Insatiable womb" from the text of the original Latin version of the* Malleus Maleficarum*. trans. Walter Stephens in* Demon Lovers: Witchcraft, Sex, and the Crisis of Faith *(Chicago: University of Chicago Press, 2003),54.*

unsuspecting human women, he chooses to make himself visible. That way the devil could rejoice in the sin of the willful, carnal action on the part of a woman. [15]

[15] *Heinrich Kramer and James Sprenger,* The Malleus Maleficarum, *trans. Montague Summers (New York: Dover Publishing, 1971), part 1 question 3.*

Protecting Deadbeat Fathers

In the late Middle Ages a culture of fear slowly emerged around the mere possibility of demonic conception. While both men and women were accused of the crime of *maleficium*, it is well documented that the witch hunts favored women by a large margin. Modern estimates put the percentages of accusations at eighty percent female, twenty percent male.[16] However, the people interrogating and bringing accused witches to trial were most *certainly* male. There is no doubt that the appearance of demonically sired children would have forced the twenty percent quite significantly higher, something the male leaders of the witch prosecutions would not allow to happen.

[16] *Laura Apps and Andrew Gow,* Male Witches in Early Modern Europe *(Manchester: Manchester University Press, 2003), 25-26.*

The simple fact is that a rise in accusations of demonic births would mean that men would be implicated as witches as well. As we know, Aquinas and church doctrine explained that demons would visit mortal men as succubi, and afterward visit mortal women in the form of incubi. Since Church doctrine allowed for the transfer of pilfered, mortal male sperm to a mortal woman via a demon, an uptick in births of children from the women accused of witchcraft would mean that the fathers of these children would have to be sought as well. If men were having relations with demons in the form of women, they would be making the same sexual pact as a woman, and thus would be equally bound to the witches' conspiracy and doomed to damnation.

Perhaps even more abhorrent to the men in charge of the witch trials was that with these demon-aided births, their very sense of self-preservation was at stake. Genesis 1:26 described the creation of man with God proclaiming, "let us make man

[17] *Gen. 1:26.*

in our image, in our likeness."[17] Children born courtesy of the devil and his minions would be the exact opposite, born not in the image of God or the child's father, but in the image of Satan himself. The men in charge of the witch trials considered themselves to be the "superior sex;" as such, they sought ways to secure themselves from blame for the crime of witchcraft and the demonic pact. This security extended to their children, living representations of themselves on earth.

Men emerged as the victims, not the perpetrators, of witchcraft. Men had to be vigilant to counteract the control women exerted over them through their sexual desires, for "through the wantonness of the flesh they have power over men."[18] Witchcraft was a female profession, and "real men" did not need it.[19] Ironically, demonological treatises from the likes of Nider, Bodin, Remy, Moliter, and even Kramer, all allowed for the possibility of male witches, and in many cases even use the masculine in describing acts of *maleficium*.[20] These same treatises allowed for the possibility of demonically inspired children. Yet men were accused far less often than women and accusations of demonic children were almost non-existent. Just because a book or treatise said it *could* happen doesn't mean the leaders of the witch prosecutions allowed it to happen in practice.

[18] Kramer and Sprenger, part 1 question 3.

[19] Apps & Gow, 128.

[20] Apps & Gow, 119.

The Right to Rites: Twisted Baptisms

Any person had free will to choose a life of witchcraft, turning away from God and giving themselves to the devil and sin. However, a baby born by the work of the devil would, "always be perverted by witchcraft."[21] Humans are given an option to accept or reject the grace of God. In Deuteronomy 30:19, God says, "I have set before you life and death, blessing and cursing: therefore choose life."[22] But in the case of a demon baby, the opportunity to commit its mortal soul to God would be taken

[21] Kramer and Sprenger, part 1 question 3.

[22] Deut 30:19.

away before it was even born. Presumably God would never allow a child to be born that was preordained to damnation, nor would he allow Satan to build up his army on Earth in such a fashion.

The late Medieval period saw a steady rise in baptisms simultaneous to the rise of the witch trials. Baptism was originally reserved only for certain seasons of the year and overseen by a Catholic bishop. By the fourteenth century it was done within eight days after birth by whomever was spiritually sound and available, most often the family's parish priest. Some theologians, Aquinas included, wanted so badly for each child to have a chance for salvation that if an expectant mother was near death he advocated Caesarian sections to extract unborn children from their womb before the children had the chance to die unbaptized.[23]

It was the commitment of the church and society to baptism that made the baptismal rites the perfect target for the devil and his legion of witches. As the image of the witches' sabbat began to take shape as a bacchanalian night gathering of dancing and carnal lust around a massive fire, an important component became parodying the traditional rites of baptism. If baptism was the public renunciation of Satan, the sabbat needed to be the opposite, the public worship and reception of Satan.

An accusation repeated frequently is that witches would take newborn babies (either their own or a stolen one) to their sabbats and after giving them to the devil, place them into a boiling pot to be stewed and eaten. In an excerpt from a fourteenth-century baptismal rite, the godparents of the child are told, "we charge you that you charge its mother and father to keep it from the fire," teaching it the laws of the church and the ways of Christ.[24] At the sabbat, the laws of Christ are turned into the laws of Satan, and the placing of the new soul into the water is replaced with placing it into the fire.

[23] *Aquinas,* Summa Theologica, *vol. 3, ed. James J. Cunningham (Cambridge: Blackfriars/ McGraw-Hill/ Eyre and Spottiswoode, 1968), 117.*

[24] *John Shinners, "Excerpts from the Sarum Rite of Baptism" in* Pastors and the Care of Souls in the Medieval England *(Notre Dame: University of Notre Dame Press, 1998), 163.*

Demonologist Johannes Nider quoted an accused witch in his 1480 *Formicarius* as saying that those at the witch's sabbat, "set our snares chiefly for unbaptized children... especially when they have not been protected by the sign of the cross and prayers."[25] While witches might set their sights on the unbaptized, many baptized babies (and baptized adults for that matter) were allegedly killed at the hands of witches, so baptism was certainly not foolproof protection against witches. All baptism could do is provide assurance that you would die a Christian with all the benefits of salvation. Your son could be killed at the hands of a witch as long as he would not grow up to be a witch himself.

[25] *Johannes Nider,* Formicarius, *trans. W. Stephens in* Demon Lovers, *241. The witches' description goes on to describe smothering the unbaptized children in their cribs, stewing the children until their flesh falls away from their bones, and making a soup that brings them both knowledge and power.*

Conclusion

It can be argued that there were so few allegations of demonic babies during the witch trials because there simply wasn't a need for them. Satan was gaining new members for his army of witches every day through the supposed cruel and overly sexual nature of women, so there was little need for the production of new witches through the birth of children. Much like a religion, converts were easy to find, and all the more welcome if they made the choice to defy God and join with the devil. However, this explanation is too easy, ignoring the prominent appearance of the phenomenon and its mechanics in witchcraft treatises and official church doctrine. All parties involved in the accusations and trials must have known that no matter how phantasmagoric the confessions of accused witches became, the birth of children already *infected* with witchcraft would overstep a fundamental boundary.

It has been suggested by some modern scholars, including Sigrid Brauner and Lyndal Roper, that during the period of the witchcraft persecutions the men and women who leveled accusations against suspected witches feared that the fertility of society was at stake.[26] Attacking the "fertility of society" consisted of imperiling all natural processes related to creation and birth, including the killing of newborn babies by midwives or mothers, the drying up of a new mother's breast milk, and the destruction of a year's crops. It would seem that the concept of a demon impregnating a human woman would be the most impressive attack on fertility possible, the corruption of the womb, the parental bond, and the process of childbirth itself. If the elite men of the late Medieval and Reformation refused to accuse or confess to such a monstrosity, then the concept, regardless of the fact that it was sanctioned by the Church, would remain a taboo impossibility.

[26] *See Sigrid Brauner,* Fearless Wives and Frightened Shrews *(Amherst: University of Massachusetts Press, 1995), and Lyndal Roper,* Witchcraze *New Haven: Yale University Press, 2004).*

ANATOMY *OR AN* OTTAMY?

Bodies on Show in Georgian London

SIMON CHAPLIN

"ANATOMY OR AN OTTAMY" SOUNDS LIKE THE START OF A TONGUE twister. The first is, of course, a familiar word: it is the one used to describe the study of the structure of the body, a practice that in the Western medical tradition was (and is) based on the dissection of the corpse. Indeed, the origin of the word lies in the Greek *ἀνατομία, to "cut up."*

But what (or who) is an "ottamy"? The simple answer is that "ottamy" (like anothomy, anothamie, anathomy, anatomie, anotomie, anotomy, notomy and atomy) is one of many variant spellings that were used in scholarly texts until the early eighteenth century and in common speech for at least another century and a half after that. For example, *The Questyonary of Cyrurgyens*, a translation of the work of the French surgeon Guy de Chauliac published in 1542, refers to the "science of *nathomy*." In 1561 the diarist Henry Machyn described seeing eighteen men and two women hanged in London (or rather, just outside London, in the village of Tyburn), one of which was "had" by the "barbur-surgens" to be "a notheme at ther Hall."[1] But Machyn's account hints at a further use of the word to describe not just the process of dissecting a body, but also the anatomized corpse itself. By the early eighteenth century, to be "ottamised" was not

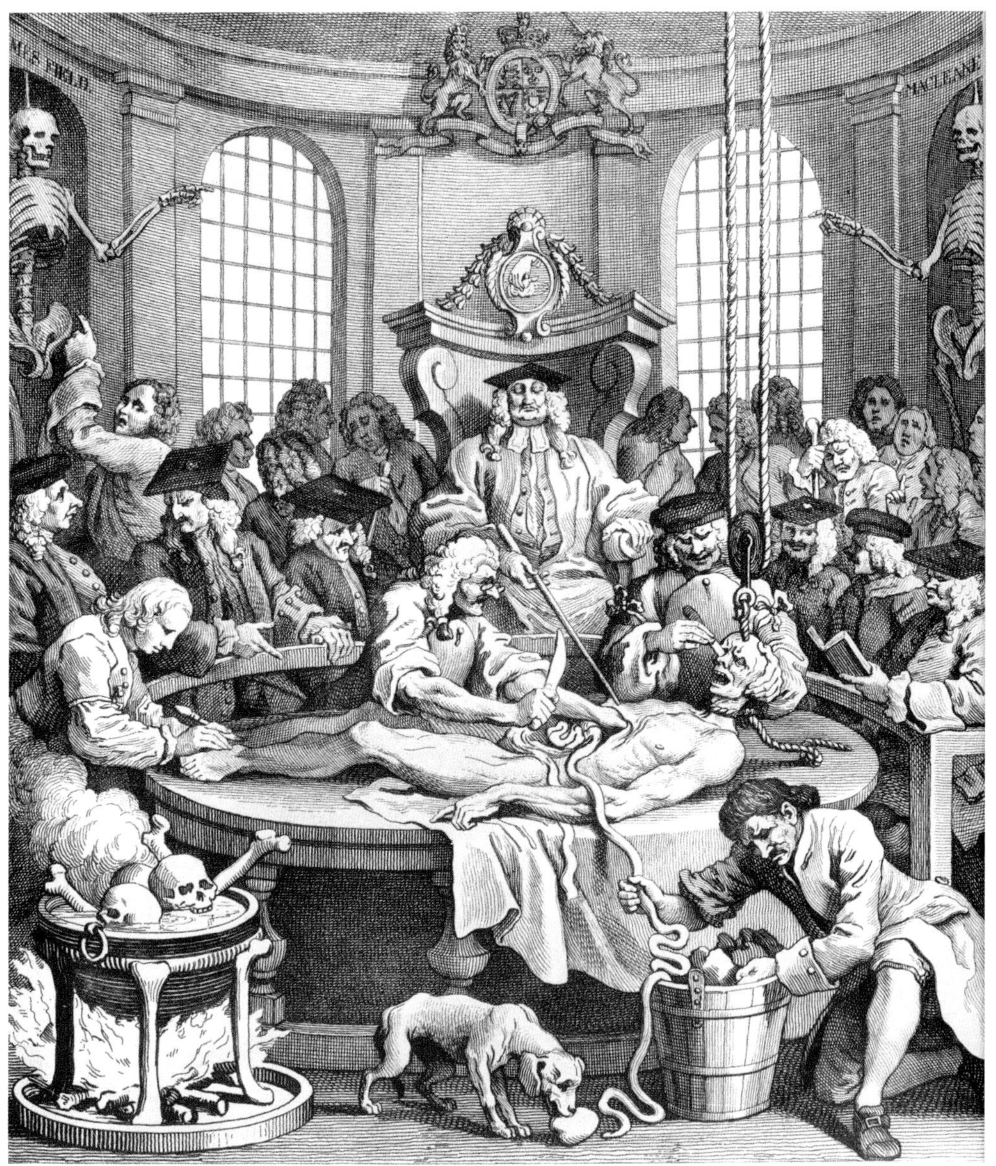

William Hogarth, The Reward of Cruelty, *1751. Published as Plate 4 of* The Four Stages of Cruelty. *The setting is a fictional composite, loosely based on the theater of the College of Physicians in London. Courtesy of the National Library of Medicine.*

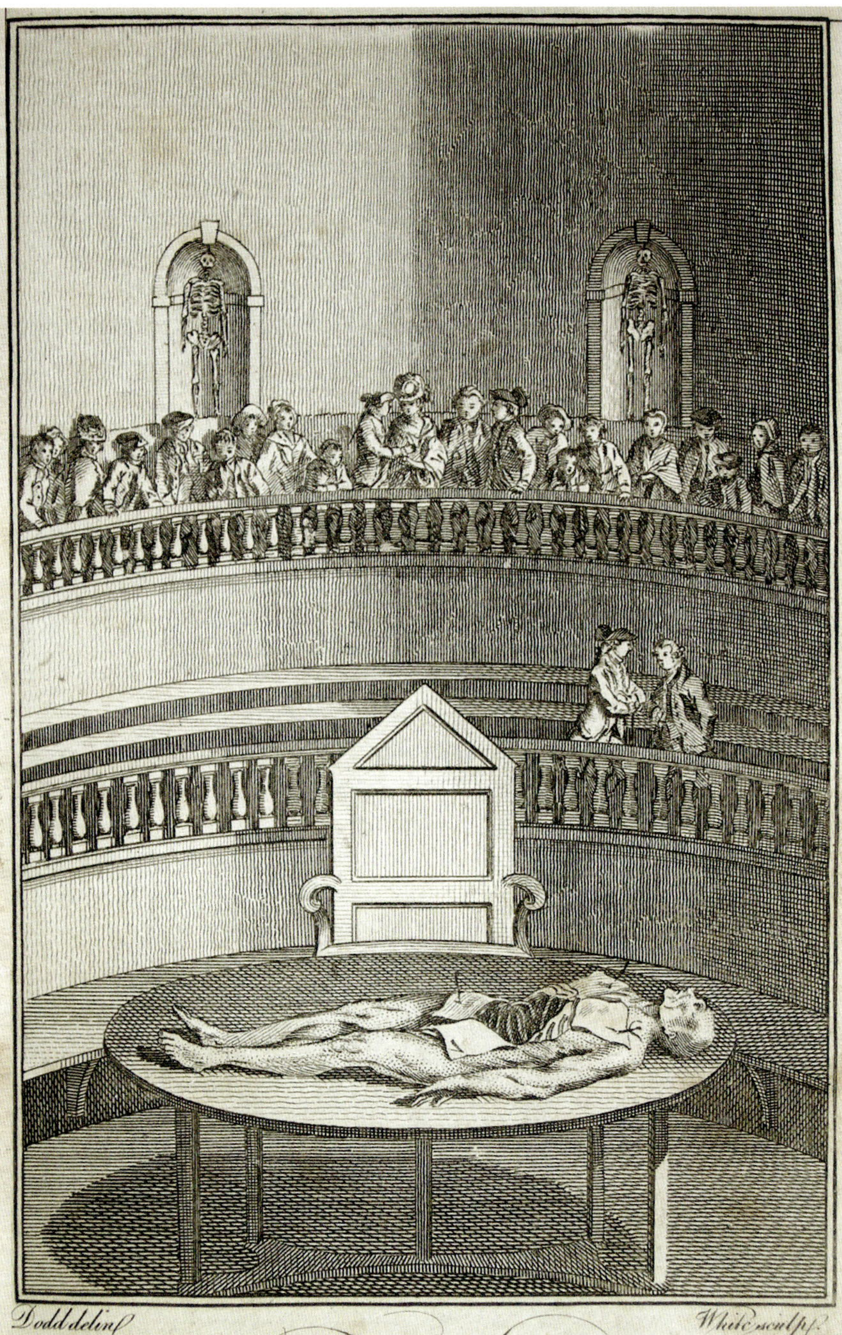

The Body of a **MURDERER** *exposed in the Theatre of the Surgeons Hall, Old Bailey &c.*

merely to be dissected, but to be preserved, most commonly as a skeleton, for further study and show. In John Gay's *Beggars Opera*—first performed at the Lincoln's Inn Theatre in January 1728, ironically on the site of what was to become the Royal College of Surgeons—this is what happens to "poor Tom," one of the robber-baron Macheath's gang. His erstwhile companion-in-crime "Matt of the Mint" recounts Tom's fate:

> Poor brother Tom had an accident this time twelve month [ago], and so clever a made fellow he was, that I could not save him from those flaying rascals the surgeons, and now, poor man, he is among the otamys at Surgeons' Hall.[2]

In Francis Grose's *Classical Dictionary of the Vulgar Tongue*, first published in 1785, to be 'ottomised' was translated as 'to be dissected': the phrase "You'll be scragged, ottomised and grin in a glass case" meant to be hanged, dissected and to have one's remains put on display.

The added fear attached to ending up as an ottamy was understandable. While dissection was itself a cruel and arbitrary fate for the condemned in the early eighteenth century, at least those bodies taken were—eventually—subjected to a Christian burial at the Barber-Surgeons' Company's expense. No such comfort was granted to those whose skeletons were preserved for display. Nor did the remains stay hidden from view, for as with the famous lecture theater in Leiden, London's Barber-Surgeons admitted visitors to see their collection. A tourist guide to London from 1708 describes at least five "ottamies," including the skeletons of Thomas Sherwood and Elizabeth Evans—"Country Tom and Canberry Bess," hanged for murder in 1635—as well as two flayed skins preserved "in imitation of Adam and Eve" (though presumably a fairly two-dimensional representation).[3]

[1] *Guy de Chauliac,* The Questyonary of Cyrurgyens, with the Formulary of Lytell Guydo in Cyrurgie *(London: Printed by Robert Wyer for H. Dabbe & R. Banckes, 1542), 252.*

[2] *John Gay,* The Beggar's Opera *(London: Printed for John Watts, 1728), 24.*

Image Left: The Body of a Murderer Exposed in the Theatre of the Surgeons Hall, Old Bailey, *ca. 1779. Courtesy of* The Royal *College of Surgeons of England.*

[3] *Edward Hatton,* A new view of London; or, an ample account of that city, in two volumes, or eight sections. *(London: printed for John Nicholson, and Robert Knaplock, 1708), 2:596-7.*

It was the fear of "ottamisation," of punitive dissection and the subsequent display of ones' remains as moral lessons to others, that helped to condition antipathy towards dissection among the London poor in the eighteenth century. Such opposition was not voiced quietly. As Peter Linebaugh has shown, at Tyburn in the 1730s and early 1740s the officers of the Barber-Surgeons' Company were sometimes fought to a stand-still by the crowd, and thus thwarted in their attempts to secure bodies. When Richard Tobin was hanged for theft in 1739, the Company was forced to pay for a posse of sheriff's men to fight off those who sought to rescue his body, although their efforts were in vain. Six years later, in 1745, at the execution of charmingly named Mary "Cut and Come Again" White, the Surgeons' officers were again beaten off by the friends of the condemned. Time and again the audit book of the Barber-Surgeons' Company reveals extra payments for men to stand guard both at the gallows and at the Hall.

The public tensions surrounding the Barber-Surgeons' Company were echoed by disputes within the corporation. In the same year that Mary White was hanged, the joint company split and a new Company of Surgeons was formed. For the next seven years no public dissections were held, and the public tension surrounding ottamisation abated somewhat. They were to re-emerge, however, in a different form in 1752. Prompted by a perceived rise in crime, and particularly by a spate of murders, a bill was raised in Parliament in 1751 to impose additional penalties on those guilty of that "most heinous crime." The Murder Act—or to give it its full title, An Act for Better Preventing the Horrid Crime of Murder—was passed the following year. It superseded the previous charters granted to the Company and the College of Physicians by making public dissection part of the judicial process. Henceforth murderers would, by default, be dissected by the surgeons, and their remains denied burial. For various reasons, not all of those convicted under the Act in either the London or the county of Middlesex between 1752 and 1832 were dissected, but a significant number did find their way to the new Surgeons' Hall at the Old Bailey (conveniently close to Newgate Prison). Between 1752 and the mid-1790s the bodies of at least eighty murderers were delivered to the surgeons to be dissected.[4] Sometimes lectures were given: these were aimed at apprentice surgeons, but many were also open to the public. Even when they were not, or when no lectures were given, the dissected bodies were ritually exposed to public spectators, in order to satisfy the terms of the Act.

[4] *Simon Chaplin,* John Hunter and 'Museum Oeconomy', *1750-1800 (PhD Thesis, University of London, 2009),* 343.

The decision to make dissection a specific punishment was not without its critics. The satirical *Drury Lane Journal* contained a scathing attack on Henry Fielding who was—with his brother and fellow magistrate John—perceived as one of the prime movers behind the Murder Act. Not content with merely dissecting murderers, the *Journal* proposed instead that:

> First, that one or more surgeons be appointed for every jail, to make ottomies of all the condemned bodies ...
>
> Two, that all malefactors, within two days after sentence of death is passed, be cut up alive in the prison yard ...
>
> Three, that while they are thus ottomising, they be tyed hand and foot... and their mouths gagged, to hinder their terrible shriekings and groans ...
>
> Four, that their flesh be roasted, boiled, broiled, fried, baked, stewed, hashed, scolloped, fricasseed, ragou'd, carbonado'd etc and at stated meals distributed to the prisoners ...
>
> Five, that their blood be made into black pudding ...[5]

[5] Have At You All: Or, The Drury Lane Journal. *London, 1752, 123.*

... and so on. Such penalties were, of course, to be applied only in the case of a first offense.

In fact—and in his defense—Henry Fielding appears to have been rather dismayed at the provision made in the Murder Act. Shortly after the act was passed he made his feelings known through the more mainstream *Covent Garden Journal*, bemoaning the fact that public execution and public dis-section were "horrid Farces": far better, he said, that such awful punishment be enacted in private, before the Court—something which he said "lily-livered" judges were keen to avoid, due to the "dis-agreeable nature" of such proceedings.[6]

[6] *Martin Battestin,* (Henry Fielding: A Life. *London: Routledge, 1989), 548.*

William Hogarth's famous prints showing the *Four Stages of Cruelty*, published the year before the Act was passed, prefigured Fielding's complaint. The final plate depicts the dissection of Tom Nero in a gruesome setting that served as an indictment of the heartless barbarity of public dissection as much as the consequences of Nero's criminality. Notably, Hogarth incorporated two ottamies or skeletons, topically named as those of highwayman James Maclaine and the boxer James Field, executed in 1750 and 1751 respectively.

Hogarth's fictional ottamies were soon replicated in fact. The first victim of the Murder Act, Thomas Wilford, was hanged on June 22, 1752. As well as paying for men to bring his body back to the Hall, and for mops and buckets for clearing up afterwards, the Company's account books include payments of one pound and five shillings for "stripping his bones," and a further two pounds and seven shillings to have the skeleton mounted for display in the Hall. Later the same year similar provision was made for the skeletons of William Descent and Randolph Branch, executed on September 22, and Abraham Ward, who was hanged and dissected in early December.

The Company of Surgeons continued to make "ottamies" of

particularly notorious criminals, and these became a significant public attraction at the Hall. Among them were the skeleton of Elizabeth Brownrigg who was hanged in 1767 after her conviction for the torture and murder of a serving girl (a trial that attracted widespread and lurid coverage in the press). Following her dissection the Public Advertiser reported that:

> ...the skeleton of Mrs Brownrigg will be fixed in the nitch opposite the front door in the Surgeons Theatre, and her name will be wrote under it, in order to perpetuate the heinousness of her cruelty in the minds of spectators.[7]

In 1777 an ottamy was made of the skeleton of Louis Mercier, also known as Louis Le Butte, and nine years later another from the bones of John Hogan. Not all of the skeletons preserved at the Hall appear to have stayed in situ. In August 1757 the minutes of the Court of Assistants noted, rather peevishly, that "the Clerk do write to Mr Moffatt [the surgeon James Moffat] to send back the bones of Mary Mussen which he took away without the leave of the Master." An écorché cast of Mussen's body was later displayed in Banjamin Rackstrow's anatomical museum and wax-works on Fleet Street. In December 1771 Asher Weil, Levi Weil, Hyam Lazarus and Solomon Porter were all hanged: Asher Weil's body was given to the Royal Academy, where the anatomist William Hunter used it to lecture to artists. The other three were dissected at Surgeons' Hall, but the skeleton of one later resurfaced in the museum of Joshua Brookes, a private anatomy teacher and museum proprietor, while the skeleton of William White, dissected in 1773, also found its way into private ownership (it ended up on public display in the museum of the surgeon John Heaviside).

[7] The Times, *September 16, 1767.*

While the dissections at Surgeons' Hall after 1752 were not entirely immune from the disorder that had attended dissections at the Barber-Surgeons' Company, for the most part the popular reaction to them was one of enthusiastic—if horrified—delight. Just as Londoners flocked to public executions, so too they thronged the Hall when dissected bodies were on display, and visited to see the ottamies when they were not. At Elizabeth Brownrigg's dissection was Sylas Neville, a young lawyer, who recorded the occasion in his diary:

[8] *Sylas Neville,* The Diary of Sylas Neville 1767–1788, *Ed. B. Cozens-Hardy (London: OUP, 1950), 25.*

> Wed. Sept. 16. After waiting an hour in the Lobby of Surgeons' Hall, got in with great difficulty, the crowd being great, to see the body of Mrs Brownrigg.[8]

In 1786, the dissection of John Hogan attracted even greater numbers of spectators:

> The crowds of the lower rank of people, who have attended for these three days past at Surgeons-hall, to see the body of Hogan, the mulatto, exposed, has made the Old Bailey almost impassable from eleven o'clock to two... .[9]

[9] The Times, *20 January 1786.*

It was the very appetite of the public for such scenes that made them problematic in the eyes of many critics. After Hogan's dissection the *Morning Chronicle* opined that:

> The exposing the bodies of murderers after their execution has not appeared to have the salutary effect expected by the Act of Parliament; but, from being frequently repeated, tends to harden the minds of the vulgar and familiarise them with spectacles of horror.[10]

[10] Morning Chronicle, *20 January 1786.*

Certainly the dissections at Surgeons' Hall did little to advance the cause of medical education. On October 4, 1759, John Taitt, Master of Anatomy at the Company of Surgeons in London, commenced a series of three public lectures over the body of the murderer Richard Lamb. He was under no illusions as to the nature and intention of his audience:

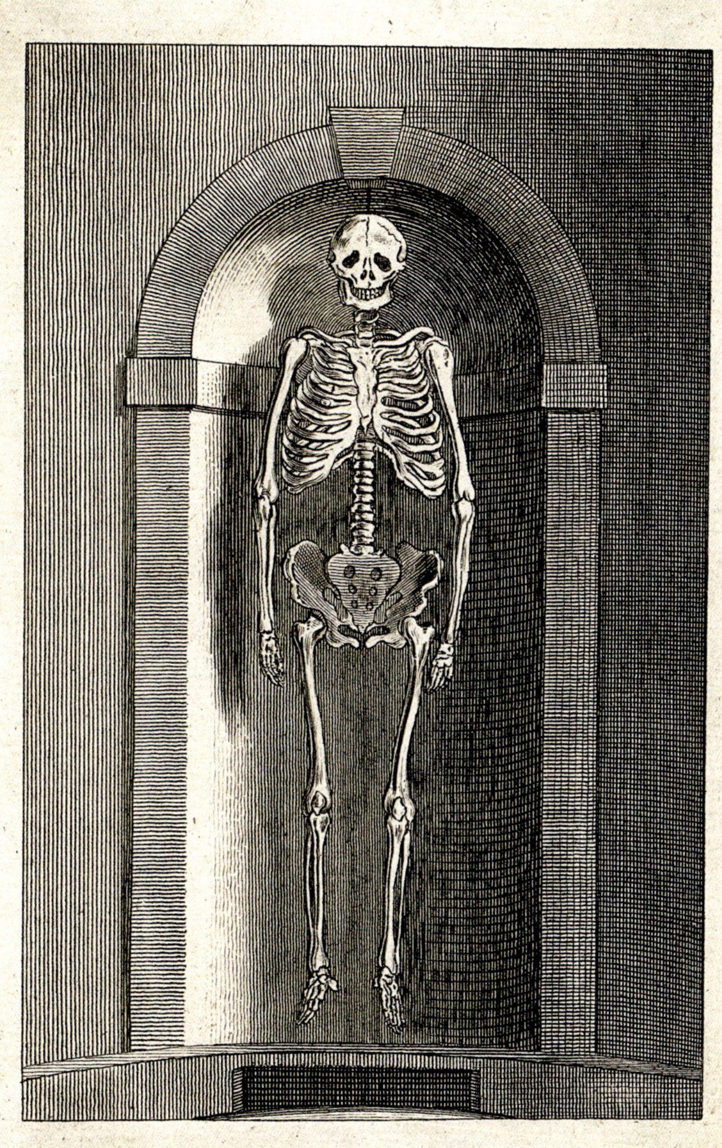

The Skeleton of Eliz[abeth] Brownrigg in Surgeon's Hall, *ca. 1779.*
Courtesy of the Wellcome Library, London.

My Wife riſen again! – thats one
Rib more than I wiſh'd to find –
What this! – arrah be easy my Dear
Devil burn me if it be not my own I know
it by the lump on the Skin here
Damn me Sir thats
– my Legg
Where's my Head
O what a smaſh among my Bottles &
Preparations! never did I suppoſe that
such a day would come
Reſtore to me my Virgin-boner did I keep it
inviolated 75 Years to have it cork'd
– up at laſt –
Prodigiouſly oblig'd to you
– Sweet Sir –
My Dear Madam I hope you are well
I am over-joy'd to see you
Lack-a-day! did nobody see an odd large Stomach
O what ſhall I do if I have left my Stomach
THE RESURRECTION
or an Internal View of the Museum in Wind-mill Street, on the laſt Day

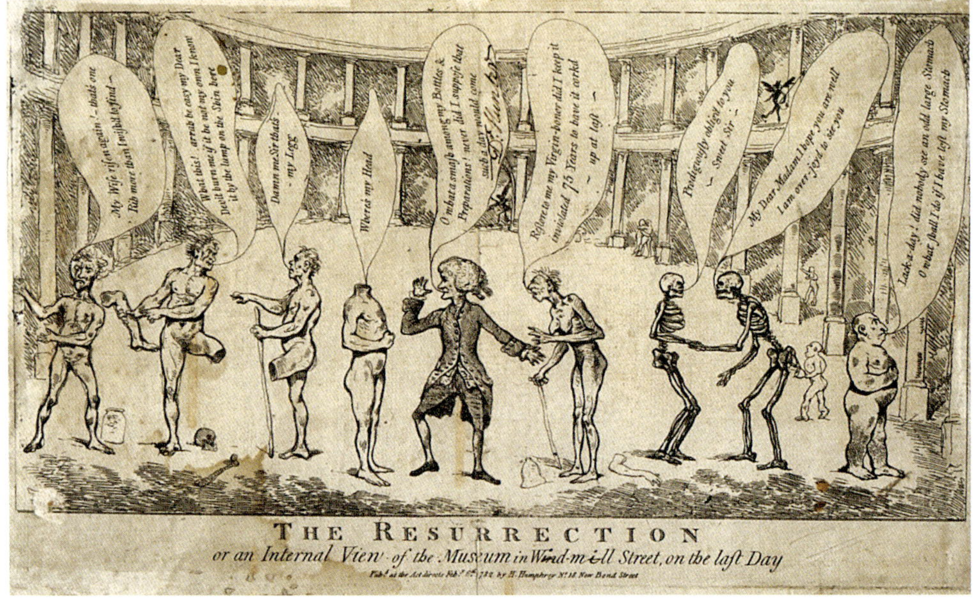

The Resurrection, or an Internal View of the Museum in W—d M—l Street, on the last Day, *published by H. Humphrey, 1782, engraving. Courtesy of the Wellcome Library, London.*

> Curiosity more than improvement has, I am persuaded, drawn the greater part of this audience together; and though such as come from mere curiosity will reap little benefit from the view of the dissected subject, yet that their time here may not wholly be thrown away, I would wish them to consider the crime which has occasioned their presence... . Let therefore the Anatomical Table in the Surgeons' Theatre be a preacher to all this audience: and should their passions run high, and the voice of reason and religion be forgotten, may this dread table present itself to their view... .[11]

The moral lessons of Taitt's ottamising made them less-than-essential viewing for those wishing to study anatomy for professional purposes.

The American medical student William Shippen Jr. (who was to become co-founder and inaugural professor of anatomy at the College of Philadelphia) was one of many who eschewed Taitt's lectures. Instead, he spent his time at work in the dissection room of William Hunter, one of London's leading private teachers of anatomy. Together with his brother John, William Hunter was one of sixty or so teachers of anatomy and surgery who worked in London between 1745 and 1800, and who made the city such a desirable destination for medical students. Unlike the public lectures at Surgeons' Hall these classes were conducted behind closed doors, with small groups of students participating directly in the dissection under a demonstrator's guidance—the direct forerunners to the classes still given in most medical schools today.

[11] *John Taitt,* Introductory Discourse to the Anatomical Lectures at Surgeons' Hall. [Bound with] The Ordinary of Newgate's Accounts for *1759 [copy at Guildhall Library, London]. London, 1759, 25-26.*

Unlike the Surgeons' Company, the private teachers could not claim the bodies of murderers. Instead they procured cadavers from other means, through collusion with grave-robbers or from hospital porters, workhouse attendants and others whose work gave access to the unclaimed corpses of paupers. Such a supply was not without problems: In 1788, Edward Howe, a messenger from the Westminster Dispensary, was arrested for trying to sell to John Hunter the body of Jedediah Thomas, who had died in an apothecary's shop in Grafton Street.[12] But while their approach to teaching anatomy differed from the Company, the private anatomists shared (and often exceeded) the Company's zeal for preserving and displaying the remains of those who had been dissected. Allied to the rise of the private anatomy schools of Georgian London was an unprecedented interest in the collecting and exhibition of preserved body parts.

[12] The Times, *14 November 1788.*

While the museums of William and John Hunter are the best known (they survive, in part, at the University of Glasgow and the Royal College of Surgeons in London respectively), similarly extensive collections were amassed by surgeons such as John Sheldon, Henry Watson, Joshua Brookes and John

Heaviside. With their ranks of jars holding preserved specimens, or skeletons and mummified bodies in glazed cases, these museums were undoubtedly important resources for teaching and research. They were also powerful tools for the public display of anatomical expertise in Georgian London. Many of them—including the museums of John Hunter, Joshua Brookes and John Heaviside—are known to have been open to the public as well as to medical guests. Joshua Brookes even provided a vivarium (an outdoor rock garden decorated with exotic animals) as an attraction to visitors, while Heaviside tempted spectators with offers of free tea and cakes. Nor was the use of preserved bodies to advertise anatomical expertise limited to those giving classes in dissection. The apothecary William Partridge was one of many who had ottamies on show in his shop. His possessions, revealed in the sale by auction of his property after his death, included "an adult skeleton, mounted, in a case" as well as the body of a child with the blood vessels injected.

While the function of such collections was to serve as exemplary medical indicators, they also excited the attention of spectators in ways similar to the skeletons at Surgeons' Hall. But if the "Dread Table" and its attendant ottamies were calculated to provide a moral warning to spectators, the remains on show in the museums of anatomy teachers, or the shops of apothecaries, appear not to have been so fearsome in their aspect. A cartoon of William Hunter in his museum, confronted on the day of resurrection by those whose remains he had placed on show, pokes fun at the idea that the retention of body parts for posthumous display was a threat to spiritual well being. One reason for this was that the preserved bodies in the private museums were not simply those of notorious criminals. In John Hunter's museum, for example, visitors could examine the preserved organs of bishops and aristocrats, politicians and actors, as well as the remains of executed felons and anonymous paupers. These virtuous ottamies were the products not only of dissections carried out for teaching, but of postmortems carried out to determine the cause of death, and conducted at the behest of (and sometimes in the presence of) the deceased's family or friends. This is not to suggest that the kind of ottamising being conducted by private teachers was beyond reproach, or universally approved of: There is of course plenty of evidence of surgeons conniving or deceiving or simply forcing next of kin to allow them to dissect their patients, and nor did the rise of consensual postmortems in any way diminish the continuing—and growing—reliance of London's anatomy teachers on the illicit supply of cadavers from burial grounds or institutions. But by displaying preserved bodies in a more overtly medical context, and by showing that dissection was not just an act of punishment, these museums helped to end the stigma of "ottamisation," and to create a common purpose to anatomical study.

By the late 1830s, the awful specter of the ottamy was starting to slip away into history. The journalist Pierce Egan, a connoisseur of London popular culture featured in "The Pilgrims of the Thames" (1838), included as a historical oddity a supposed letter from a condemned highwayman to his lover, Peg. In it, the luckless robber wrote:

> But you know the traps [officers] first nippered me, the beaks [Magistrates] then lumbered [imprisoned] poor Bob, the Big-Wigs [Judges] knocked him down [sentenced him to death], which rendered your fancy man of no use to you, Peggy, or any body else, and the nubbing chit [executioner] will finish the innings by changing poor Bob into a stiff 'un! But let me be put to bed decently, for you know, Peg, I never was a shabby or a mean fellow in my life; and, therefore, I

Image following page: John Howship, Interior of John Heaviside's Museum, *1814. Courtesy of Hunterian Museum at the Royal College of Surgeons.*

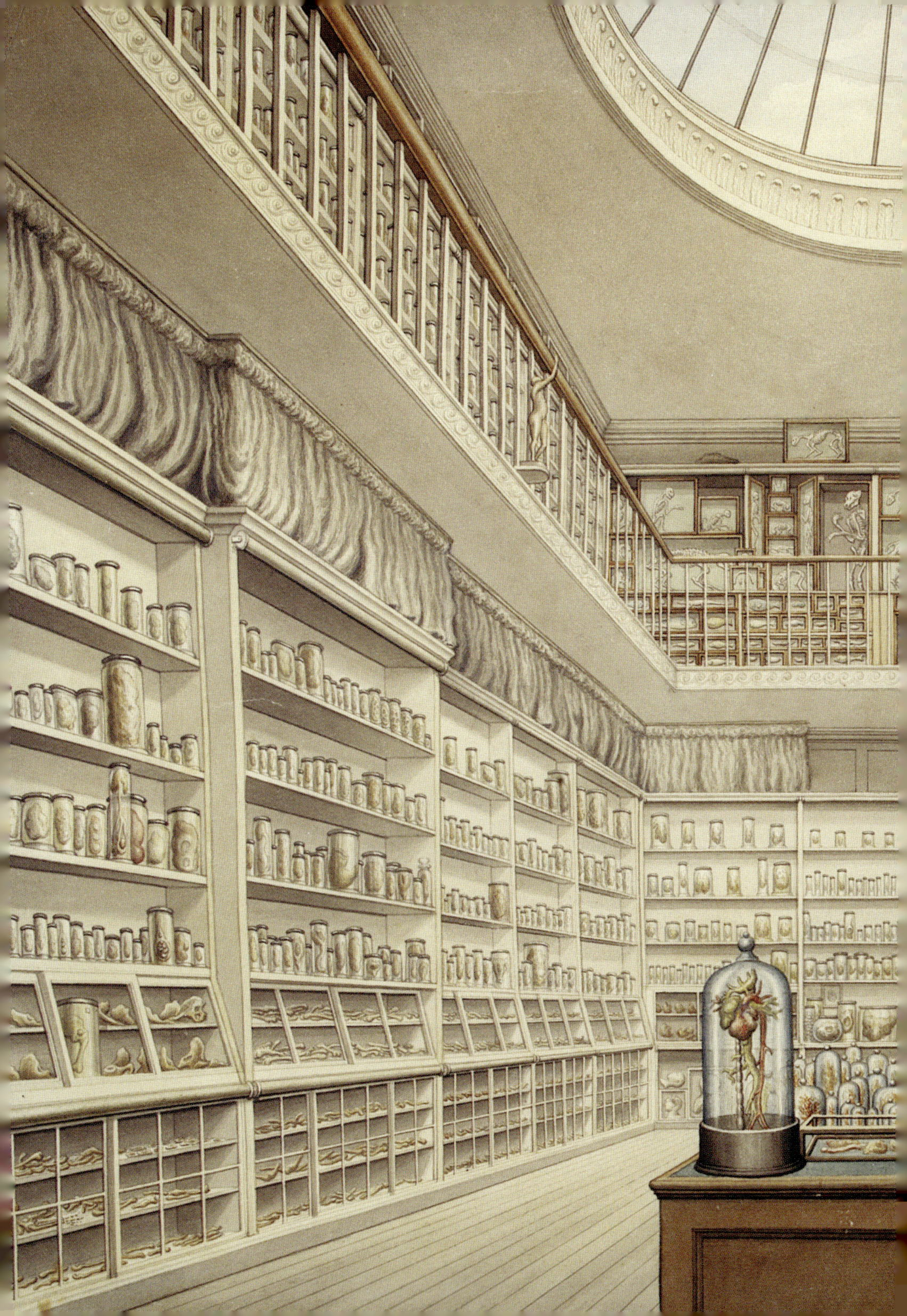

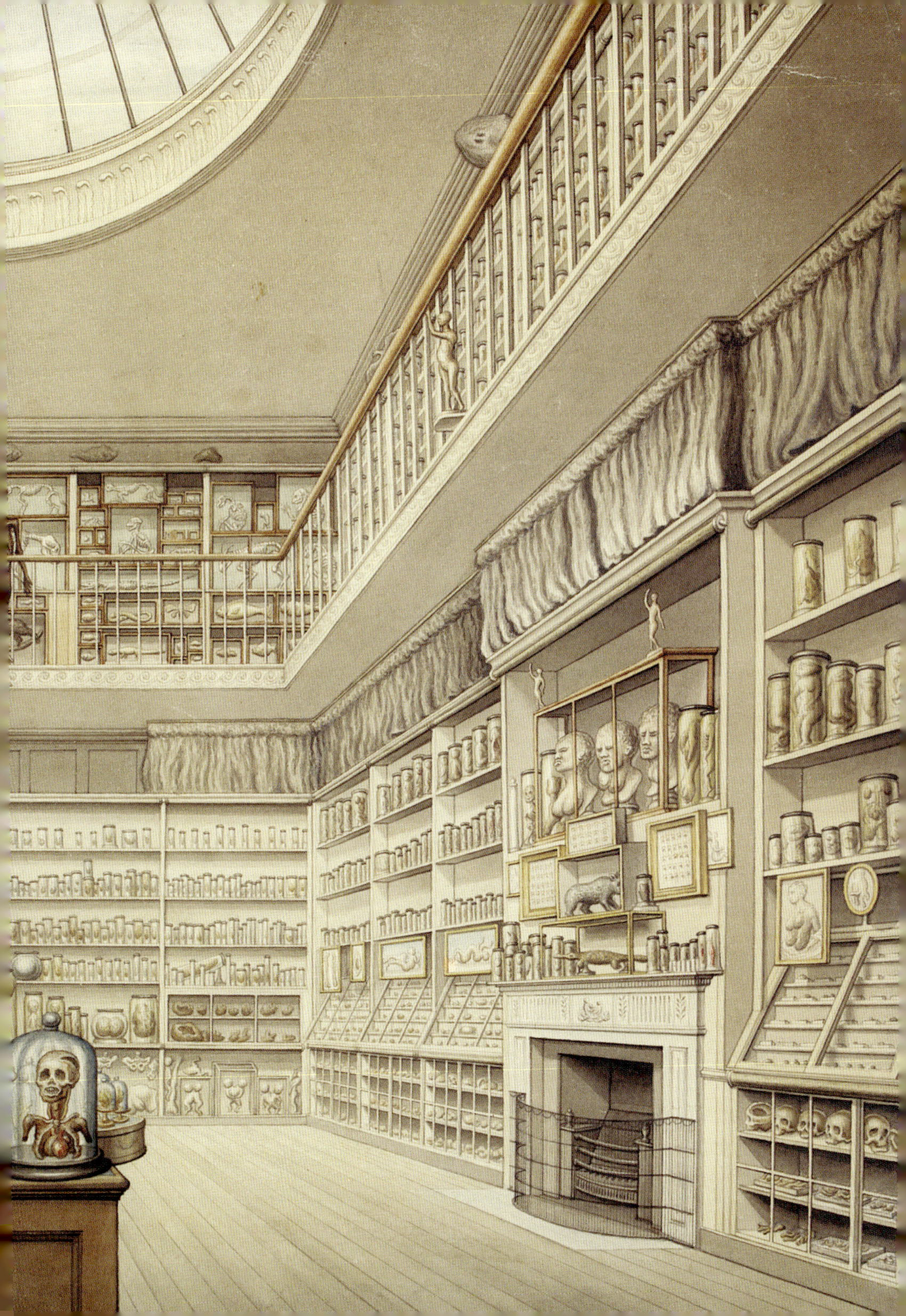

> should like the tie-up of Poor Bob to be nothing else but good. I am sure some of my old pals will watch in turns, throughout the darky [night], to prevent the body-snatchers from selling me for an Ottamy.[13]

In truth, judicial dissection and bodysnatching were no longer the pressing concerns they had been a hundred years before. The age of the ottamy was over: anatomy ruled supreme.

[13] *Pierce Egan,* The Pilgrims of the Thames, in Search of the National *(London: W. Strange, 1838), 123.*

STAGING SCIENCE *AT* WELLCOME COLLECTION

Anatomical Models in Context

KATE FORDE

IN 2009, WELLCOME COLLECTION STAGED AN EXHIBITION ENTITLED "Exquisite Bodies," inspired by the popular anatomical museums of nineteenth-century Europe. The exhibition was visited by over 50,000 people, and received national and international attention in the press. It was by no means unique in its focus on anatomy—in recent years Gunter von Hagen's *Body Worlds* and Roy Glover's *Bodies* have attracted millions to their exhibitions of plastinated cadavers and body parts, while ostensibly more academic exhibitions have set anatomical models and illustrations into a wider art historical context, aiming to elevate them beyond the status of mere medical curiosities.[1] What was unusual about Wellcome's exhibition was that it emphasized the contemporary *locations* within which objects including wax models, preserved specimens and anatomical illustrations were originally shown. By tracing the movement of such collections from the dissecting theater to the private museum to the fairground, the exhibition considered the range of associations and fantasies they originally inspired, examining their popularity (in some cases notoriety) and their ultimate demise. In this brief essay I

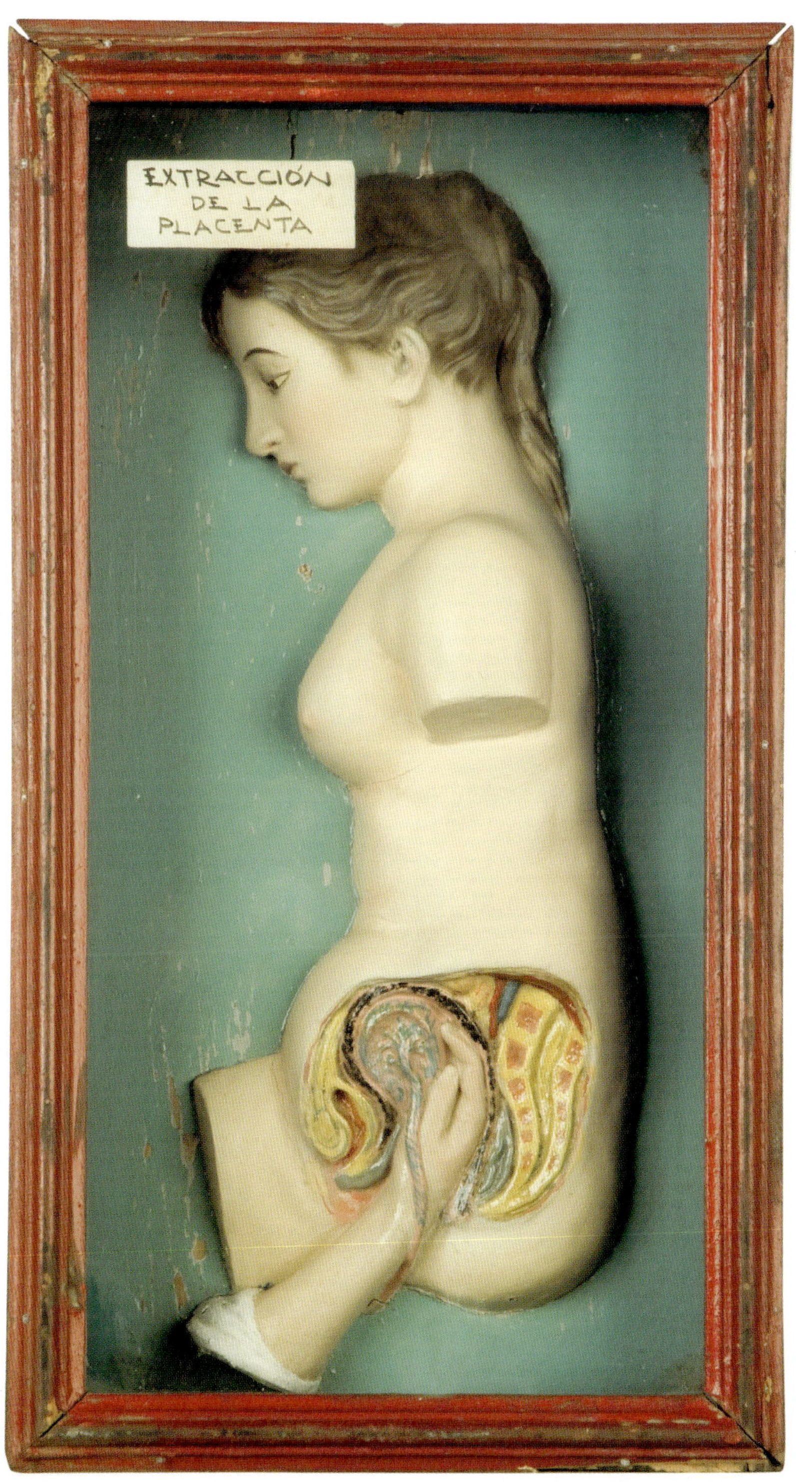
EXTRACCIÓN
DE LA
PLACENTA

will look at a selection of material included in the show, and say something about the meaning of displaying such objects within an institution dedicated to exploring medical science.

Wellcome Collection opened in 2007 as the public venue of the Wellcome Trust, one of the world's largest biomedical research charities. Describing its goal to provide "radical insights into the human condition," director Sir Mark Walport focused on Wellcome Collection's potential to forge "imaginative links between the disciplines of science, humanities and the arts."[2] This interdisciplinary approach was in part the legacy of Sir Henry Wellcome's own extraordinary collection. Begun with his discovery in childhood of a Neolithic stone arrowhead, Wellcome's passion for accumulating evidence of the past was enabled and shaped by his later success as a pharmaceutical magnate. Following the death of his business partner Silas Mainville Burroughs in 1895 until his own death forty years later, Wellcome developed a plan to create a "museum of man" that would illustrate all aspects of humankind's medical evolution and facilitate new forms of research and discovery. Thus was begun an endless project.

Traveling extensively himself and sending his agents across the world to gather source materials, Wellcome amassed a collection which was as remarkable in scale as it was breathtaking in variety. At one point numbering more objects than the Louvre, the now somewhat diminished collection ranges from a unique etching of Dr. Gachet by Vincent Van Gogh to hundreds of thousands of pharmaceutical jars; from ancient votive offerings to amputation saws, waxwork models, and medicine chests; and hundreds and thousands of rare books on subjects as diverse as witchcraft, alchemy and anthropology. It is this radical, eclectic, and somewhat unconventional approach to the history of medicine that informs Wellcome Collection's own approach

[1] *Two notable examples from the United Kingdom were "The Quick and the Dead: Artists and Anatomy" (1997), curated by Deanna Petherbridge and Ludmilla Jordanova, and Martin Kemp and Marina Wallace's* Spectacular Bodies: The Art and Science of the Human Body from Leonardo to Now *(2001), both produced by the Hayward Gallery.*

[2] *Mark Walport, "Open to Explorers of the Human Condition," (London: Wellcome Trust, 2007).*

to programming. To date it has presented exhibitions devoted to subjects like the relationship between war and medicine, the mysteries of sleep, the history of London's skeletons, and the role of mind-altering drugs in culture.

Image previous page: Extraction of the placenta: Plaster relief from a series illustrating the stages of childbirth, undated (c. 1900). Courtesy of the Collection Family Coolen, Antwerp.

The decision to develop the "Exquisite Bodies" exhibition was originally inspired by the miniature diagnostic dolls and "puzzle-boxes" in the form of pregnant women which feature prominently in Wellcome's collection of medical artifacts. Dating from the seventeenth century, most are fashioned from ivory and come from Germany (although the collection also includes examples from Asia). These objects raise interesting and apparently contradictory questions about the nature of scientific scrutiny—were they, as has been argued, teaching tools used by obstetricians and midwives to reassure pregnant women? Or, as in an example from China, were they used by women of affluent families to indicate where their symptoms lay, as they were forbidden to undergo physical examination? Or was the "medical" appearance of these objects ultimately of less importance than their status as toys or curiosities?

Their mysterious nature led me to consider the history of our relationships with surrogates, from life-size, eighteenth-century Italian Venuses molded in wax to the Surrealists' love of mannequins, to contemporary crash-test dummies and therapeutic diagnostics used in psychiatric therapy. I was intrigued by the ability of these objects to teach and to titillate, and by their sometimes startlingly life-like appearance. While I anticipated it would be virtually impossible to borrow the famous wax figures made by Clemente Susini which form the centerpiece of "La Specola" (at the Museo di Storia Naturale dell'Università di Firenze), Wellcome Collection does include a miniature version thought to be from the same workshop. Like her sisters, this model presents a rather idealized kind of human

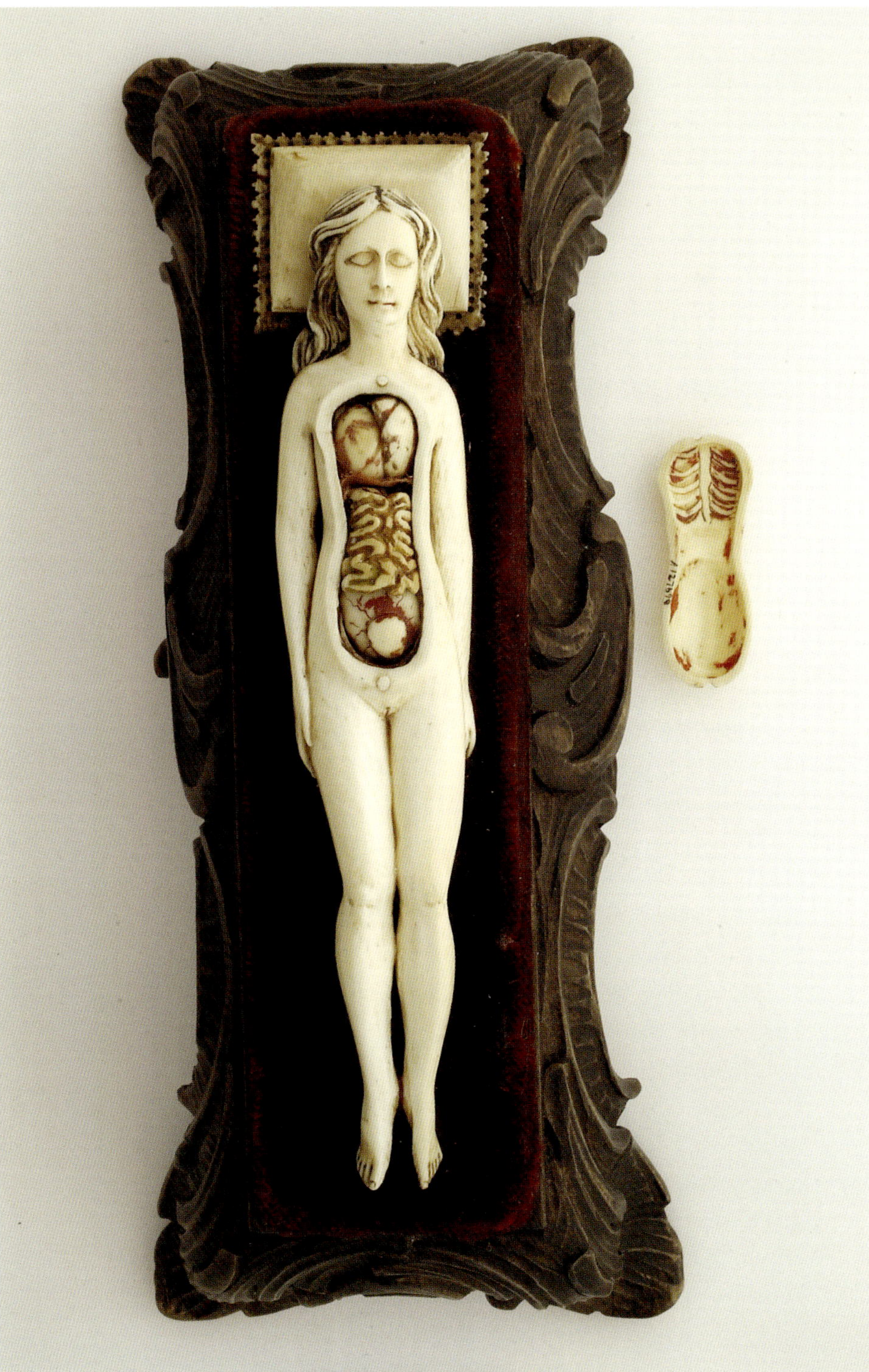

anatomy complete with real hair, sensuously parted lips and lambent skin; like them and despite her reduced size, several layers of dissection can be exposed by removing the wax parts, beginning with the superficial muscles and ending with the uterus wall—whereupon a fetus is exposed. It is obvious that this object owes as much to classical portraiture and religious iconography as it does to the dissecting theater, and that despite the graphic information it conveys, its erotic allure is at least a partial distraction from the disturbing physical reality of death. Displayed as an early highlight of the exhibition, it demonstrates that wax figures, for all their 'scientific truth,' could still communicate Christian-inflected ideas about the divine architecture of the body in a way that real bodies might not.

Image left: Seventeenth century dissectible ivory figure; Wellcome Collection / Science Museum. Courtesy of the Wellcome Library, London.

Ironically enough, it was a destroyed collection of anatomical waxworks which provided the rationale for the exhibition. An 1863 handbook for Dr. Joseph Kahn's Museum in the Wellcome Library advertised a collection of models showing the development of the human fetus, life-sized dissectible models of the "Apollo Belvedere" and "Venus de Medici" and numerous specimens illustrating the "diseases of imprudence."[3] To complement these displays, Kahn (a medically trained doctor from Alsace) gave lectures daily on a number of subjects, including diet, embryology and sexual health. From the research of Dr. Alan Bates in particular, I was intrigued to learn that Kahn's museum was just one of many anatomical museums that were vying for trade in London from the 1820s until the 1870s. These small museums generally charged a shilling entrance (a not insignificant sum), and were open to men—and, somewhat controversially, to women (though usually on separate days). Kahn's museum, located in Leicester Square, was one of the most famous, attracting two thousand visitors a week during the peak of its popularity, and initially attracting

[3] *W. Snell,* Handbook of Dr Kahn's Museum *(London, 1863).*

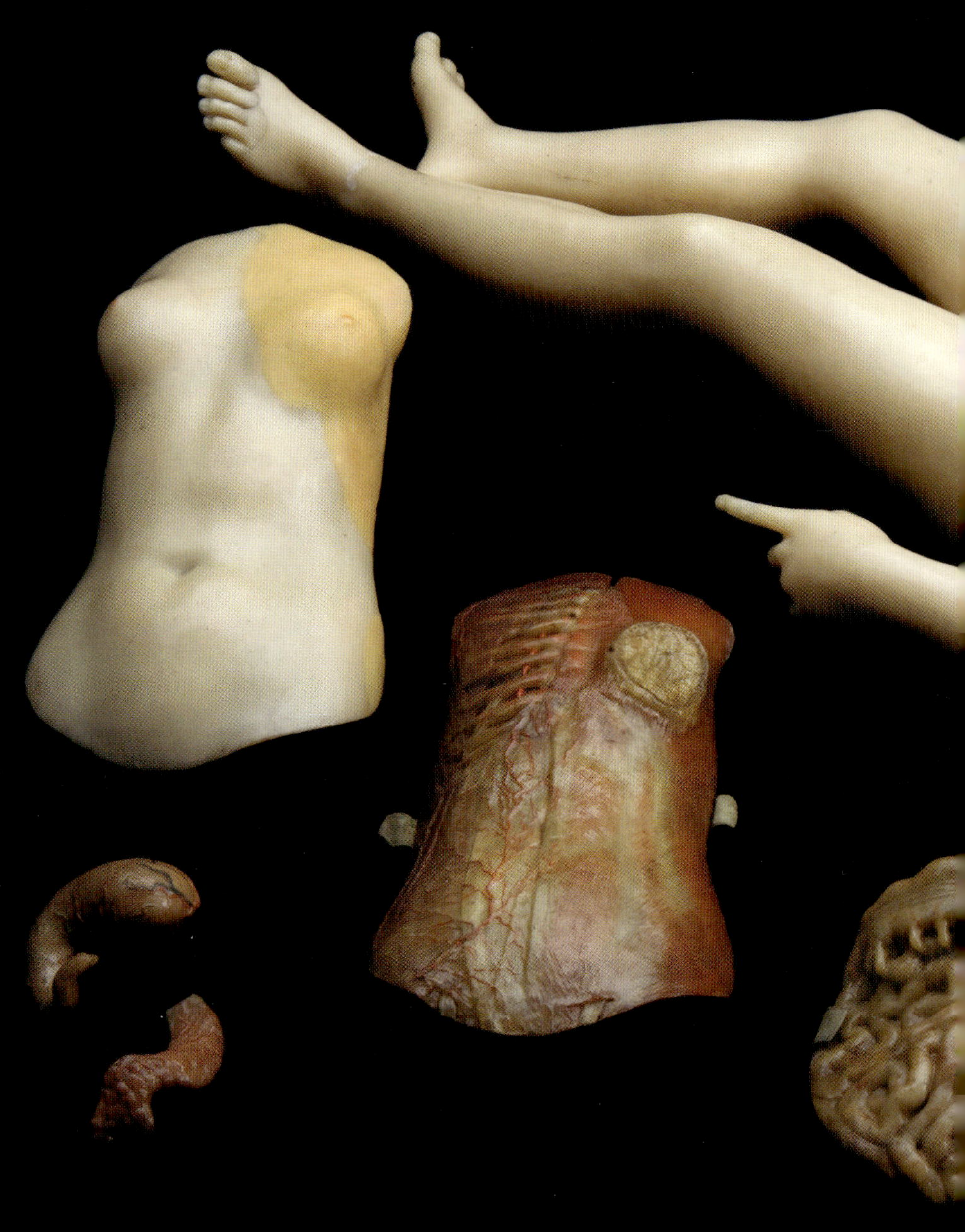

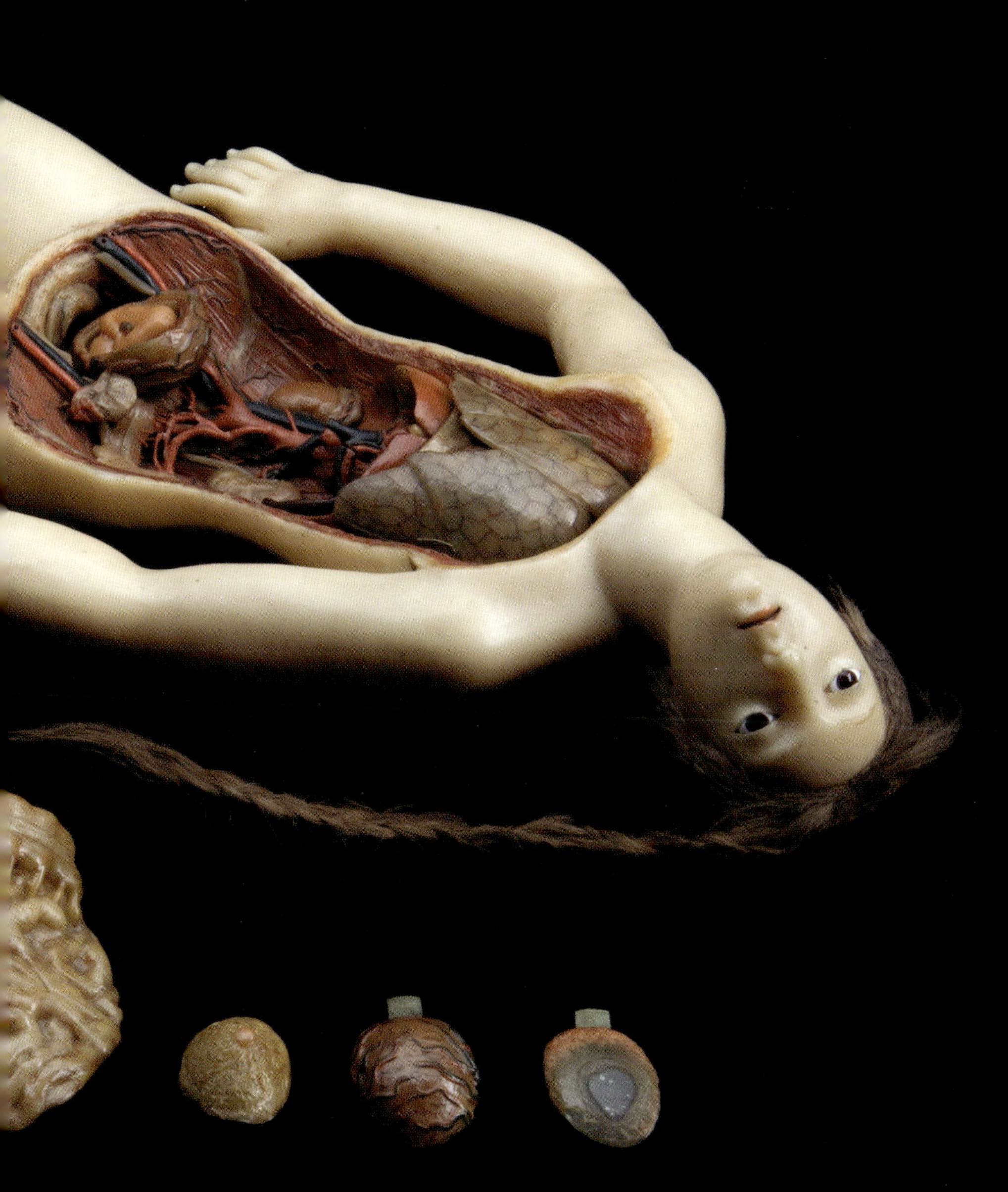

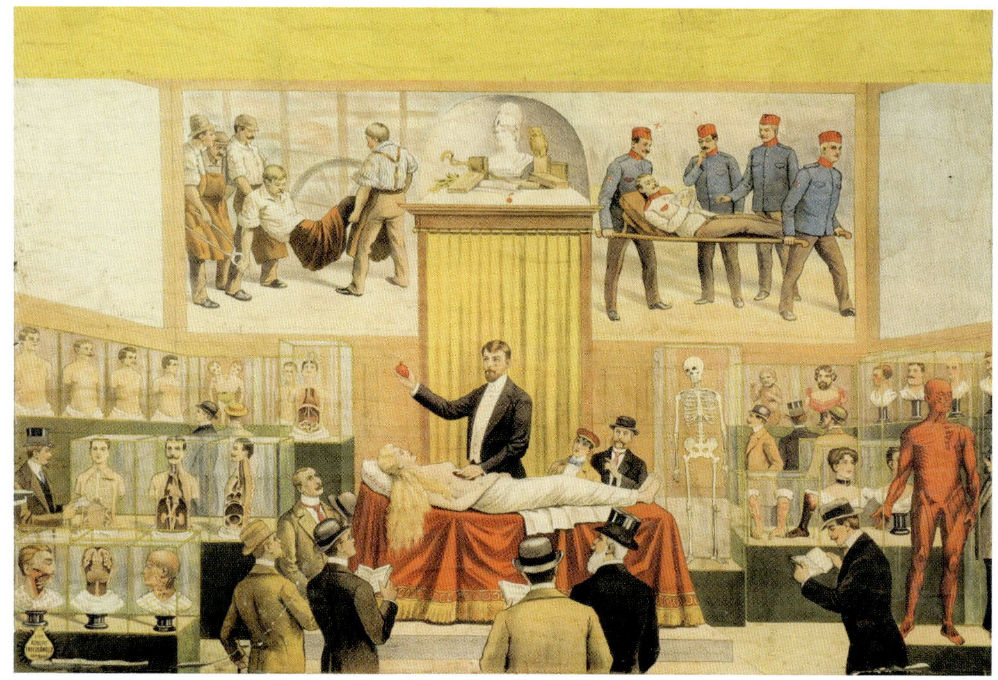

Above image: Poster from the Roca collection, circa 1900. Courtesy of the Collection Family Coolen, Antwerp.

positive reviews from the medical establishment. By the latter half of the nineteenth century, however, Kahn's museum had fallen into disrepute, and in 1873 his exhibits were prosecuted as "obscene publications" and were smashed to pieces by police officers from Her Majesty's Constabulary. On the face of it, Kahn's reputation was undermined by those concerned by his partnership with Perry and Co, producers of quack "cures" for venereal disease. Bates argues convincingly, however, that the increasing professionalization of doctors during this era led to the desire for a medical monopoly on anatomy and resulted in deliberate attempts to categorize it as knowledge from which laypeople could be excluded on moral grounds.[4]

Though dramatic, the rise and fall of Kahn's anatomical museum was not untypical. Across metropolitan Europe from

[4] *A. W. Bates, "Indecent and Demoralising Representations": Public Anatomy Museums in mid-Victorian England" in* Medical History *52 (2008): 1–22.*

the mid-nineteenth century, museums of anatomy achieved a brief but significant period of success. In London, Paris, Brussels and Barcelona, visitors seeking an unusual afternoon's diversion could visit displays that mixed serious science with spectacle, and used remarkable (sometimes hair-raising models) to convey information about the body's internal structure, its reproductive capacity, and its vulnerability to disease. In this way, those with relatively little means could gain access to knowledge that was formerly the privilege only of the nobility or to those studying medicine. At a time when there was concern over the practice of cadaver dissection, displays of artificial human surrogates seemed to offer a bloodless solution. Even doctors sometimes recommended these museums, acknowledging that they allowed students more extended study than was possible in the dissecting theater where specimens quickly decomposed. Ultimately, however, they were attacked by moral campaigners and those involved in the anti-quackery movement, and many were destroyed (including Kahn's collection). Those that survived fetched up in a new realm of entertainment: the fairground.

Image previous spread: Miniature wax "Anatomical Venus" attributed to the workshop of Clemente Susini and Francesco Calenzuoli Italy, 1776–1780. Wellcome Collection / Science Museum. Courtesy of the Wellcome Library, London.

Le Grand Musée de l'Homme was one such attraction and a regular feature at fairs in Brussels from the end of the nineteenth century to the late 1950s. During this period, the fair was seen as a place of education as well as entertainment. Here the facts of normal anatomy, serious operations, childbirth, vaccination and major epidemics were presented alongside traditional amusements. At a time when a large proportion of the population was illiterate, such fairground museums were an important way of communicating public health information, often about subjects that were considered taboo such as sexual reproduction and venereal disease. Graphic representations of disease were felt to be a powerful way to promote the message "prevention is better than cure"—particularly to young military recruits who were given reduced entrance to the museum. Some of the most disturbing models in the show came from this collection (on loan from la Musée de la Medicine in Brussels): a series of disembodied loins exhibiting the advanced stages of sexually transmitted diseases, including syphilis and gonorrhoea. Similar displays were to be found at Le Grand Musée Spitzner, probably the most famous anatomical collection of them all (and unfortunately not represented in the Wellcome show). From its founding in 1856 until a century later, Pierre Spitzner's museum toured France, Germany, Belgium, and Holland together with a team of doctors and nurses who interpreted the models and gave lectures on the various diseases they illustrated.

[5] *For more information about the Roca collection see Patrick Allegaert,* Kermis of Kennis: Wassen beelden uit de Roca-collectie / Circus or Science: Wax sculptures from the Roca Collection *(Ghent: Museum Dr Guislain, 2008).*

One of the best represented collections in the show was from the Museo Roca—a waxworks museum originally established in the heart of Barcelona's Barrio Chino (the city's Red Light district) around 1900.[5] Señor Roca was a successful fairground entrepreneur whose family had been touring attractions around Spain for decades. The "Parade of Monsters," as his enterprise was known, originally contained a mechanical wizard, a "house of murders," and a selection devoted to human oddities, alongside its embryological and anatomical models and jars of preserved human parts. This diversity indicates that the contents were originally amassed from several European collections, some of which were probably designed for medical teaching, for instance the models showing the positions of the child during delivery made by Jules Talrich, the official model maker for the Faculty of Medcine in Paris; others however were clearly intended for audiences better acquainted with visiting live freak shows.

Image right: Bearded lady Undated (c.1900). Courtesy of the Collection Family Coolen, Antwerp.

The location of the Roca Collection in an area where there was a great deal of prostitution and sex-oriented trade was by no means accidental. Several of the models were devoted to what were at the time termed the "social diseases," such as

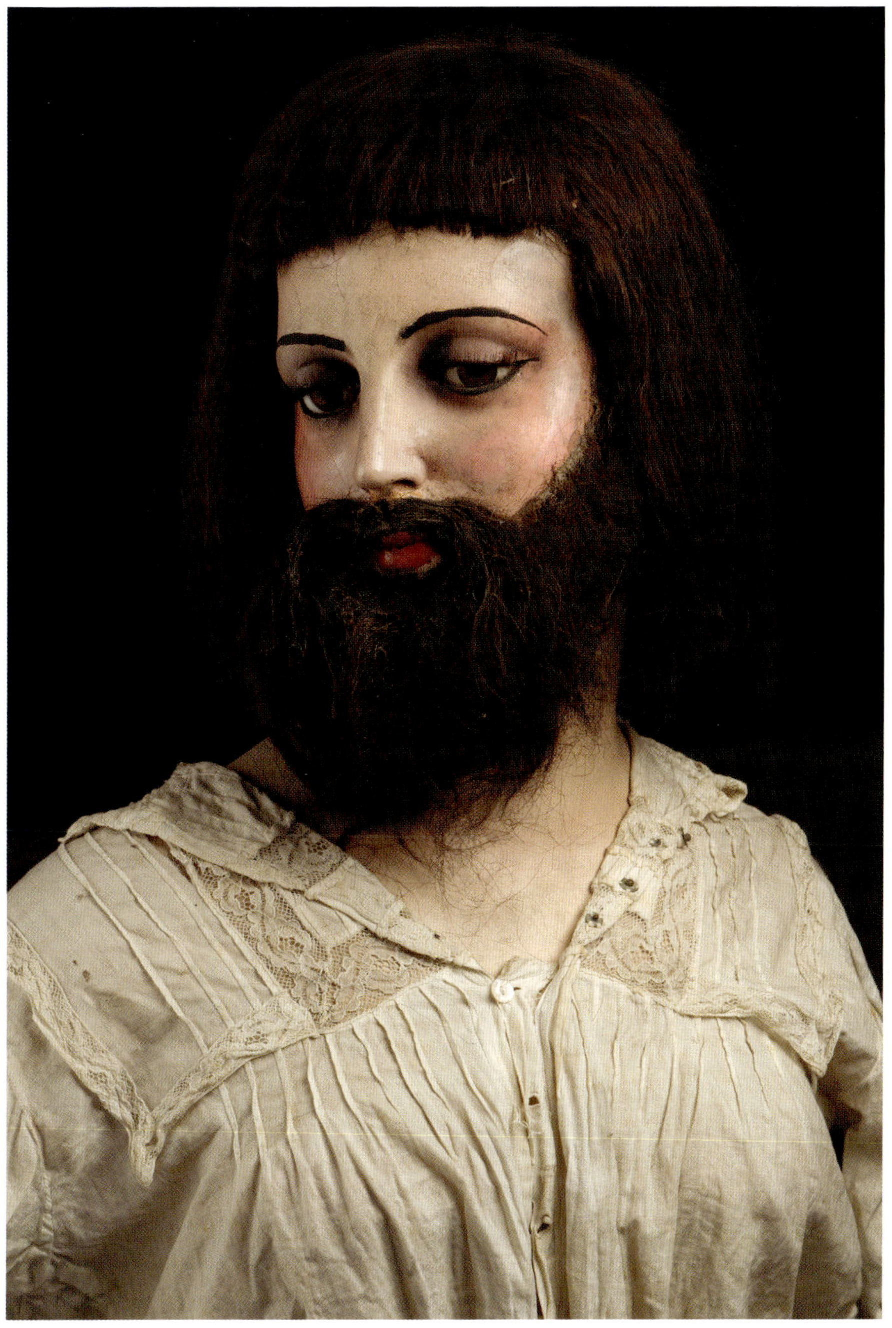

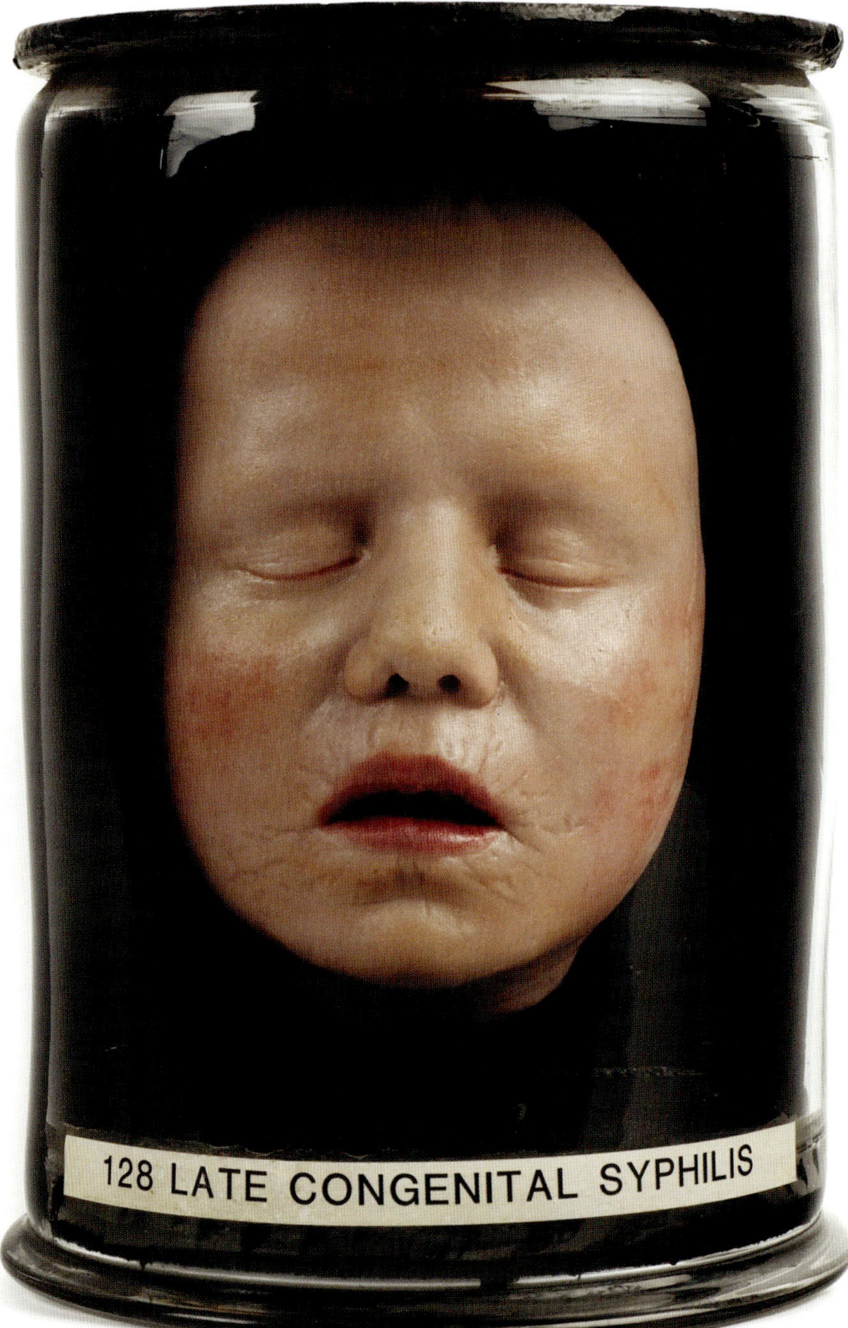
128 LATE CONGENITAL SYPHILIS

syphilis, tuberculosis, even leprosy, as well as alcoholism and drug addiction. These diseases were thought to originate in the poor and insalubrious districts of the city, and were usually stigmatized and regarded as punishment for degenerate behaviour. At a time when there were few effective cures, and public discussion of such matters was considered unacceptable, the Museo Roca's exhibits were on one level quite radical in that they helped to communicate information about the transfer and prevention of disease. As well as illustrating the impact of such infections, the Museo also provided information about the importance of personal hygiene and the need to live a moderate and balanced lifestyle. Intriguingly, the Museo Roca was for a while run under the auspices of the Red Cross, in a move that must have highlighted its pedagogical mission. Unfortunately this patronage failed to prevent the museum from having to close its doors to visitors in 1935, for reasons that remain unclear.

Image left: Wax model depicting the face of a child with late congenital syphilis, Joseph Towne London, c. 1827–79. Courtesy of the Gordon Museum, King's College, London.

One collection of anatomical models that have remained in their original context are the shockingly realistic waxes belonging to Guy's Hospital in the borough of Southwark in Central London. Made by British moulager Joseph Towne, these models, based on actual dissections, were made over a period of fifty years.[6] Towne was hired in 1826 when he was just nineteen years old, and by the time he died had made over one thousand works, several of which won him prizes at the Royal Society of Arts and at the Great Exhibition of 1851. Calling himself a sculptor, Towne was praised by scientists and artists alike who admired both the rate of his output and the "exquisite skill" with which he created unflinchingly realistic depictions of the dissection process and of pathological anatomy. Towne collaborated closely with the surgeons and physicians at the hospital whose cases he reproduced, but he evidently kept his working methods to himself—allegedly plugging the keyhole

[6] *Samuel J M M Alberti, "Wax Bodies: Art and Anatomy in Victorian Medical Museums" in* Museum History Journal *2, no. 1 (January 2009): 7–36.*

to his workshop with wax and hiding under a cloth while applying colour to the models. Unlike his Italian predecessors, Towne's waxworks did not present his audiences with an idealized version of the body. Instead, they remained uncannily faithful to the individual cadavers and patients they represented. Admired at the time for their "rigid regard for truth," his models became an important part of London's medical establishment: the dermatological examples in particular are still used today to illustrate lectures at the Gordon Museum in Guy's Hospital.

Naturally we can only speculate about the kind of reception anatomical models and museums received in past eras, our theories pieced together from surviving accounts of visitors and reinterpreted for twenty-first century purposes. Due to conservation requirements, the models shown in "Exquisite Bodies" were displayed behind glass and roped off, when originally they may have been handled, disassembled and smoked over. Nonetheless the exhibition did succeed in drawing attention to a singular chapter in medical history, one that is sometimes regarded as sensational and unworthy of serious attention. Indeed, the responses of contemporary visitors faced with these remarkable things clearly demonstrated their enduring power and ability to generate debate. On the one hand, the waxwork figures illustrate modern scientific interest in empirical knowledge, while on the other they reveal extremely complex attitudes towards reproduction, disease and death. It was frequently their three-dimensionality that both disturbed and delighted visitors, the opportunity for encounters with bodies and bits of bodies that seemed at once familiar and strange. It is interesting to consider that, despite our access to sophisticated x-ray technologies, something profound might have been lost in the gradual shift towards modern two-dimensional representations of the body.

Image right: Wax model of a dissection of the head of a baby showing full brain & dissection of the head of a baby with partially dissected brain Joseph Towne London, c. 1827–79. Courtesy of the Gordon Museum, King's College, London.

What then was the intention of displaying such material within a museum dedicated to medical science? Seeing these models through the prism of history was not an invitation to "commune" with ghosts, nor by implication a way to set up contemporary science as objective truth. Instead, "Exquisite Bodies" offered a chance to explore our predecessors' experiences of life, health, suffering and disease so that we might better understand our own.

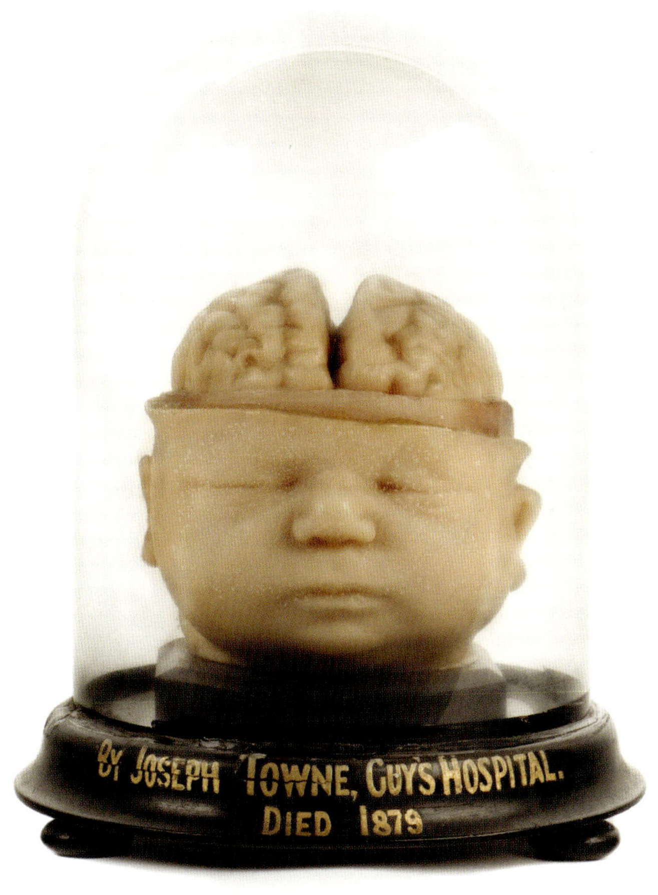

SOAP STORIES

The Mysterious Life & Dreadful Afterlife of the Mütter Museum's Adipocere Body

RICHARD FAULK

IN LIFE, SHE WAS CALLED ELLENBOGEN. BORN IN PHILADELPHIA sometime around 1730, much of her tenure among the living was caught up in the violent and uncertain spasms that midwifed our democracy. A citizen of the nation's capital before there was a nation, she might have stood among the sweaty patriots that gathered at the building now known as Independence Hall one July day to hear proclaimed for the first time the formal case for our separation from Great Britain. But probably not: Morbidly obese, Mrs. Ellenbogen lived a sedentary life. A recluse, perhaps, or an invalid, she might have observed from a darkened parlor or bedroom window, one other summer, the arrival of delegates, who were not yet known as the Founding Fathers, come to argue out a document that was not yet the Constitution. She survived her city's occupation by hostile forces of the crown and lived to see the thirteen colonies of her childhood emerge from their rebellion, improbably enough, victorious and unified. A venerable sixty-something when she finally succumbed to yellow fever, Mrs. Ellenbogen died toothless and decrepit in 1792, the same year that saw the advent of both the U.S. Postal Service and the New York Stock Exchange.

That is the meager biography that was passed down. No list of deeds, no known friends, not even an address. What Ellenbogen descendants might walk the earth today are unknown. Indeed, the only reason anyone still knows about this Mrs. Ellenbogen at all is for the celebrity she gained after her death: For 138 years, she has been one of the star attractions of Philadelphia's Mütter Museum, the United States' premier collection of medical oddities.

Having undergone a peculiar and spontaneous type of mummification, the body of the late Mrs. Ellenbogen looks like a statue crudely rendered in unfired clay. The color of lichen overgrowing misshapen knobs of raw-umber and sienna, her head is tilted back slightly and her mouth lolls open impossibly wide, toothless jaws frozen as if in a perpetual shriek at some horror visible only to her eyeless sockets. Gruesome as she is to look at, this prodigious corpse has nevertheless not withered or decayed in more than a century of display, and it is to her lumpy, yellow-waxy appearance that she owes her new name, the Soap Lady.

Since the 1940s, several rounds of increasingly rigorous forensic investigations have been conducted in hope of shedding more light on the life and the posthumous fate of the Soap Lady. What they unintentionally revealed are the corners that are sometimes cut in the headlong race for knowledge: The findings have overturned the entirety of Mrs. Ellenbogen's official biography. Everything, including her name.

The one thing we do know with complete certainty about the Body Formerly Known as Ellenbogen is the fact that most strains credibility: She really is a soap lady.

You're Not Being Soft Soaped

The misidentified Mrs. Ellenbogen is a remarkable example of *adipocere*, a phenomenon that connoisseurs of the bizarre have been documenting with morbid fascination for centuries. Descending to us through the delicate indirection of the French tongue, the term literally means "fat-wax." Some people prefer to use the straightforwardly English expressions "grave wax," or "corpse wax." But by whichever name you choose to call the phenomenon, there is a case of mistaken identity at work—for the substance in question is not wax at all: It is soap. Human soap.

Soap is nothing more than a special form of fat. (It's the salt of a fatty acid, for those of you keeping score.) In principle, soap making, or saponification (from *sapo,* the Latin for soap), is quite simple. Just take fat trimmings from your leftover steak, mix them with lye (in a ratio of about one part lye to five parts fat, by weight), and boil in water. Skim and collect the fatty goo that bubbles to the surface, and, when it cools, you will have soap—a very nasty, harsh soap, but soap nonetheless.

From the most rustic farm-caldron lye soap to the silkiest, cucumber-scented spa moisturizing bar, all soaps derive their cleansing property from the same peculiar molecular structure. One end of a soap molecule is hydrophilic—that is, it bonds readily to water—while the other end is hydrophobic, or repelled by water. When you lather up in the shower, the hydrophobic molecule tips bond with the oils on your skin. This greasy emulsion is then rinsed down the drain when water from the tap grabs on to the soap molecules by their hydrophilic end and carries the mess away.

Given the right environment, saponification can occur from beyond the grave. Modern forensic science has ascertained how: In the anaerobic environment of the tomb, heavily alkaline soil can react with the fat of an interred body. A catalytic jolt from enzymes provided by *Clostridia*, microbes that normally live inside our guts, helps the process along; a little extra moisture doesn't hurt, either, although there is generally sufficient water in a human body to do the trick. As the muscles of the decomposing corpse start to wither, the newly formed adipocere oozes into the nooks and crannies, where it solidifies. This led the early observers of soap corpses to mistakenly believe that the entire body had been transformed. Actually, the process is more like colonization, where the grave wax migrates into spaces that other tissue is retreating from. This incursion continues until the supply of corpse wax runs out. Accordingly, saponification occurs most thoroughly in obese individuals, who have more fuel, so to speak, to keep the chemical reaction going. Naturally gifted with generous fat reserves, babies and women are more prone to adipocere formation than men.

It was the French chemist Antoine François de Fourcroy who coined the term adipocere in 1791. He was also the first to advance the theory that the substance was soap and not wax. Which makes one wonder why he decided to call it "fat-wax" in the first place. Etymologically confused he may have been, but Monsieur de Fourcroy's chemical intuition was substantially correct—but this is not to say that every adipocere body is genuine soap.

Readers with a more technical bent might recognize that saponification consists of two distinct chemical processes: hydrolysis and hydrogenation. (If you are not technical minded, keep reading anyway: This gets cool in just a second, I promise.) In the first stage, water dissolves the chemical bonds in the fat molecules; and in the second, the so-called free fatty acids now bond with hydrogen and solidify. Only certain varieties of reconstituted fat will form genuine soap, however. If the requisite ingredients are out of whack (in the strictly scientific sense, of course) what you will have is not soap but a whole bunch of hydrogenated fat—aka trans-fat, aka human margarine, or Oreo filling minus the sugar. You can recognize a hydrogenated corpse by its creamy texture and rancid-ammoniac smell. The fat also aerosolizes readily, coating nearby surfaces in a grease film, just like bacon does during your Sunday brunch.

True adipocere, to the contrary, is brittle and flakey, and it has no odor. Since insects and microbes won't touch it, adipocere—and the fleshy tissue it encases—is also practically immune to decay. Saponified corpses can endure for centuries. In fact, the greatest danger to a soap-corpse is breakage from mishandling.

Grave Violations

Having cracked the code of adipocere formation, twentieth-century chemistry laid to rest the mystery of the Soap Lady. However, the riddle of "Mrs. Ellenbogen"—that is to say, who the Soap Lady was in the world of the living, and when and how she exited it—has proven a harder knot to unravel.

Something we do know with unimpeachable confidence is that the Soap Lady first emerges in the year 1875—remarkably enough in the company of a Soap Man, and in the possession of one Dr. Joseph Leidy of Philadelphia. It is Dr. Leidy who acquired and then divided the soap couple—donating the woman to the Mütter Museum and the man to the University of Pennsylvania (which later handed him over to the Smithsonian, where he remains to this day, off display and in a special protected environment). It is Leidy too who provided the original biography of "Mrs. Ellenbogen."

Professor of natural history at Swarthmore College, distinguished professor of anatomy at the University of Philadelphia, and chair of the Board of Curators of the city's Academy of Natural Sciences for forty-four years, Dr. Leidy was a formidable figure in early American intellectual circles and precisely the sort of person you'd expect to have a saponified cadaver or two on hand.

Dr. Leidy was the quintessential natural philosopher: a man of keen observation, inexhaustible energy, and boundless capacity for facts, but with no patience for theorizing and utter indifference toward the growing fad for clinical experimentation. For him, the call of the scientist was to observe and record nature's boundless plenitude—which he did in countless medical illustrations of striking detail and precision. Counter to type, however, Dr. Leidy was also so gentle in manner and generous of spirit that, even in the notoriously prickly world of scientific publishing, he was regarded universally with affection.

Despite his celebrity, Dr. Leidy was already something of an anachronism, scion of the dying breed of polymath naturalists. Biographer Leonard Warren elegiacally dubbed him the last man who knew everything—and that is almost not an exaggeration. Leidy gave up a medical practice to study dinosaur fossils and other New World novelties, and he was one of the founders of American vertebrate paleontology. He named hundreds of species of plant, animal, and fungus. He was the first to identify canine heartworm and the nematode in raw pork that causes trichinosis. An early champion of microscopy, too, Leidy was the world's first CSI agent: In 1846, he became the first person to use microscopic analysis of bloodstains to identify a murderer.

Well-respected, well-loved, and very well-connected, Dr. Leidy received tributes of unusual specimens from acolytes across the globe and wrote volubly about them. On the subject of the soap couple, though, he remained singularly coy. And this stands to good reason: Respected as Dr. Leidy was and valuable as the soap couple were to the pursuit of human knowledge, none of this altered the fact that he was in no way legally entitled to them. In the eyes of the law, Dr. Leidy would have been regarded a common grave robber.

The only firsthand testimony we have about the acquisition of the soap couple comes from an associate, Dr. William Hunt, who gave his side of the story in a funeral address following Dr. Leidy's death in 1891:

> The only instance I ever knew of Dr. Leidy's departure from strict truth was, to a medical man's way of looking at it, a very amusing one. Some years ago he came to my house in quite an enthusiastic mood, and said, "Dr. Hunt, do you know that they are moving the bodies from a very old burying-ground down town to make way for improvements?" "Yes," I said. "Well," he went on, "two bodies turned into adipocere are there.... They have been buried for nearly a hundred years, an old man and an old woman; nobody claims them, and they would be rare and instructive additions to our collections. Now, I think I can get them, and if you will take one for the Mütter Museum, I will take the other for the Wistar and Horner Museum." ... So down Leidy went, full of the idea of securing the prizes. When he spoke to the superintendent or caretaker of the ground, that gentleman put on airs, talked of violating graves, etc.; so the discomfited doctor was about going away quite chapfallen. Just then the caretaker touched him significantly on the elbow and said, "I tell you what I do; I give bodies up to the order of relatives!" The doctor immediately took the hint. He went home, hired a furniture wagon, and armed the driver with an order reading, "Please deliver to bearer the bodies of my grandfather and grandmother."
>
> This brought the coveted prizes, and one is now in each of the museums, and the virtuous caretaker was amply compensated.
>
> But they all do it... .[1]

[1] *William Hunt,* An Address upon the Late Joseph Leidy *(Philadelphia: Collins Printing House, 1892), 27-28. A receipt at the Mütter Museum, signed in Dr. Leidy's hand, discloses the caretaker's ample compensation: "Expenses in the Procural of an Adipocere Body — $7.50."*

Aside from its direct relevance to the story of the Soap Lady, Dr. Hunt's anecdote provides an amusing account of a pair of dilettante body snatchers getting schooled in the art of resurrectionism and—more tellingly—an insight to how casually corpse theft was once regarded within the scientific community.

As picturesquely gothic as it sounds to us today, grave robbing was still very much a real thing in 1875. Although the supply of medical cadavers was becoming more reliable, chronically undersupplied medical schools still occasionally resorted to extralegal means to meet their need, as they routinely had fifty years earlier during the bodysnatching boom years. Additional pressure was coming from another direction: Medical research museums, such as the Mütter Museum and Washington's nascent Army Medical Museum (now the National Museum of Health), were vying to assemble the most comprehensive collection of human injury and dysfunction. Consulted by physicians just like real-life, walk-in reference books, these so-called pathological cabinets—ghoulish assemblages of twisted limbs, mutant babies, and syphilitic brains afloat in jars of preserving formaldehyde, of articulated skeletons, and of detached skulls arrayed to illustrate the relative worth of the "Five Races of Man"—presented an insatiable demand for medically intriguing human remains.

Although there were laws regulating the acquisition of bodies for research and display, they were observed largely in the breach. Consequently, as Dr. Hunt alludes at the end of the quoted passage, museum shelves were chockablock with dubiously sourced specimens plucked off battlefields, plundered from cemeteries, and pilfered from Native lands. When necessary, legal-ish documentation could always be arranged.

Whether events played out exactly as Dr. Hunt recalled—or, for that matter, whether Leidy had given him all the facts—the two conspirators understood what they were up to. To create the fiction of legality over an act that, however laudable in intention, was clearly criminal, the identities of Wilhelm von Ellenbogen and Mrs. Ellenbogen were invented.[2] Both were in their 60s when they died of yellow fever in 1792, and they had been exhumed from a cemetery at Fourth and Race streets that was being moved on account of some undefined urban renovation. Some of this is clearly information that Leidy believed, but some is deliberate misinformation to ensure the bodies were never properly identified.

[2] Leidy, who spoke German, would have known that "Ellenbogen" is a variant of ellbogen (elbow). Was it an inside joke, perhaps alluding to the caretaker's meaningful tug at Leidy's sleeve? We can only wonder. Perhaps it was merely a coinage of opportunity, like Jan Brady's invented teen lover, George Glass.

It is more than likely that, when the soap people were delivered to their new homes, all parties understood that the documentation might be worth somewhat less than the paper it was written on. But succeeding generations, eager to forget the sins of medicine past, were apt to take things at face value. It wasn't until 1942 that Dr. Joseph McFarland, then curator of the Mütter Museum, decided it was time to test the Soap Lady narrative. McFarland was just old enough to have attended some of Dr. Leidy's lectures at Penn, where it was an open secret among the students that the elder scientist had engaged in a ruse to obtain soap couple. But McFarland wondered how much Leidy really knew about their provenance.

Not very much, it turned out. Acting more as a gumshoe than a scientist, Dr. McFarland pored over city directories, legal documents, death notices, ship passenger lists trying to authenticate the Soap Lady's documentation. While he did establish that there had indeed been a cemetery near Fourth and Race, there was no yellow fever outbreak of 1792. That came in 1793, and there were no Ellenbogens among the victims. In fact, there was no one of that name in Philadelphia at all before 1836.

Cutting Through the Soap Film

Dr. McFarland's research cleared away some false leads, but it offered little in its place.[3] And that is the highly dissatisfying point where our knowledge of the soap couple remained—until the end of the twentieth century, when high technology was at last brought to bear on the puzzle. In 1987, the Mütter Museum requisitioned a portable X-ray machine, and, taking great pains not to crumble their precious specimen like a block of feta cheese, made a radiographic analysis of the Soap Lady. The images revealed, embedded in her adipocere, two buttons, dating probably to the 1820s or 30s, as well as seven straight pins of a design that was not manufactured in the U.S. until 1838. Thus the Soap Lady's time of death had to be adjusted downward by at least 46 years. By the look of her bones, too, she was younger that Dr. Leidy had claimed—perhaps forty years old. Radiographic analysis of the Soap Man in 1994 came up with similar evidence that corroborated the Mütter's findings.

In 2001 and 2008, the Mütter Museum repeated its radiographic analysis—the first time with a CT scan and the second with new and powerful X-ray equipment—in an act of what curator Anna Dhody calls hardcore "archaeo-forensics." Since irradiation poses no threat in her present state, instead of using a standard medical X-ray device, the Soap Lady was zapped by an industrial machine designed for peering into things with less water content than a human body— like, say, a huge bar of soap. The high-resolution images, along with evidence that could be collected without damaging the body—fallen hairs and fibers, adipocere peelings that had sloughed off—were sent for analysis at an independent laboratory. The study has not yet been completed, but the information released so far, like everything else in this story, is both highly suggestive and disappointingly inconclusive.

There's no telling whether the Soap Lady is German, but she probably is white and is most definitely a lady. The X-rays show that the bones in her skull are fused, which means she

[3] Dr. McFarland did venture to contribute to the dataset by asserting that the Soap Lady was "probably ugly"—an opinion that seems somewhat unscientific and wholly unkind. Nevertheless, those who have studied her most thoroughly tend to concur, including current Mütter curator Anna Dhody, who has compared her unfavorably to cornrow-enthusiast and equine-rights advocate Bo Derrick. But then again, who among us can compete with a perfect 10?

cleared her early 20s. But she didn't make it much further: The complete absence of joint wear indicates that she died in that brief sweet-spot between maturation and the moment when the decay starts to show—somewhat before 40. The presence of gallstones (though no evidence of an attack) would put her toward the upper limit. Let's say she died in her midthirties—about half the age ascribed to Mrs. Ellenbogen.

It turns out that teeth were a serious a red herring. The Soap Lady has absolutely none, which made everyone initially assume that she had died elderly. But far from the toothless crone once imagined, radiography reveals the Soap Lady as a toothless...nubile? But if age did not remove her chompers, then what did? After all, even with their minimum of oral care, most Victorians contrived to hold on to at least some teeth through middle age. Until a more intensive investigation is completed, the mystery of the Soap Lady's toothless howl must remain an eerie enigma—an unhappy variant of the Mona Lisa smile.

As for how she became the Soap Lady, we have made some progress there. The pins and fiber traces argue that she had been wrapped in a funeral shroud, but there is no evidence of any more elaborate funeral preparations. This might indicate that she died in poverty and was buried in a mass grave: A pit would have been dug, lye strewn between successive layers of the stacked indigent, and the grave topped off with soil. This would create all the necessary conditions for adipocere formation—airlessness, an abundance of alkali, the possibility of moisture, and no barrier of a coffin to impede the reaction. In such a felicitous environment, it would be surprising not to have found a few soap corpses. Interment in an unmarked grave would also explain why no one came to claim the soap couple, who could have been dead for no more than 37 years when Dr. Leidy obtained them under false pretenses.

Now for the real surprise. To become as thoroughly saponified as the Soap Lady demands a good deal of fat, hence the assumption that she had been morbidly obese. But her weight is concentrated overwhelmingly in her midsection. A thirty-five-year-old dead woman, fat around the middle, but otherwise in reasonable health—the conclusion is inescapable: Could the Soap Lady have died in childbirth?

Despite the many and enduring gaps in our knowledge, the new forensic evidence nevertheless gestures toward a very different and more poignant vision of the Soap Lady's last mortal days than Dr. Leidy in all good faith must have imagined for her. Exhausted and prematurely aged, did she die in a final delivery, the grim terminus in the succession of births that, for many of her nineteenth-century sisters, was the inevitable trajectory of wifehood? We know now that she missed the nation's heroic age, but the era she witnessed was no less transformative, or turbulent. Laid to rest in a pauper's grave, had she come in from the frontier wilderness only to end her days in an urban slum? And the baby she left behind, was its fate to be factory-fodder in Philadelphia's burgeoning industrial revolution?

Or was there even a baby? For all its novelistic allusiveness, the underlying hypothesis is not confirmed and cannot easily be. After all, by what non-invasive means can you confirm that a two-hundred-year-old corpse, whose organs are fortunately preserved but encased in a thick layer of soap, died in a miscarriage? How close can we get to the truth of this anonymous woman without destroying the Soap Lady she has become? These are questions that Dhody and her colleagues at the Mütter are asking as they prepare for yet another bite at the elusive apple of knowledge.

[This essay has been adapted from the author's book Gross America: Your Coast-to-Coast Guide to All Things Gross. *New York: Jeremy P. Tarcher, Penguin, 2012.]*

[SELECTED BIBLIOGRAPHY]

Aufderheide, Arthur C. *The Scientific Study of Mummies*. New York: Cambridge University Press, 2003.

Conlogue, Gerald, et al. "Radiographic Evaluation of the Soap Man Mummy." *Radiologic Technology* (May/June 1997).

Dohdy, Anna. Interview with author on February 12, 2013.

Hunt, William. *An Address upon the Late Joseph Leidy*. Philadelphia: Collins Printing House, 1892.

Warren, Leonard. *Joseph Leidy: The Last Man Who Knew Everything*. New Haven: Yale University Press, 1998.

PART IV

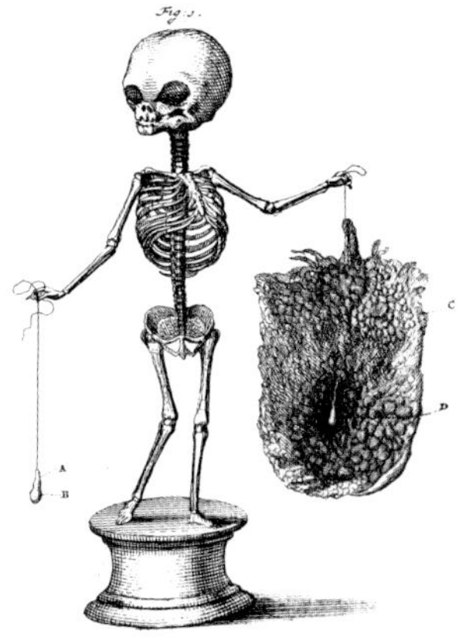

THE FALSE ATRIUM

Notes on Mourning

COLIN DICKEY

> *We can no longer speak of everlasting memory and the veneration of our forebears. On the contrary: the dead must now be cleared out of the way as quickly and comprehensively as possible. What mourner at a crematorium has not thought, as the coffin moves into the furnace, that the way we now take leave of the dead is marked by ill-concealed and paltry haste?*
>
> —W. G. Sebald[1]

"FIRST WEDDING NIGHT. BUT FIRST MOURNING NIGHT?" SO BEGINS Roland Barthes' *Mourning Diary,* a collection of scraps and orts, fragments and unprocessed jottings he began to keep the day after his mother's death. He was sixty-one, she had been eighty-four; her death destroyed him. Eventually he was able to channel this grief into his late masterpiece on photography, *Camera Lucida,* but it is in these notes (posthumously published in 2009), that we see his naked confrontation with grief and death.

From the beginning, he wrestled with the problem of mourning's length, and its intensity. "Everyone guesses," he wrote a few days after his mother's death, "the degree of bereavement's intensity. But it's impossible (meaningless, contradictory signs) to measure how much someone is afflicted." A few days later, ironically, he wrote out: "The *measurement* of mourning. (Dictionary, Memorandum):

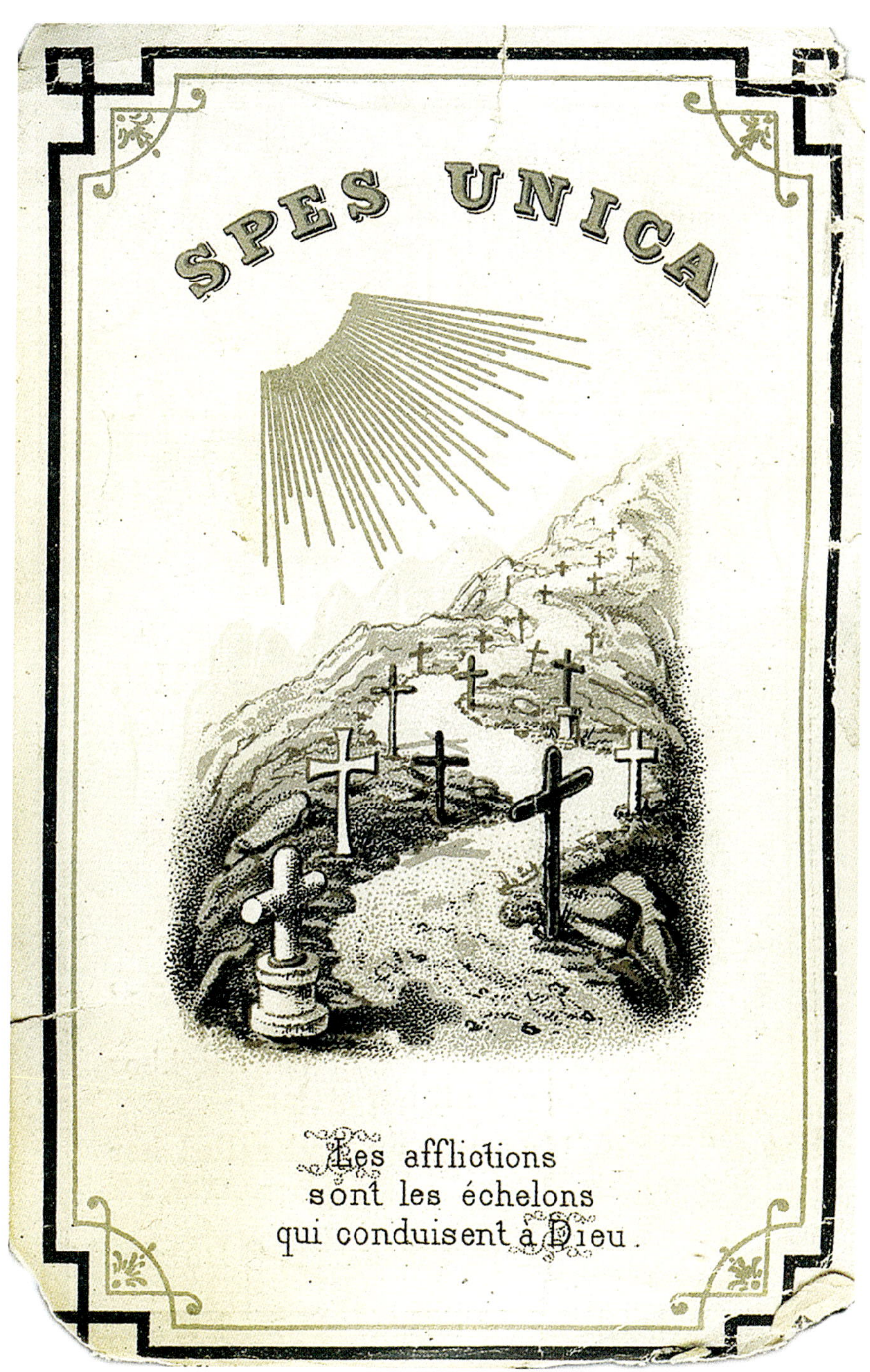
SPES UNICA
Les afflictions
sont les échelons
qui conduisent à Dieu.

eighteen months for mourning a father, a mother." From the outset, Barthes was not interested in a specified window of time in which he could experience grief and then move on. "It is said that Time soothes mourning," he wrote that March. "No, Time makes nothing happen; it merely makes the *emotivity* of mourning pass.... Emotion (emotivity) passes, suffering remains."[2]

Throughout his diary, Barthes constantly returned to these questions, of the duration of mourning, and the experience of time for the bereaved. In February he wrote, "Mourning: I've learned that it was immutable and sporadic: *it does not wear away,* because it is not continuous." A few months later, he clarified: "(Mourning) Not Continuous, but Immobile."[3] Grief breaks the continuity of time, ruptures the linear progression of life. It has no distinct beginning nor end, and it cannot be accommodated by our usual concepts of time, psychological evolution, and personal development.

And it is precisely this reason that it is so problematic, why so many societies and cultures have developed elaborate rituals in order to contain and confine it in some way. Mourning—unpredictable, unquantifiable, inexplicable—must be given shape, form, direction. "All *judicious* societies," Barthes wrote the following June, "have prescribed and codified the externalization of mourning."[4]

[1] *W. G. Sebald,* Campo Santo, *trans. Anthea Bell (New York: Random House, 2005), 31-32.*

[2] *Roland Barthes,* Mourning Diary, *trans. Richard Howard (New York: Hill and Wang, 2010), 3, 10, 11, 101, 103.*

[3] *Ibid., 95, 137.*

[4] *Ibid., 155.*

How do we define our relationship to grief? Is it a thing external to us, alien to us, a thing to be slowly eradicated? Barthes himself wrote that July, with reference to the possibility of being medicated for depression: "Impossibility—indignity, actually—of entrusting to a drug—on the pretext of depression—my

Image previous page: Mourning card from the collection of The Morbid Anatomy Library, dated 1885.

suffering, as if it were a disease, a 'possession'—an alienation (something that makes you alien)—whereas it's an essential, an intimate part of yourself...."[5]

Across the Atlantic, the American Psychiatric Association (APA) was coming to a radically different conclusion. The Diagnostic and Statistical Manual of Mental Disorders (DSM) had been around since 1952, and had already gone through two editions, but with the DSM-III (compiled and edited between 1974 and 1980), the book moved away from vague theories of psychoanalysis towards an objective, rigid picture of mental health. Gone were poorly defined words like "neurosis," and in their place lists of symptoms: if a patient was suffering from one symptom in column A, or three in column B, and had none of the mitigating factors in column C, then she or he could be diagnosed as having a specific condition and treated accordingly (or, put another way, the treatment could be reimbursed by insurance companies).

This strategy prevented individual doctors from asserting personal biases and incorrect beliefs, but its exclusive focus on visible, external symptoms created other problems. As Gary Greenberg outlines in his book *Manufacturing Depression* (2010), the DSM-III's definition of a Major Depressive Disorder (MDD) relied on symptoms that were all equally present in those who'd recently been bereaved—calling into question whether this new system could differentiate between persistent depression and temporary bereavement.[6] The DSM-III's solution was to carve a caveat into the MDD diagnosis, the Bereavement Exclusion: if a patient was suffering from the depressive symptoms within two months of suffering the loss of a loved one, that patient was instead suffering from "uncomplicated bereavement," which doctors could treat if they wanted to, but for which treatment they would likely not be reimbursed by insurance companies.[7]

[5] *Ibid., 163.*

[6] *Gary Greenberg,* Manufacturing Depression: The Secret History of a Modern Disease *(New York: Simon and Schuster, 2010), 246-248.*

[7] *Beyond MDD, the DSM-5 proposes another disorder, Complicated Grief Disorder (CGD), which is the result of persistent and debilitating grief that lasts longer than six months. The DSM is moot on the status of one's grief during that gray area from two weeks to six months, but more to the point, I can think of no one who's experienced the loss of a loved one who wouldn't describe their emotions at six months out as "uncomplicated." Grief is always complicated.*

The Bereavement Exclusion became a way of medically differentiating between uncomplicated grief and MDD, an uneasy and problematic compromise, but one that has tenuously worked for the past thirty years or so. But as work began on the new latest edition of the DSM (the DSM-5), the question of grief, and its relation to depression (and thus the question of medicating it) has returned once again. Some psychiatrists argued that the exception associated with bereavement should be expanded to include things that don't necessarily include the loss of a loved one (the loss of a job, for example, or a divorce); others argued that the bereavement exclusion ties their hands, that thoughts of suicide and other severe symptoms need immediate treatment.

The end result has been that with the new revisions to the DSM-5, the window for the bereavement exclusion has become vanishingly small: two weeks now, instead of two months. Writing in the *New York Times,* Allen Frances (chair of the DSM-IV committee, and now a vocal apostate against the DSM-5) excoriated the new decision. "Turning bereavement into major depression," he wrote, "would substitute a shallow, Johnny-come-lately medical ritual for the sacred mourning rites that have survived for millenniums."[8] Even though the previous window of two months was in many ways just as arbitrary (implying that the normal progression of grief is identical for the entire population), it's begun to seem that we have an increasing impatience when it comes to grieving, and a strong desire to "cure" the bereaved of this condition.

"No," Barthes himself wrote, "bereavement (depression) is different from sickness. What should I be cured of? To find what condition, what life?"[9]

[8] *Quoted in Gary Greenberg,* The Book of Woe: The DSM and the Unmaking of Psychiatry *(New York: Blue Rider Press, 2013), 155.*

[9] *Barthes, 8.*

—⁂—

This isn't the first time a powerful organization has tried to downplay and minimize, if not outright eradicate, grief and mourning. Early Christian writers were aghast at public displays of mourning, and cautioned against any overtly emotional display at the loss of a loved one. Saint John Chrysostom (347–407) threatened excommunication for those who "hired women, pagans, as mourners to make the mourning more intense, to fan the fires of grief, ignoring the words of Saint Paul." The canons of the patriarchate of Alexandria likewise recommended against public displays of emotion: "Those who are in mourning must remain in the church, monastery, or house, silent, calm, and dignified, as befits those who believe in the truth of the resurrection."[10] By the ninth century, Christian authorities were still warning against excessive or pagan displays of grief: The St. Hubert Penitential dictates that if "anyone lacerates himself over his dead with a sword or his nails, or pulls his hair, or rends his garments, he shall do penance for forty days."[11] If one genuinely believed not just in heaven but in the bodily reunion of the dead on the day of Christ's Second Coming, this reasoning went, then it was highly inappropriate to weep for the dead, since you were bound to see them again soon enough.

The Church, and the Church alone, dictated proper mourning. "The penance for the wailing of a woman after [the death of] a layman or a laywoman," an Irish canon dictates, is "fifty days on bread and water."[12] In order to affirm the truth of the Resurrection and the dogma of the clergy, mourning had to be suppressed, standardized, and limited. For the APA, this minimizing of grief is different—it's about returning the bereaved to "functionability," as though the human mind were a machine that was prone to malfunction. If we expect our citizens to be productive members of society (emphasis

[10] *Philippe Ariès,* The Hour of Our Death, *trans. Helen Weaver (New York: Vintage, 1981), 144.*

[11] Medieval Handbooks of Penance, *eds. John T. McNeill and Helena M. Gamer (New York: Columbia University Press, 1938), 294.*

[12] *Ibid., 121.*

on productive), then it's important that they don't waste too much time grieving for the dead. As Barthes suggest, judicious societies must always legislate mourning; it is perhaps their prime task.

The *Corrector* of the Burchard of Worms recommends up to twenty days bread and water for those who mourn inappropriately, but while the Church could dictate funeral rites and demand penance for transgressions, its real power lay in the ground. Only those who were buried in consecrated ground within the walls of the church and its cemetery (its "atrium") could be guaranteed resurrection and an immortal soul, and only those who submitted to the church were allowed access to hallowed ground.[13] If the APA's attempt to control mourning is temporal, for the Church it was often topographical. Those who died outside the church's protection were condemned to be buried in fallow fields, in what Alain de Chartier described in the early fifteenth century as "the false atrium":

[13] *"Every Christian of either sex, after attaining years of discretion, shall faithfully confess all his sins to his own priest at least once a year, and shall endeavor according to his ability to fulfill the penance enjoined him.... Otherwise he shall both be withheld from entrance to the church while he lives and be deprived of Christian burial when he dies."* Medieval Handbooks of Penance, *413*.

> It is a kind of false atrium
> And there they throw the bodies of the damned.
> I saw more than four of them,
> blackened, rotting, left to life
> On the ground, without a grave.[14]

[14] *Quoted in Ariès, 43.*

For those in the False Atrium, no mourning was allowed; the best hope was to try to convince the bishop for a posthumous reburial in consecrated ground. Philippe Ariès writes of coffins being surreptitiously laid in the trees above cemeteries, a last-ditch attempt at redemption for the apostate and for families desperate to mourn.[15]

[15] *Ariès, 45.*

Human cultures have long known the perils of a death unmourned, or improperly mourned. Eastern European folktales speak of the dangerous potential of those who died alone, those who were improperly buried, and those who died without anyone to grieve for them. In Hungarian and Bulgarian folklore, for example, these dead are precisely the ones who are most likely to return as vampires. Long before Bram Stoker's *Dracula* fixed the vampire myth for Western cultures, and set in stone the sexual metaphor of the vampire bite as the primary mode of transmission, legend suggested that the vampire was born of a dead body that wasn't properly mourned. Bachelors, illegitimate children who died stillborn, whole families who died at once and left no one behind to grieve—these all became vampires. As far back as the ninth century, the corpses of unbaptized children were taken to out-of-the-way locales and staked to the ground, lest "the little child would arise and injure many."[16] Vampirism, Laurence A. Rickels writes, "always covers the need to mourn. That the vampire is someone who was buried improperly also meant, still to the point, that this special someone was not mourned properly."[17]

[16] Medieval Handbooks of Penance, *339*.

Not just these unfortunates, but also robbers, murderers, prostitutes, apostates—those explicitly denied proper burial by the Church were also thought to return as vampires. Suicides, condemned by the church and denied burial in consecrated ground, were buried instead at crossroads, because it was believed that if the suicide's corpse rose from the dead, it wouldn't be able to determine which road led back to town. Banished to the False Atrium and denied mourning, the exiled dead return with a vengeance. The myth of the vampire, one could say, involves our anxieties of an all-powerful institution that claims to hold dominion over who can be mourned and how. Vampire mythology suggests that a need for mourning, for grief, is far

[17] *Laurence A. Rickels,* The Vampire Lectures *(Minneapolis: University of Minnesota Press, 1999), 4.*

Image right: from Monro, Alexander, and Sue's Traité d'ostéologie traduit de l'anglois de M. Monro ... *Paris: Chez Guillaume Cavelier, 1759. Courtesy of the New York Academy of Medicine Library.*

more universal, far more primal, than a religious or scientific authority that claims superiority—and that if this primal need to grieve is ignored or suppressed, the dead will linger in our consciousness. The undead monster, at its core, is a metaphor for the way the dead continue to haunt us in the absence of proper burial customs.

Incorrect, pagan funeral rites have been replaced by illnesses like Complicated Grief Disorder, but we are once again faced with an institution trying to convince us that mourning is a thing that can be regularized, controlled, hidden away. The rhetoric underlying the APA's decisions regarding depression, grief and bereavement in the DSM-5 suggest a philosophy that mourning is a temporary aberration, one that can be dispensed with using pharmaceuticals, and is at best a minor obstacle on the individual's path back to proper functioning. In a hyper-accelerated landscape, perhaps a quick two weeks of grief is enough, sufficient to placate the dead.

But those who cannot be properly honored in such a short time may be banished to lie fallow in the False Atrium, outside the purview of this new regime of bereavement, haunting us from the margins. Perhaps, then, it should come as no surprise to us that our pop culture is overrun with vampires and zombies, from *Twilight* to *True Blood* to *Pride and Prejudice and Zombies* to *The Walking Dead.* These hip and sparkly updates of age-old mythologies may perhaps bear the traces of a darker fear: that the dead are not yet done with us—that in hiding our own grief we have done them a terrible disservice, and that we cannot expect to go on living if we cannot properly bury our dead.

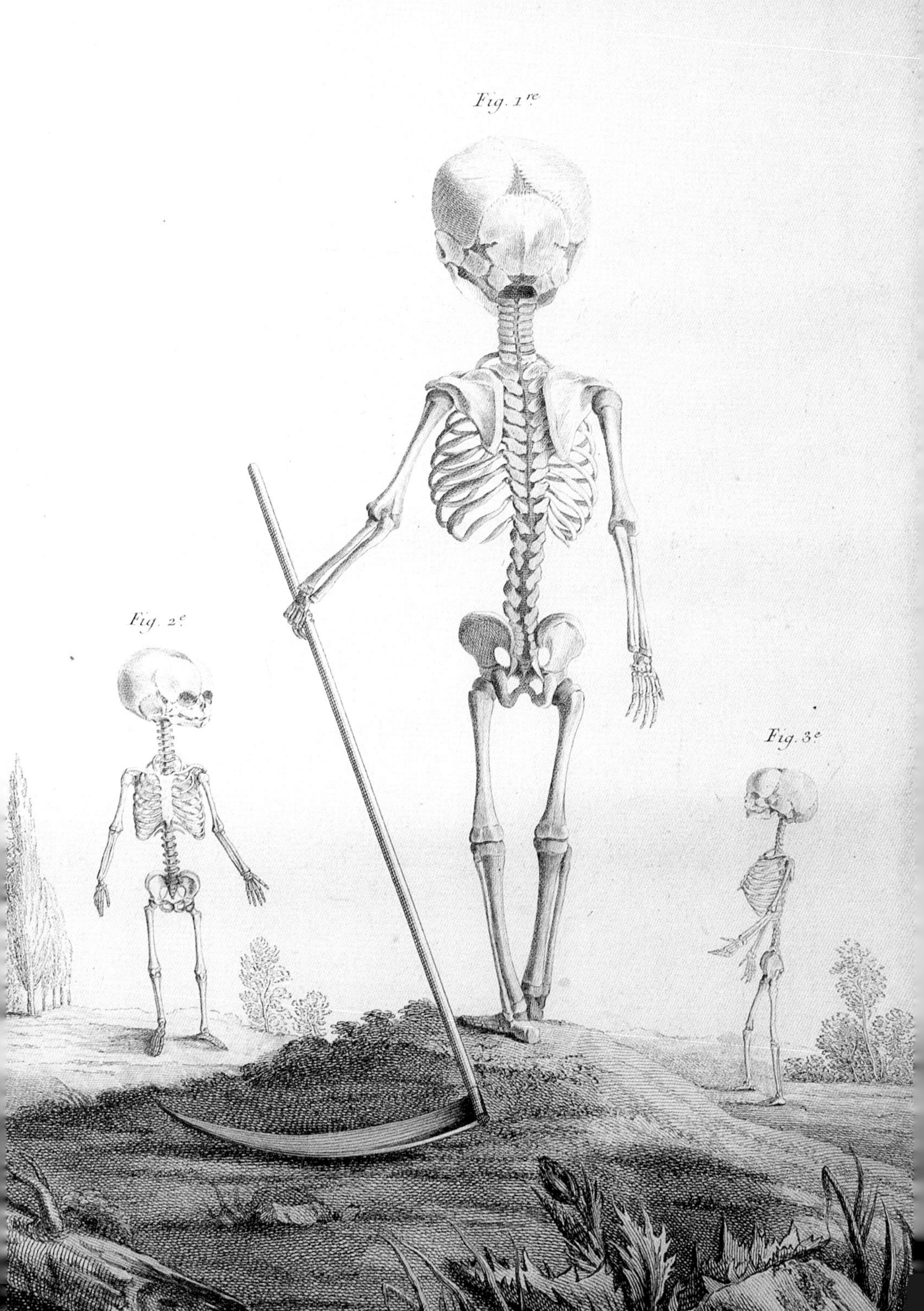
Fig. 1re
Fig. 2e
Fig. 3e

SKULLS & BIG RIGS

The World's Strangest Truck Stop

PAUL KOUDOUNARIS

SEVERAL HOURS SOUTH OF LIMA, PERU, AS THE HAIRPIN TURNS OF the Panamerican Highway straddle desert and beach, sit the small towns of Pescadores and La Planchata. They are fishing villages specializing in anchovies, and their processing plants ensure that the roadway is perpetually covered in a bridle of putrid smoke that is intolerable to anyone who has not grown up here. In a country that counts tourism as one of its major industries, this area sees no outsiders. The only traffic on the highway consists of long-haul truckers, who stop just north of the villages, at kilometer 744. For the drivers on their lonely routes, kilometer 744 is a pilgrimage site—it is akin to their version of Lourdes, a place where they are blessed, purified, and kept safe from harm. This is the *Santuario de Calaveritas* (The Shrine of the Little Skulls), a small chapel where God provides for truck drivers. "This is our holy place," explains Jose Alarcón, a poultry delivery driver, "this is where miracles happen"—miracles that are so numerous that the local parish priests say it is impossible to even keep track of them.

A crude stucco sanctuary, the site is named for its three enshrined *calaveras*, or skulls, which are the source of its power, and the souls of the deceased trio act as intercessors with God on behalf of the truckers. Makeshift altar tables are plastered in a mishmash of religious

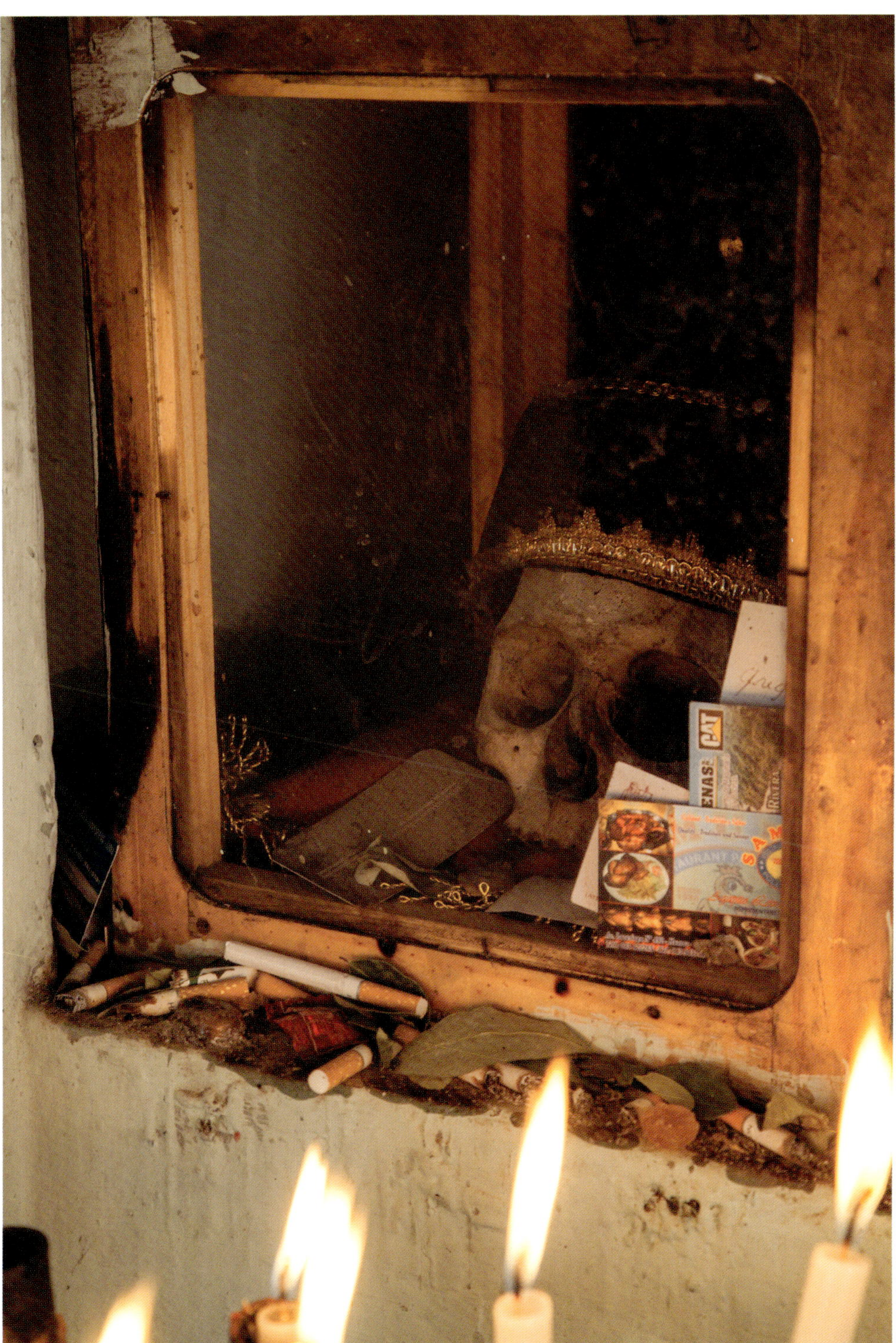
CAT

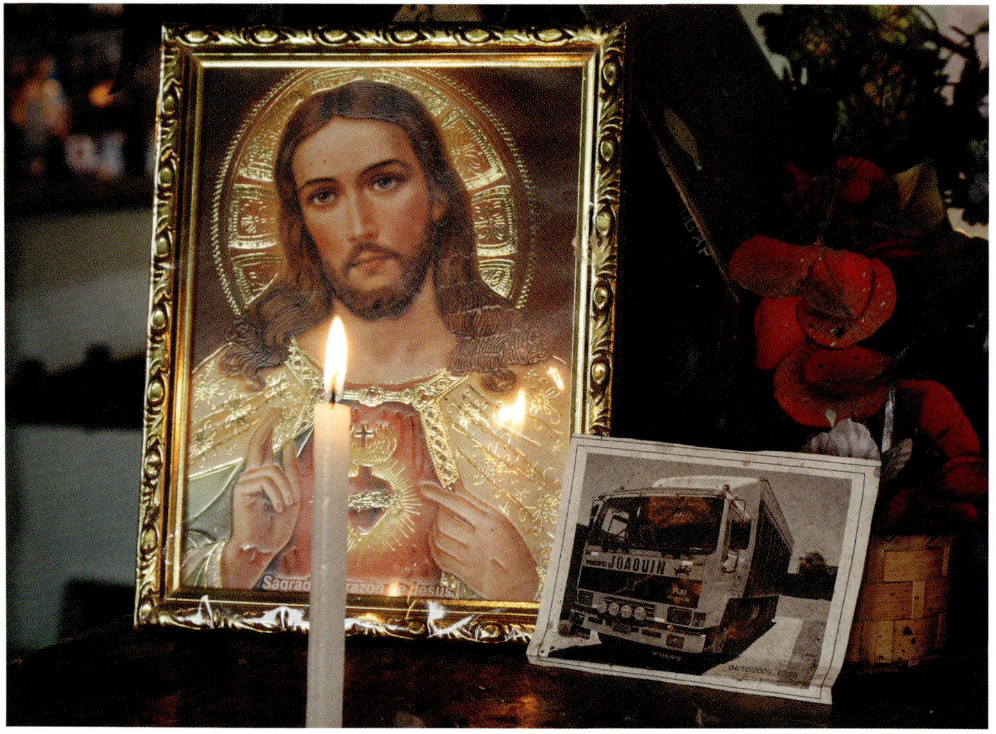

All photographs by the author.

votives and photos of trucks left as gifts from thankful drivers, while the walls hold hundreds of testimonials to the supernatural powers of this place. It is certainly the world's strangest truck stop, but while its adherents are obsessively devoted, the origin of the skulls is a mystery. A popular account holds that the skulls are those of Peruvian soldiers who were killed in battle against Chilean troops; blessed by God for their patriotic sacrifice, their spirits acquired supernatural powers to aid those who traveled along the coast. According to an alternate history, the skulls are those of three nuns, who died in the desert after becoming lost en route to their convent. Because of their exceptional virtues, their souls were allowed to remain at this spot, and shepherd other travelers so they would not meet a similar fate.

However the skulls wound up among the shifting sands of the Peruvian coast, they were found in the early twentieth century by road workers, and a small, wooden shrine was built to contain them. Since it was located in the middle of a long and barren stretch from Lima to Arequipa, Peru's second-largest city, it became a popular place for truckers to break their journey. It became customary for drivers to give prayers as an offering to the souls of the unknown deceased—but in this case, the deceased began to offer services in return. The first important miracle associated with the site occurred in the 1940s. A driver hauling fish pulled over to find that at a previous stop, a large portion of his cargo had been pilfered. Panicked by the discovery and afraid that he would lose his job if he arrived at his destination with less than a full load, he prayed to the skulls and beseeched whatever assistance they could provide. When he returned to his truck, he found that not only was the full load restored, there was a loaf of bread marked with a cross set atop his cargo—this was seen as an emulation of the miracle of the loaves and fishes, and created a sensation when word reached other drivers.

Truckers soon swarmed the roadside shrine, asking any number of favors—which the skulls continued to grant. Since this part of the site's history is passed down only through oral accounts, it will always be murky, but among the famous feats also attributed to the skulls in the 1940s are granting a trucker named Juan Encarnacion a new set of tires (which manifested themselves on his truck while he was driving); miraculously replacing the head gasket and water pump on a overheated truck owned by a driver whose last named is recorded as Padilla; and curing of any number of physical ailments. One of the souls even accompanied a driver named Miguel Mamani all the way to Nazca—taking one of the treacherous local turns

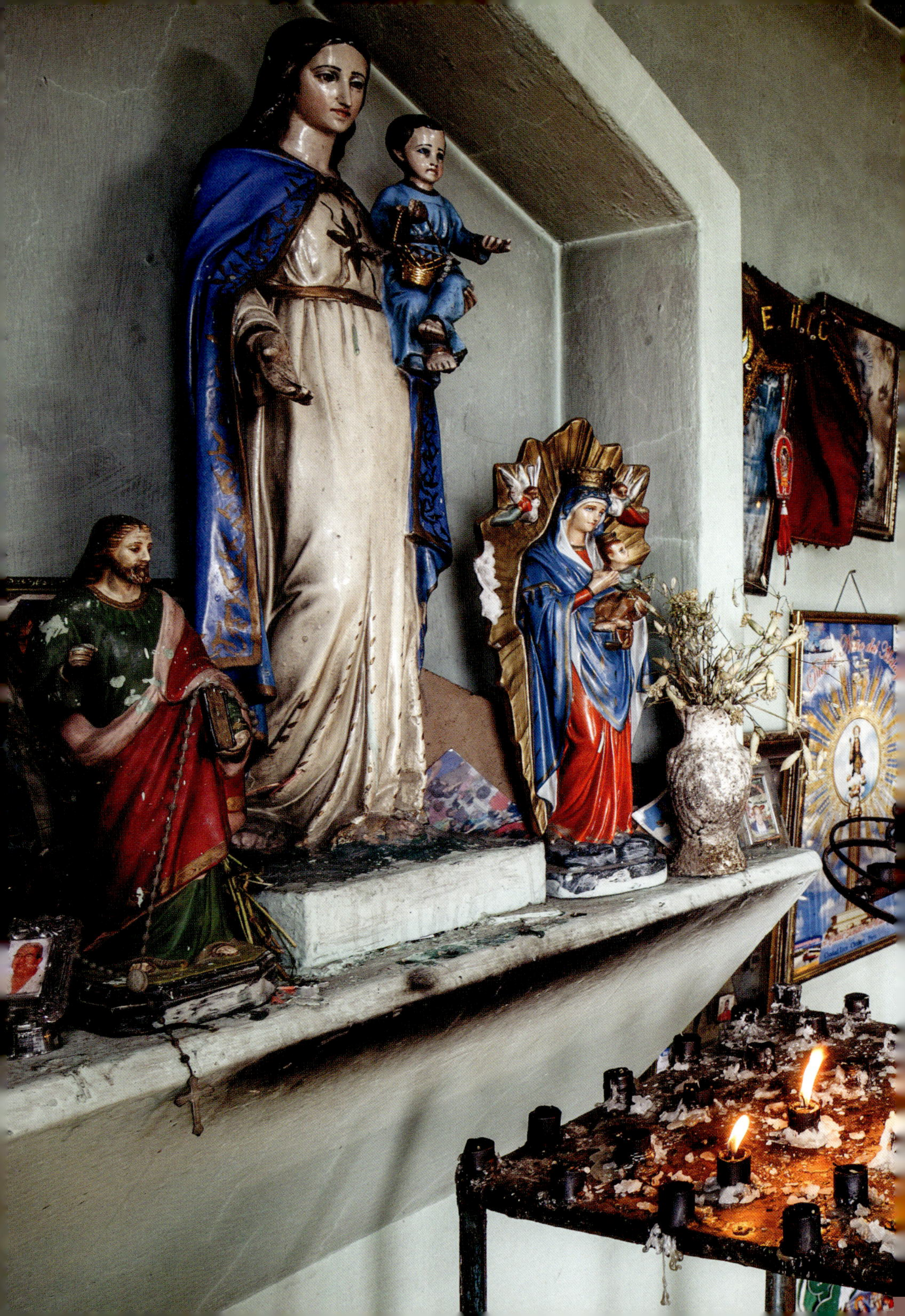
E. H. C

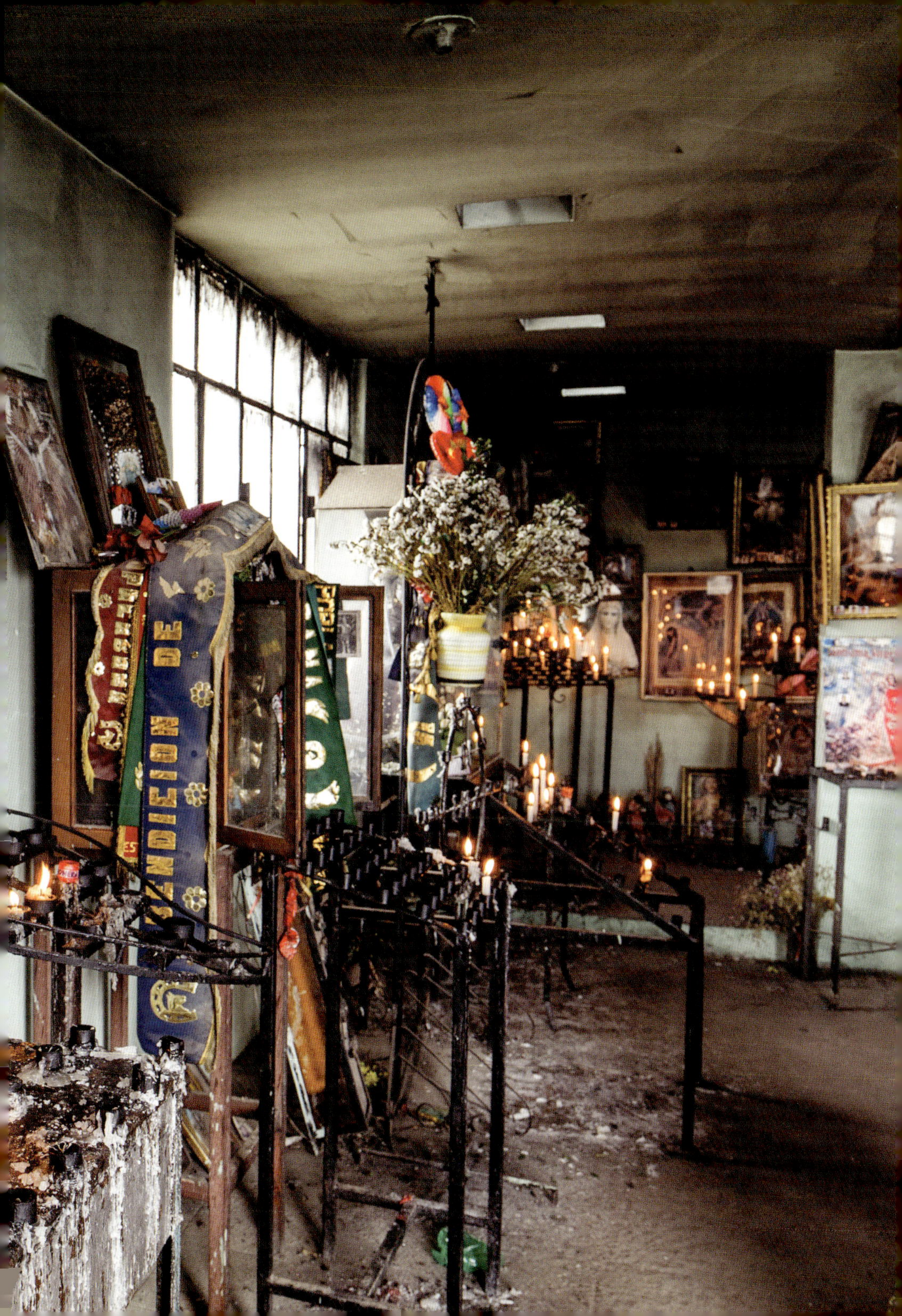

too hard, Mamani was thrown against the door of his truck and fractured his arm, but when he beseeched assistance at the shrine, a spectral apparition appeared and rode by his side, to maneuver the gear shift on his behalf.

Such impressive displays of supernatural power ensured that the three skulls assumed a position as something along the lines of patron saints of truckers, who by the 1950s desired to return the favors by offering donations. The problem was that the site was without any administration, so there was no one to whom they could donate. Since Pescadores and La Planchata are very small towns, the miraculous skulls were placed under the jurisdiction of the parish priests of Ocoña, a city of some ten thousand residents lying twenty minutes south on the highway, and a more formal sanctuary was built. The early gratuities left by drivers were sufficient at first to fund the construction of a grotto for the skulls in 1956. This was enlarged several times until it was finally reconstructed as a full-fledged chapel in 1995, paid for by donations from drivers and trucking companies, with additional funds provided by truckers' unions, who realized the benefits the skulls had been providing their members. Continued gifts allowed for an enlargement to the chapel a year later, and a reconstruction of the building's façade in early 2011. A small café was also added to feed the pious visitors.

There is no way to tabulate how much has been donated to the site, but Jose León, a driver who plies the coastal route, said that he spoke with a union representative who estimated that the total since the 1950s must have been over a million U.S. dollars. "We are a poor country," he said, "but the skulls deserve it, for what they have provided." He recounts his own tale—going around a treacherous bend outside of Ocoña a couple of years ago, he blew out a front tire. As his truck lurched towards the cliff wall, León explains, he called on the skulls in desperation.

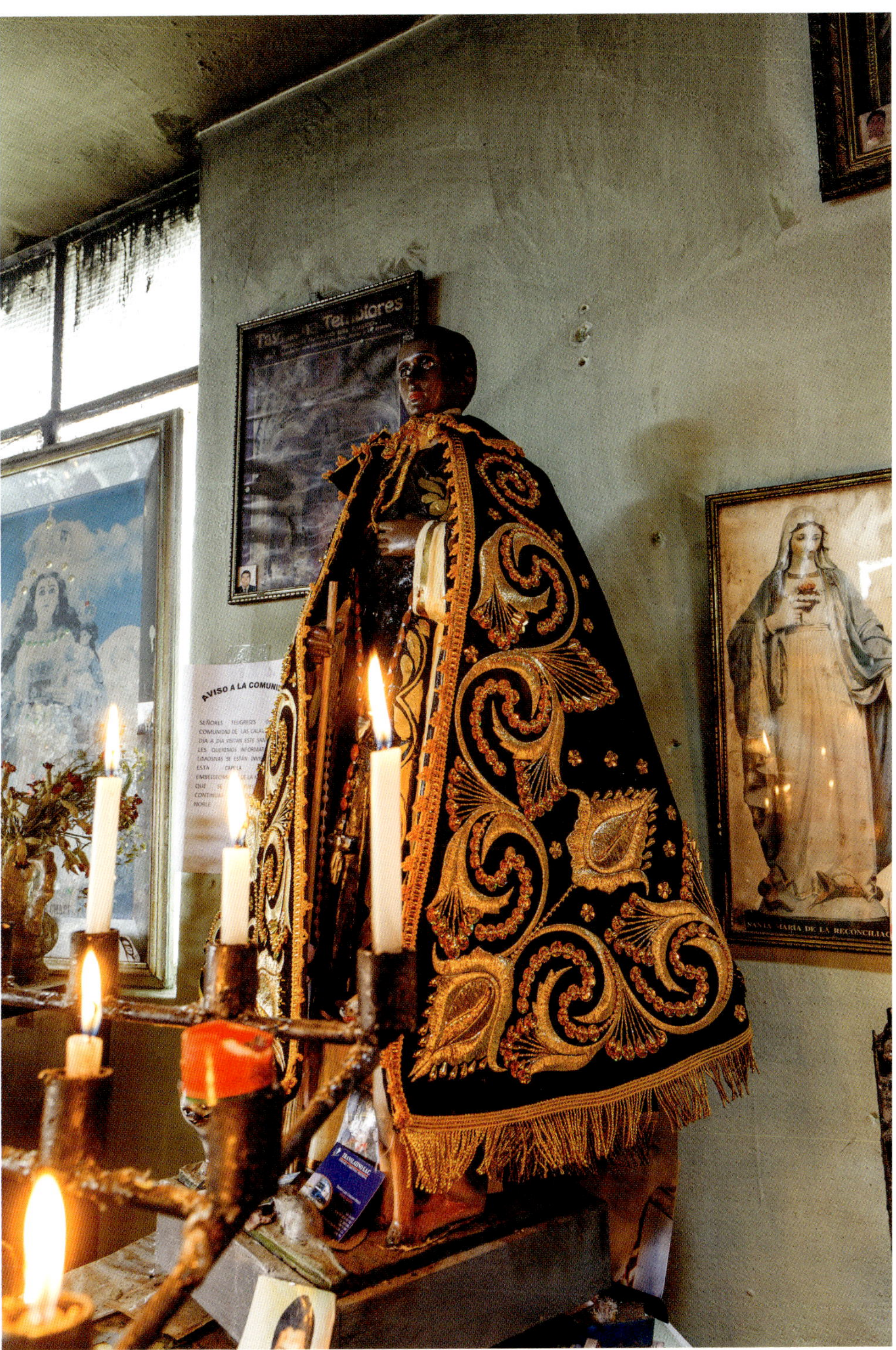
AVISO A LA
DE LA

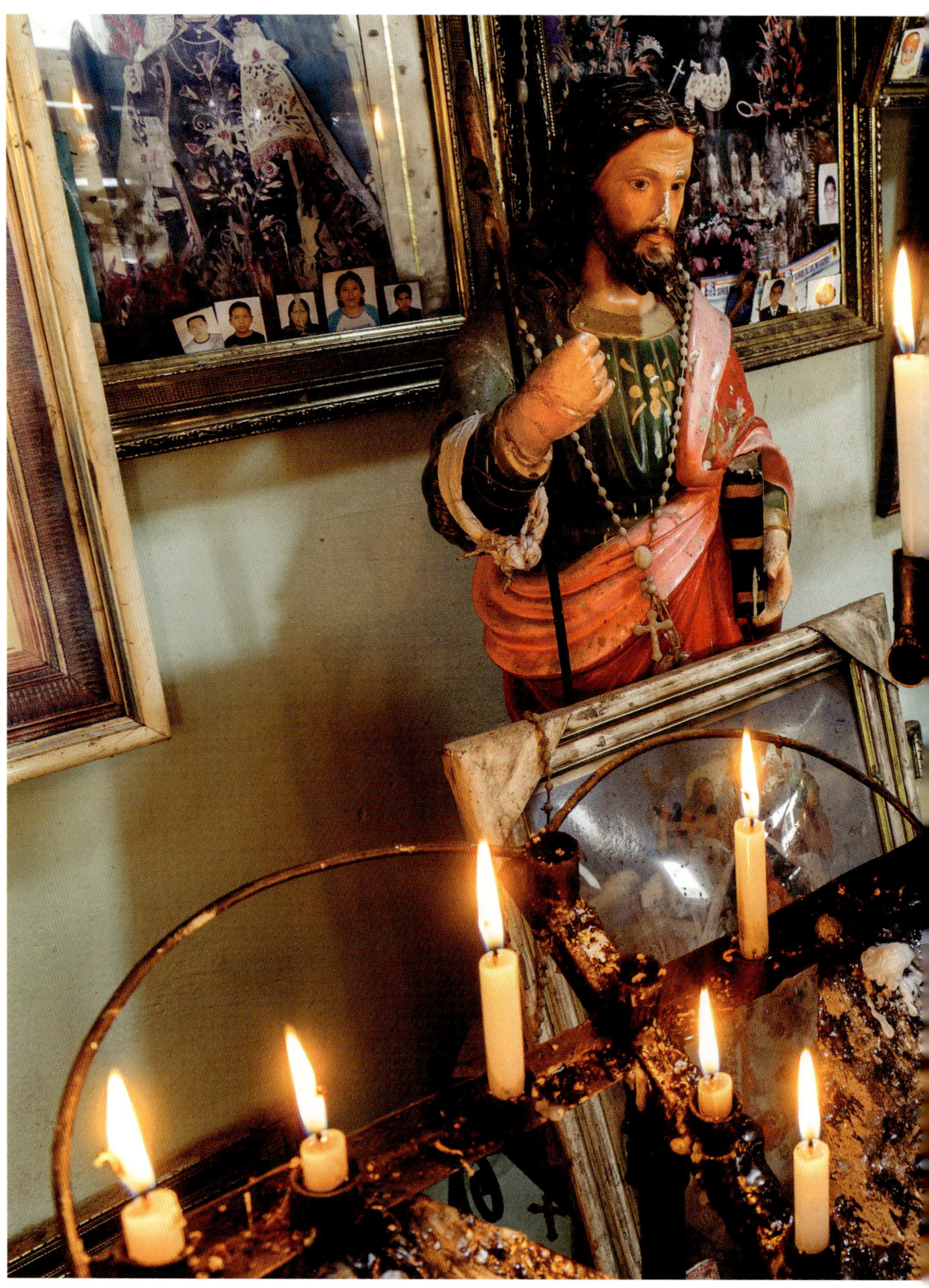

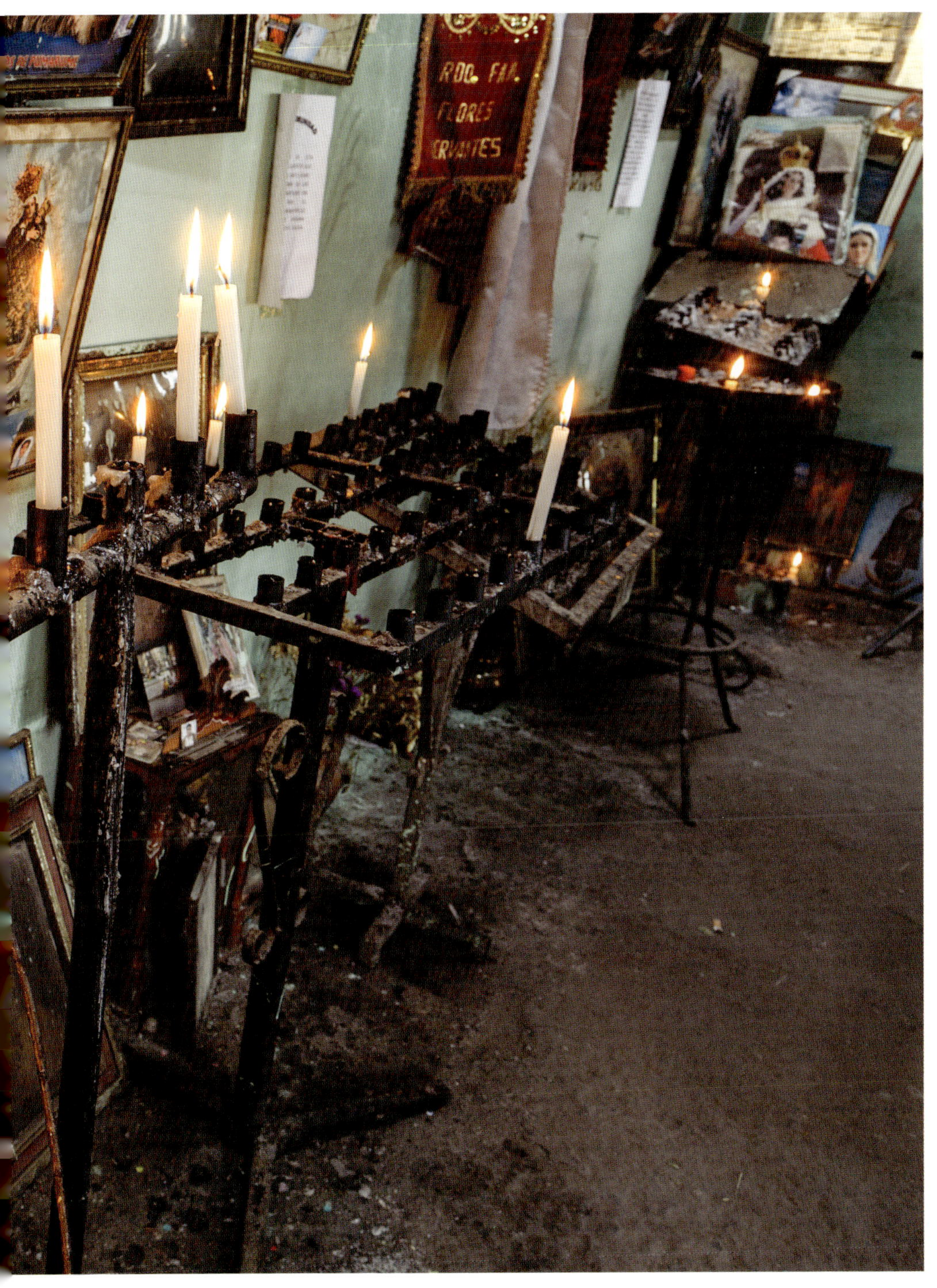
FLORES

Regaining control of the vehicle, he brought it to a stop, and jumped out to inspect the tire. It was no longer flat, and in fact had been miraculously reinflated. He credits the skulls with saving his life: "What price is that worth? The power of this place is real, all of the drivers believe this."

The drivers believe it enough that the chapel's walls are inlaid with plaques attesting to miracles associated with the skulls. February, 1955, is the earliest dated testament—while the specifics of the event are no longer known, the memorial was offered in the name of "J. Pacheco J." as thanks for assistance provided him at that time—and the plaques then document an ensuing half century of devotion and service. Among the most recent is one dated June 21, 2011, from Empresa Transportes, thanking the skulls for ensuring the protection of drivers from the mines at Secocha near Arequipa. Do the skulls really provide such a service? Absolutely, according to Carlos Pomata Cano, a former employee of Empresa. "That road is very dangerous," he explains, "and there were numerous accidents and fatalities on it. But you never hear of them anymore, not since the skulls were asked for their protection."

The rest of the interior is crammed full of devotional images in every style and medium imaginable. Naturally, the place of honor goes to the three crania, which are set on a makeshift altar. They are encased in crude wooden boxes, inscribed with the identity of the driver who provided them, Flores Levano from Nazca, and surrounded by holders for votive candles. It is typical to light candles in honor of the skulls, and according to some drivers they expect it. Chasco Huanco, a trucker from Tacna, relates a story of how he came to the shrine "with only two candles, so that is all I could light, even though there are three skulls. I turned to leave, but the door slammed shut and I was trapped inside. I broke one of the candles in two and lit

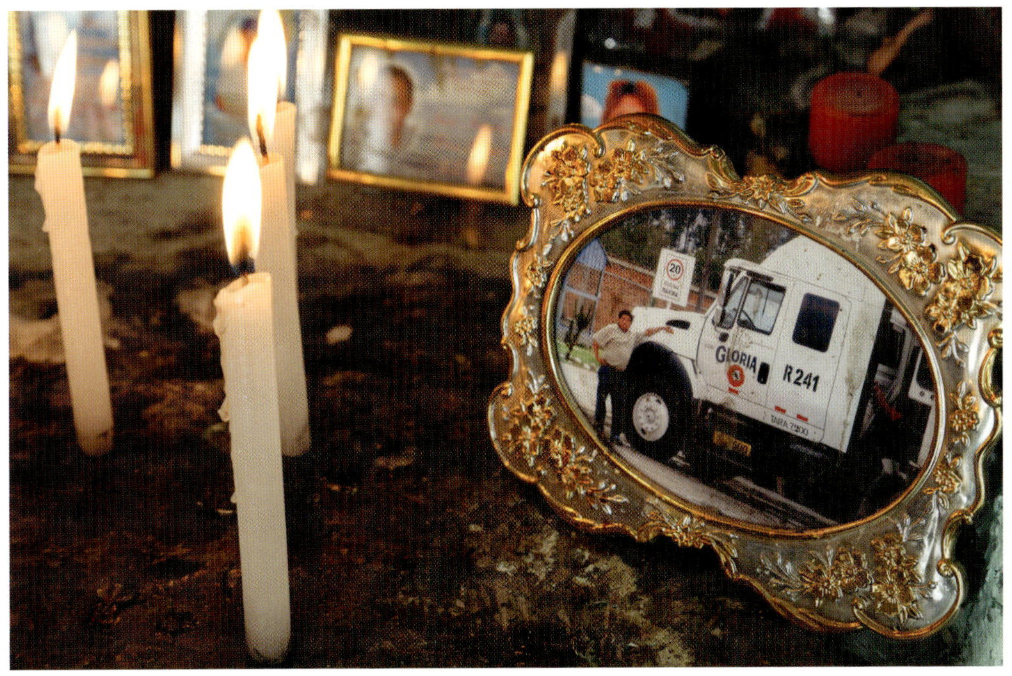

both halves, and the door opened. Now I always make sure to have three candles in my truck when I come this route."

Drivers are also known to leave statues of their own favorite Catholic saints, so they can venerate them at the shrine, as well. The native Peruvian saint Martin of Porres is particularly popular and is present several times, as is the Virgin of the Immaculate Conception. The most numerous offerings, however, are the photos of trucks and business cards for individual drivers and trucking companies. The shrine is especially littered with the latter. Some of the cards—set into the frames holding pictures of Christ, or attached to statues—are left to record the identities of those who donated gifts to this hallowed ground. Others are intended simply as votives, to ensure that the power of the skulls will continue to protect those named from afar. One

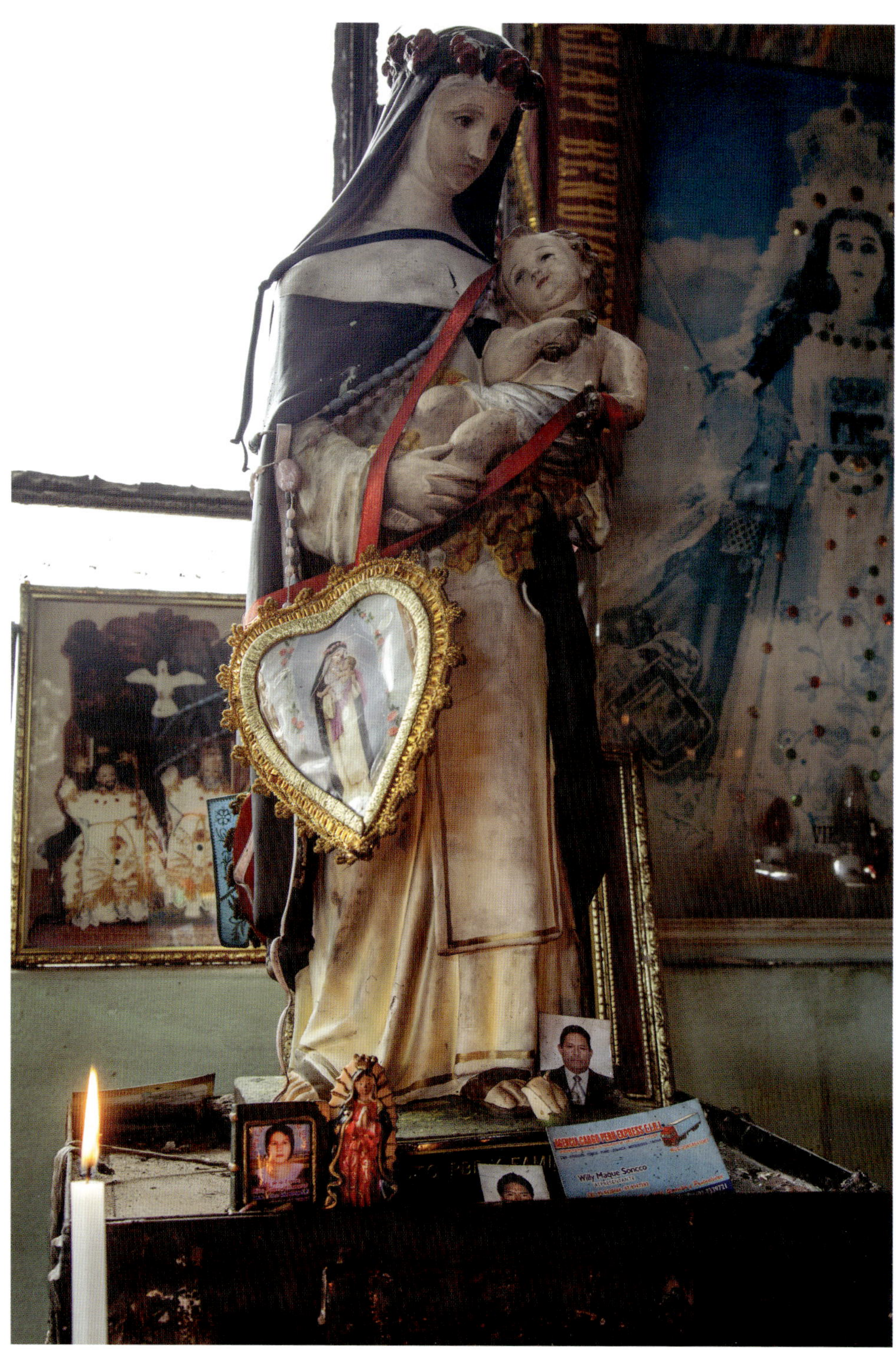
Willy Maque Soncco

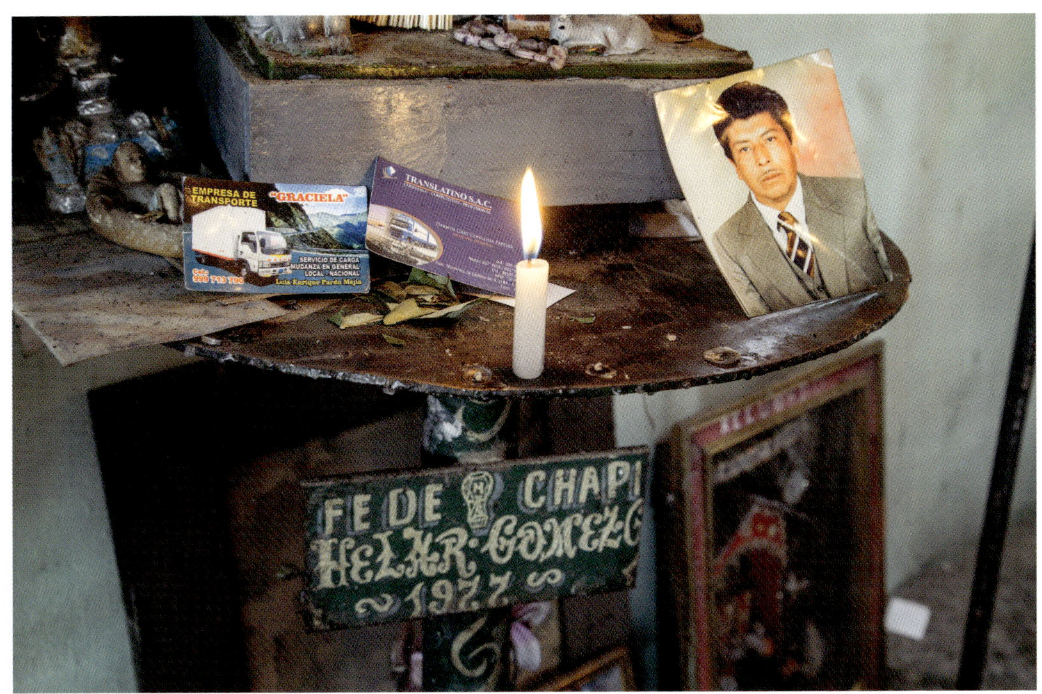

of the chapel's statues of Martin of Porres, for instance, is marked by cards from Empresa de Transporte Graciela and Translatino SAC; another bears the placard of the poultry distribution company, Distribuidora de Pollo Rosita. Meanwhile, a card for the cargo company Agencia Largo Peru Express is attached to the feet of the Virgin Mary. Finely embroidered velvet cloths are also found draped around sacred objects—likewise gifts from the faithful. A red velvet shawl over the Nazarene, for example, is embroidered with the names of the drivers Flores, Cervantes, Teofilo, and their families, and notes that it was a gift presented on the occasion of Christmas, 2010.

The miraculous skulls remain under the jurisdiction of the church office in Ocoña, and the current father, Victor Vilca Añasco, realizes that there is a certain awkwardness with what goes on at the shrine. Praying to human skulls as intercessors with God is not exactly standard Catholic practice, and in fact attributing miraculous power to them directly would be a *de facto* heretical belief. Nevertheless, he finds the truckers to be of exemplary Christian faith, and chooses to believe that God works through the skulls. He comes to the shrine every Saturday at 3 p.m. to provide a weekly Mass for whichever truck drivers happen to be passing through, and to keep tabs on any newly reported miracles. These fall into several different categories, he reports, but the most common nowadays involve health issues. "There are frequent stories of drivers who have taken ill and are unable to complete their journey. They are often cured after pulling over and praying to the skulls." Father Añasco believes power at the Santuario is a divine reward for prayers offered to the souls of the deceased trio in purgatory, but admits that he cannot say with certainty how the miracles occur. "But I know they do," he affirms, "especially involving health, because I am one of the people who was cured. I had suffered for many months with severe ulcers—until I stopped here several years ago and prayed to the skulls for assistance. The ulcers stopped within days and have never returned." Thus convinced, the Father himself has been devotee of the sanctuary ever since, rewarding the skulls with incense, prayers, and votive candles whenever he comes to their shrine.

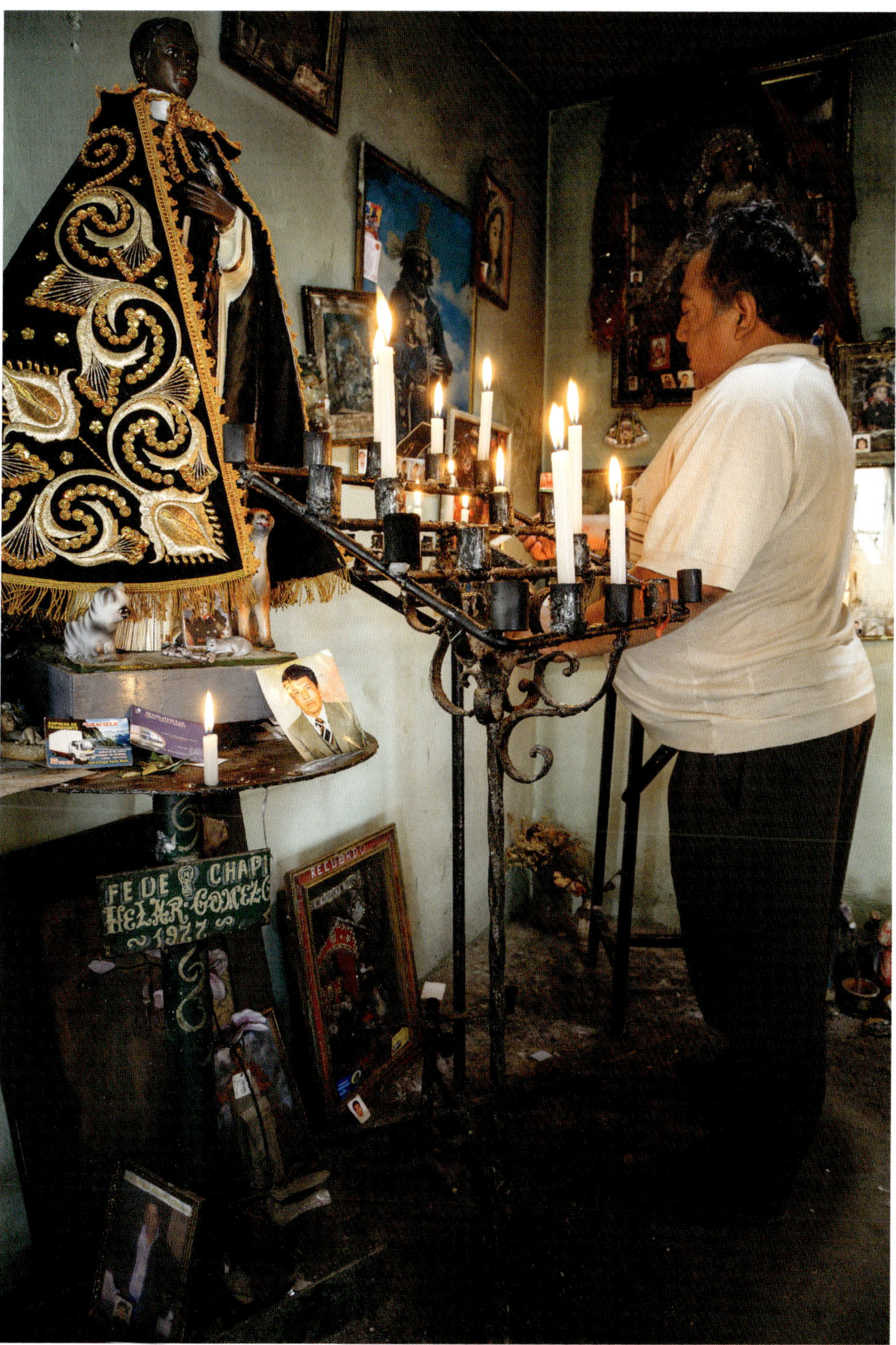
FE DE CHAPI
HELAR·GOMEZ
1977
RECUERDO
GRACIELA

EMPRESS & LOVER

Personifying Death in Mexico

SALVADOR OLGUÍN

Death is the Lady

MEXICO'S POPULAR CULTURE SEEMS TO BE INFUSED WITH AN uncanny fascination with death. Death imagery is so pervasive in the country it has become a major component of the national stereotype. Cartoonish sugar skulls and papier-mâché skeletons, typically associated with Día de los Muertos, spread out across street markets and retail stores all year long, delighting tourists and nationals alike. During the twentieth century José Guadalupe Posada's *Calaveras*, rescued from the penny press and popularized by Diego Rivera and other artists after the Mexican Revolution of 1910, quickly gained iconic status in the country.† Representations of death were also

---

† *Posada's Calaveras first appeared in Mexico City's newspapers and gazettes at the turn of the twentieth century. These engravings representing skeletons and skulls in various activities were produced in order to turn a satirical eye on the country's social inequalities during the regime of president Porfirio Díaz. Though popular, they were quickly forgotten due to the cheap nature of the periodicals in which they appeared. After the Mexican Revolution of 1910, Diego Rivera and other intellectuals became interested in Posada's work. Rivera included Posada's "Calavera Garbancera" in one of his major works. Originally meant to represent poor chickpea merchants who had indigenous ancestry, but rejected their traditions and imitated French customs and fashion trends, this Calavera was renamed "La Catrina" by Rivera, and quickly became an icon of Death personified in the country. Bellas Artes, 1997).*

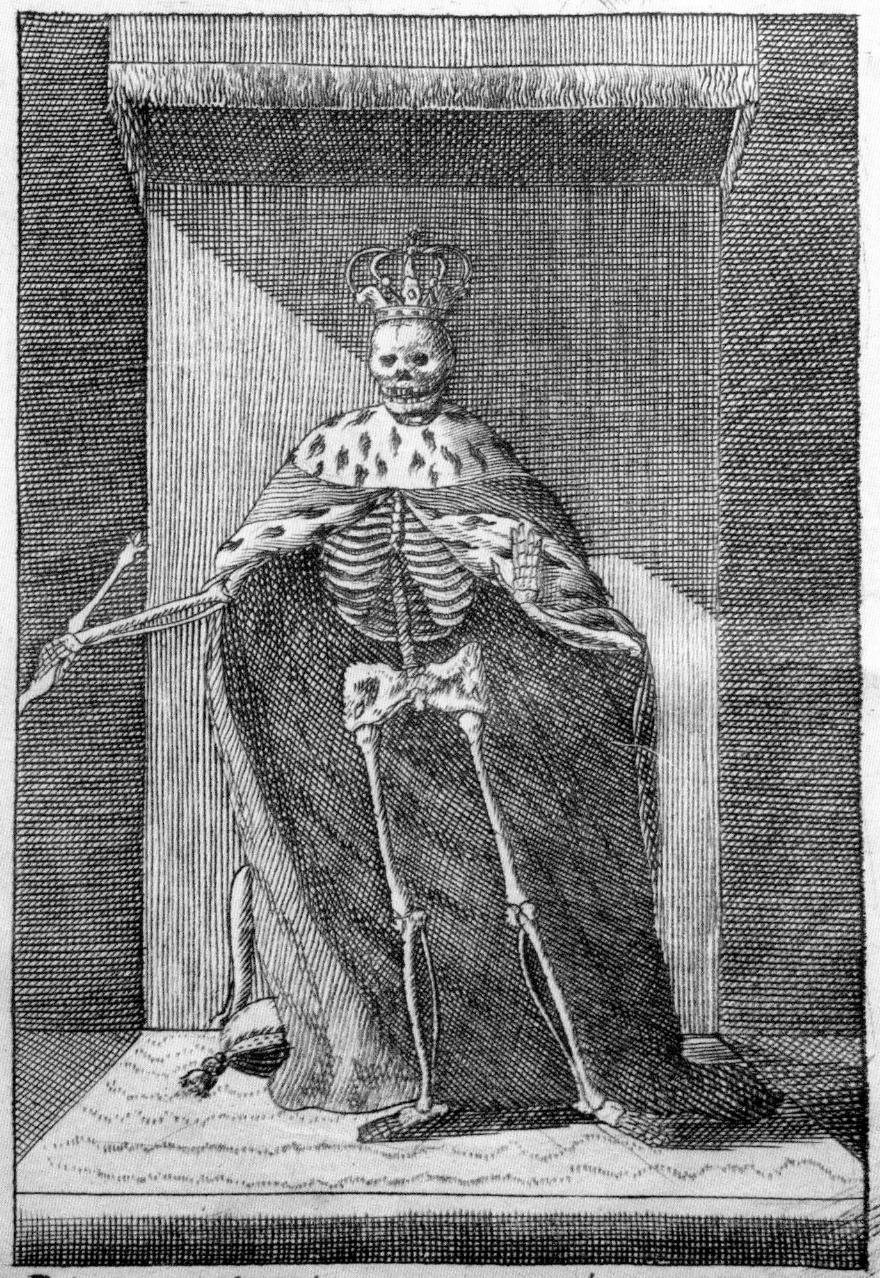

*Dixit: Cogitationem suam in eo esse ut om-
nem terām suo Subjugaret Imperio: Judit. cp. 2.*

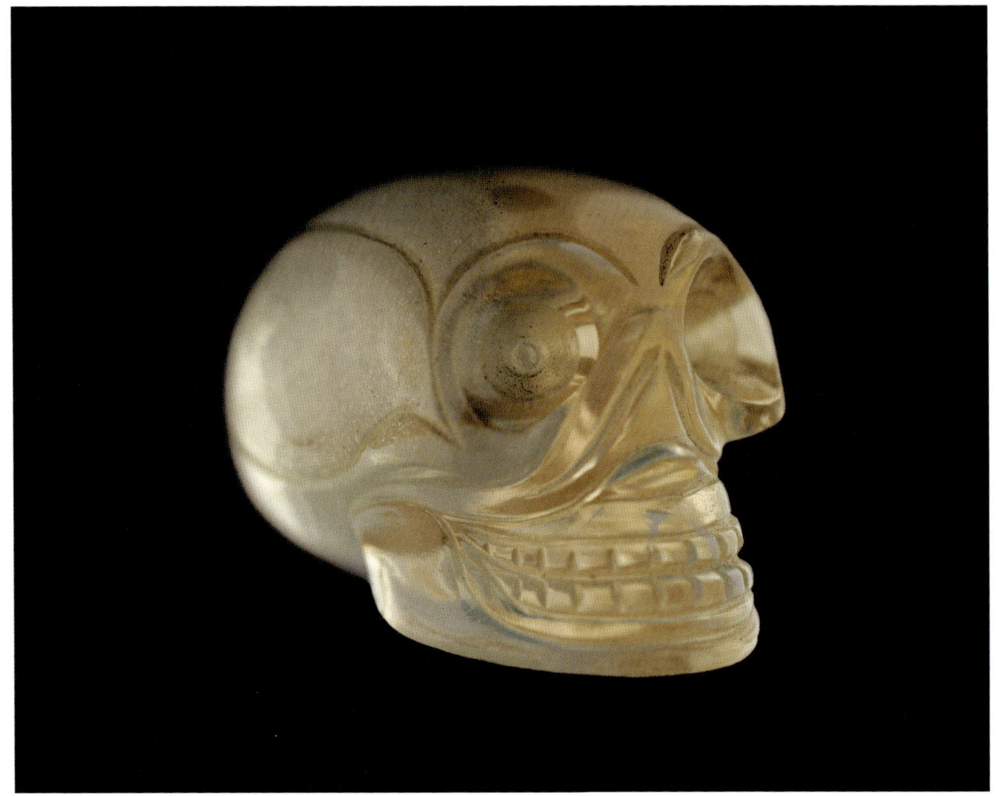

Image above: Skull made of pure quarz rock crystal. Courtesy of the Museo Nacional de la Muerte (National Museum of Death), Aguascalientes, Mexico.

present during the colonial period, and are a prominent feature of Aztec art; the pre-Columbian art of death is still quite visible in contemporary Mexican culture, regarded as a valuable part of the country's cultural heritage.

In *Death and the Idea of Mexico* (2005), Columbia University professor Claudio Lomnitz entertains the notion that death could be considered Mexico's "national totem," echoing a phrase first uttered by Guatemalan intellectual Luis Cardoza y Aragón.[†] But ideas about death in Mexico are as

---

† *Claudio Lomnitz-Adler,* Death And The Idea Of Mexico *(Brooklyn: Zone Books,*

diverse as the country itself, something that can easily be confirmed by examining the different traditions associated with Día de los Muertos across the country and in the United States. The different attitudes Mexicans have had towards this celebration throughout history, mapped meticulously by Lomnitz while he weaves a cultural and political history of representations of death in Mexico, are also very diverse. Attempting to provide a univocal explanation for this abundance of death imagery runs the risk of oversimplifying a rather rich and multilayered cultural phenomenon, and Lomnitz's genealogical approach is testament to this fact. His work and that of others like him indicate the need to look back and revisit the country's archives in search for new clues that may illuminate the origins of this proverbial fascination, especially at a time when the topic of death in Mexico has taken a truly somber meaning.

Image previous page: from Bolaños, Joaquín. La portentosa vida de la Muerte: emperatriz de los sepulcros, vengadora de los agravios del Altisimo, y muy señora de la humana naturaleza. *México: Impresa en la oficina de los herederos del Lic. D. Joseph de Jauregui, 1792.*

One aspect of this fascination is particularly ubiquitous: the tendency to project human attributes on death, to think of death as a character subject to human passions and, moreover, to portray her as a woman. This "Lady Death" is a character that haunts the country's imagination. She appears time and again in songs, illustrations, poems, proverbs and colloquial expressions. There are dozens of names for her; "la flaca" (the skinny one) and "la pelona" (the bald one), two of the names used to refer to La Santa Muerte ("Saint Death" or "The Holy

---

2005). Though ambiguous, this notion reflects the appropriation of popular and folk death imagery by ideological and political groups who have used it as a way to instigate nationalist sentiments in the country. Mexico's relationship with death has been presented as essentially different from that of every other culture and, therefore, a source of national pride by all sorts of groups in the country, from left-wing activists to tourism officers. Like other icons such as the Virgin of Guadalupe, which was used by one of the country's founding fathers to rally the masses during the first uprisings against the Spanish crown, nationalist groups, proponents of indigenismo, radical left-wingers and conservative Catholics alike have claimed this unique relationship with death and used it as a tool to put forward their own ideologies and agendas.

Death"), a folk saint worshipped in some areas of Mexico and the United States,[1] though they have been used by Mexicans to designate this mysterious female character long before the folk saint first appeared on the horizon. It is difficult to trace the origins of this Lady Death, but one of the first literary pieces devoted entirely to the personification of death in the country was Fray Joaquín Bolaños' *La Portentosa Vida de la Muerte* (*The Astounding Life of Death,* 1792), a biographical account of Death's life from cradle to grave.

[1] *For a study in English about the devotion to La Santa Muerte, see* Andrew Chesnut, Devoted to Death: Santa Muerte, *the Skeleton Saint (Oxford: Oxford University Press, 2012).*

Though perhaps it would be far-fetched to state that Bolaños single-handedly created this character that now haunts the imagination of an entire country, especially if we consider the hazardous history of the reception of his book in Mexico, it is nonetheless true that his was a very early prototype of it. In *La Portentosa Vida de la Muerte*, Joaquín Bolaños tells the life story of Death from a very human perspective: His protagonist has flaws, she is temperamental, and she often succumbs to her passions. The book is written in satirical tone and in it, Death herself flaunts her good sense of humor on many occasions. She is also portrayed as a salacious lover; she has romantic affairs with numerous characters, and her beauty is said to be proverbial. But she can also be treacherous, and show her ugly side. Bolaños' Death truly displays all the characteristics of a trickster. Remarkably, these traits introduced by Bolaños appear also in later works featuring Death as a character, all of which became part of the popular characterization of Death in the country.

La Portentosa Vida de la Muerte was first published in Mexico City in 1792. A little known engraver named Francisco Agüera Bustamante produced a series of illustrations to accompany this edition. The book would not be reprinted until 1983, when

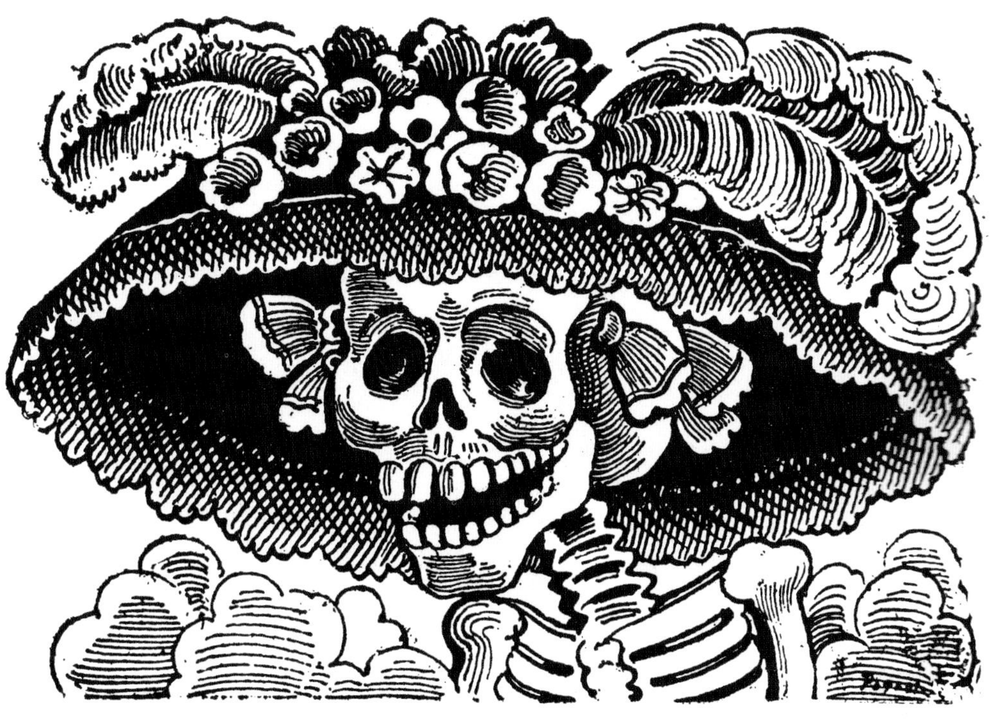

"Calavera Garbancera," circa 1913, etching by José Guadalupe Posada.

Mexico's National Institute of Fine Arts and Literature published it in an edition of 1,500 copies, with only a brief introduction. Prior to that edition the book had been all but forgotten, except for a few excerpts that were published in 1944 under the supervision of Mexican novelist Agustín Yáñez, whose commentary on the text was as dismissive as it was lackluster. The first critical edition of *La Portentosa Vida de la Muerte* had to wait until 1992. It was prepared by professor Blanca López de Mariscal, and published by El Colegio de México. It's the only critical edition of the book to this day.

Little is known about Fray Joaquín Bolaños' life. He was a Franciscan monk, and in the book he identifies himself as an "Apostolic Preacher of the Seminary College For The Propagation of the Faith of Mary Most Holy of Guadalupe."

When he wrote *La Portentosa Vida de la Muerte*, he was living and working in the city of Zacatecas, in the province of Nueva Galicia, in northern Mexico. We also know he was associated with the seat of the bishop's diocese in Monterrey, Nuevo León, and that part of his job as an Apostolic preacher was to ensure the conversion of the tribes that lived in the northern regions of New Spain, now northern Mexico and the southwestern United States. He published a few other minor titles, but beyond these sparse details most of what we know of him involves his most singular literary creation.

La Portentosa Vida de la Muerte was one of the first novels ever to be published in Latin America. Since it first appeared in 1792, Mexican literary critics and the country's cultural bureaucracy have dismissed it either on literary or moral grounds. The book was harshly criticized by José Antonio Alzate, a prominent priest and intellectual of that time, only months after its publication. Alzate wrote about *La Portentosa Vida de la Muerte* in his *Gaceta de Literatura de México* on three different occasions, in January, February and March of 1793. Besides being a theologian, Alzate was also a scientist. He was a corresponding member of the French Academy of Sciences and the Royal Spanish Academy. The main targets of Alzate's critique of the book were Bolaños' baroque style, the lack of a unifying plot, and the lightness with which he handled one of life's greatest mysteries. In fact, Alzate gave his critique the title of "Sancta Sancte Sunt Tractanda," which roughly translates as "Holy Matters Should Be Treated With Sanctity." His review of the book is meticulous; he quotes Bolaños profusely, and he provides moral and literary arguments against him. His tone is bitter. At some point, he complains he might have made a few mistakes while commenting on some of the passages, a fact he attributes to "the severe disturbance I experienced in my brain the first time

I read such an outlandish work."[2] He even comments on the illustrations, calling them "puerile allegories."[3] After Alzate's critiques of the book were published, *La Portentosa Vida de la Muerte* was quickly surrounded by silence and Fray Joaquín Bolaños stopped writing fiction.[4] Later intellectuals and literary critics in the country followed Alzate's example, dismissing Bolaños' book as a rarity in the best of cases. Even Blanca López de Mariscal, who praises the value of the book as well as of Agüera Bustamante's illustrations, and criticizes the excessive harshness of Alzate's review, echoes some of his prejudices.

Nevertheless, Mexico's popular representations of Death display traits that mirror Bolaños' picaresque style. Mexican personifications of Death seem to paint her with the colors of Bolaños' main character. The country's visual death imagery even resembles the style of Francisco Agüera Bustamante's engravings, as can easily be seen by comparing his work to that of José Guadalupe Posada.

La Portentosa*: A Seminal Text*

The true seminal nature of this book can be better explained by a brief examination of its contents. In the prologue of the book, Fray Joaquín Bolaños writes that he conceived *La Portentosa Vida de la Muerte* as a moralistic piece of literature to remind its Christian readers that death was a topic worthy of pious meditation. But he also confesses that his work is satirical, and that he wishes to portray Death as an empress whose majesty is rather ridiculous. Hence, Bolaños is clear about the fact that the tone of the entire book will be characterized by ambiguity, by a constant tension between seriousness and humor.

In spite of this ambiguity and Alzate's later condemnation, Bolaños' book received all the proper authorizations by the secular government and the Inquisition when it first appeared. It

[2] *Joaquín Bolaños,* La Portentosa Vida De La Muerte *(México, D.F.: INBA, Premia Ediciones, 1983), 360.*

[3] *Ibid.*

[4] *This explains the fact that so few copies of the book exist today. But various private collectors preserved copies of the book, some of which may still be out there. Since 1992, when Blanca López de Mariscal published her critical edition of* La Portentosa Vida de la Muerte, *more copies of the book have been discovered, some in Mexico and at least one in the United States.*

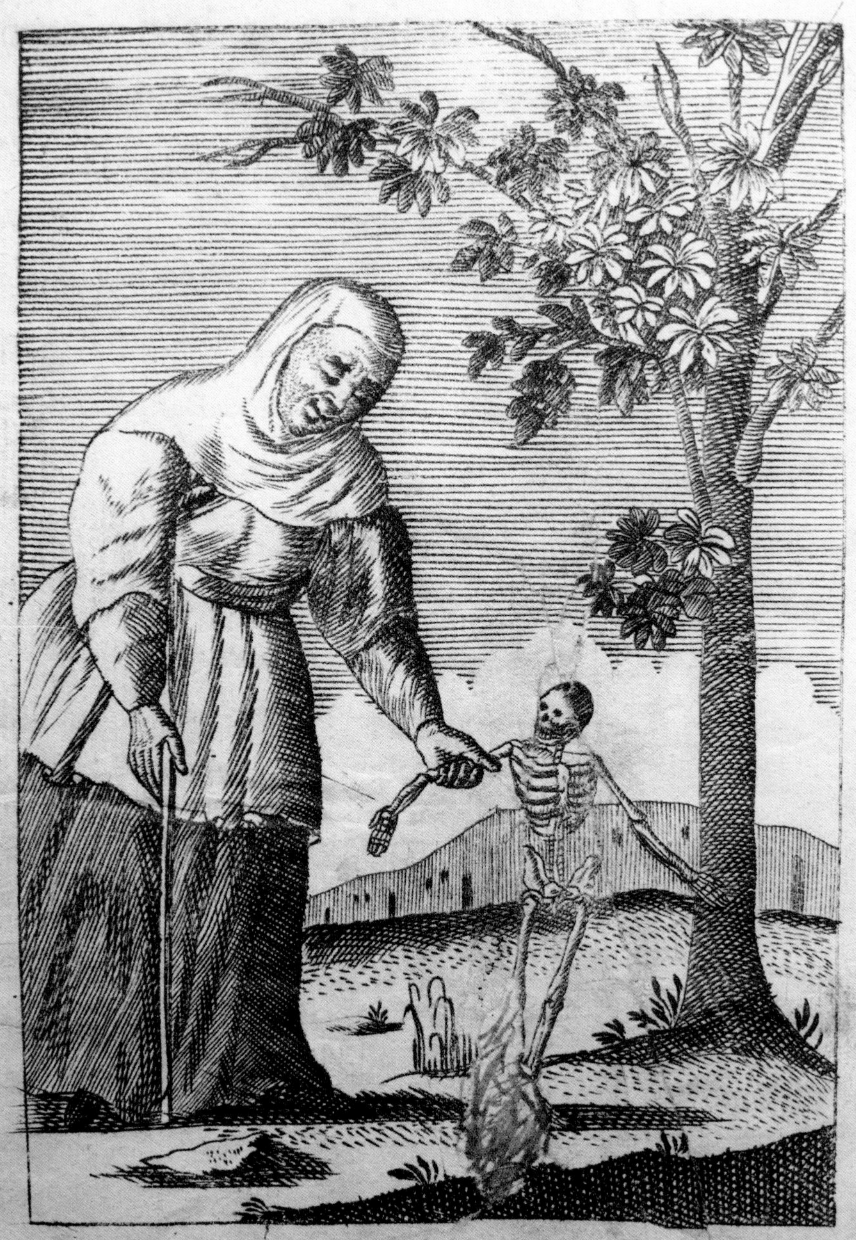

Concupiscentia cum conceperit p̄rit peccatum, peccatum vero generat mortem, Jacobi. ep.1.

is perhaps surprising that the Inquisition allowed it to be published in the first place, given the laxity and irreverence of Bolaños' treatment of death. Moreover, he constantly interprets the Bible and the writings of the Church Fathers in a rather indulgent way—something not always viewed with good eyes by the Catholic Church. The book is accompanied by an introductory "Censorship" written by Ignacio Gentil. This "Censorship" was a letter of authorization that customarily appeared in the first pages of a publication during that time. Ignacio Gentil was a "Calificador del Santo Oficio," an officer of the Inquisition, and as such, his job was to make sure no questionable material ever made it to the press. Gentil's "Censorship" clearly states that the book does not "contain anything that opposes our Holy Faith."[5]

After praising Bolaños for having chosen such a pious topic, and without further commenting on the content of the book, Gentil uses his "Censorship" as an opportunity to criticize the ideas of some of the European philosophers of his time, especially Voltaire and other intellectuals of the Enlightenment. He particularly complains about the wickedness of their deism, their lack of piety, and their mechanistic views about God and the universe. Due to his sudden change of subject and sparse commentaries on *La Portentosa*, it is difficult not to suspect that Gentil did not read the entire book, and chose to trust on Bolaños' moral integrity instead. The fact that Bolaños dedicated *La Portentosa Vida de la Muerte* to Manuel María Trujillo, another officer of the Inquisition, was probably one of the reasons why he was given the necessary authorizations.

Throughout the book, Bolaños is less interested in religious orthodoxy than in revealing private and extravagant details about Death's life. He relies heavily on passages from the Bible and the Church Fathers in order to support his biographical reports. One of the first things that concern him is establishing

Image left: Young death with "Concupiscence," her grandmother. Bolaños, Joaquín. La portentosa vida de la Muerte: emperatriz de los sepulcros, vengadora de los agravios del Altisimo, y muy señora de la humana naturaleza. *México: Impresa en la oficina de los herederos del Lic. D. Joseph de Jauregui, 1792.*

Lady Death's ancestry. Her father, he claims, was Adam's sin; her mother, the guilt experienced by Eve after the original sin. Since no family is complete without a grandmother, Bolaños deems it necessary to find out who is the grandmother of Death, dedicating all of the fourth chapter to the question. After carefully studying the scriptures, he comes to the conclusion that the true grandmother of Death is a lady by the name of "Concupiscence": an enticing and seductive old woman whose main attribute is that she gives birth to sin in the hearts of men. She is like "a household dog that bites the people of its own house without barking," writes Bolaños. In the end, he adds, "her own Granddaughter will avenge our grievances, putting out the fires of concupiscence in the midst of the frozen ashes of the Sepulcher."[6] Agüera Bustamante charmingly illustrates this chapter portraying a very young Death, a child-sized skeleton held by the wise hand of her grandmother while they seem to be out for a stroll. Like some kind of parody of a biblical writer, Bolaños bases his genealogy of Death in a verse from the Epistle of James, and later in the chapter he mentions Saint Ambrose, Saint Thomas Aquinas and Saint Augustine to give more credit to his findings.

[6] *Ibid.*, 29.

Bolaños' technique of structuring his tale around loosely interpreted Bible verses and isolated passages from the Church Fathers becomes less careful as the book progresses. He improvises. His interpretation of the Bible becomes more daring. For example, when writing about the death of a certain sinner, Bolaños recalls the parable of the ten virgins from the Book of Matthew. The Church teaches that foolish sinners can be compared to the five virgins who were not prepared for the arrival of the husband. The Church also teaches that the husband in the parable is none other than Jesus Christ himself. But according to Bolaños, the real mystery of the parable of the ten virgins is the identity of the bride. He knows the virgins are not waiting to marry the husband, as this would make Jesus a polygamist. The virgins from the parable are actually the bridesmaids. After explaining all this, Bolaños puts forward his own hypothesis: "for me, Death is represented in this Bride."[7] He goes on to say that in the End of Days, Death will follow her husband's command and bring doom to all sinners before being thrown into the Lake of Fire herself. But suggesting that Death is the bride of Christ is something Bolaños is not ready to defend, so he immediately makes it clear he doesn't mean to change the literal meaning of the parable, and that he leaves the matter to the consideration of wiser, holier men.

[7] *Ibid.*, 46.

In another passage Bolaños finds a similarly suggestive connection between Death and God the Father. Bolaños is writing about how beautiful Death can look when her task is to collect a soul that is pure. Taking a verse in Psalm 16 as his point of departure, Bolaños tells the story of a certain righteous man who passed away after a life of good deeds. Since this was a special occasion, "Death appeared so radiant, so peaceful, so pretty, so unusually fine-looking, so graceful and so beautiful, that God himself was left enamored (*enamorado*: "in love") by her wonderful beauty."[8] This is Bolaños' way of explaining what the Bible means when it says the death of a saint is precious to the eyes of God.

[8] *Ibid.*, 112.

These and other episodes stress the character's femininity as a very important component of Death's personality. As a lady, she is definitely ahead of her time. She enjoys and seeks the company of men—she is said to be particularly fond of doctors. But in spite of having several friends and lovers, Bolaños portrays her as a strong and independent female character—she is, after all, an empress. She is said to have married many men throughout her life, but since all of her husbands died before the marriages were consummated, she is always free to marry someone new if she feels like it. In *La Portentosa Vida de la Muerte*, Death is not merely a female version of the Grim Reaper. She is not the Great Equalizer either. On the contrary: she has her favorites, and even though she fulfills her duty with diligence, she mourns the deaths of some and rejoices on the deaths of others. She's bound by God to do her job of taking the souls of the mortals, and she complies; but she also conspires with the devil and even seeks out his help when she is trying to expand the reach of her ominous "Empire in the Americas."

La Portentosa Vida de la Muerte is truly a seminal text, not only because of its irreverent treatment of the topic, but because many of the traits that make up the personality of Bolaños' character can still be found in today's Mexican personifications of death. One of the most peculiar ones is her gender: still to this day, death is usually personified in Mexico as an intriguing woman. There are some notable exceptions to this—Bruno Traven's tale "Macario" is one of them.[9] But from La Catrina to La Santa Muerte, death is almost always conceived as a woman. This is not necessarily due to the fact that *muerte* is a female noun in Spanish. As Karl S. Guthke suggests in *The Gender of Death* (1999), assigning death a gender has more to do with complex cultural and historical tendencies than with grammar. In his book, Guthke gives many examples of how the norm for assigning a gender to death varies regardless of the grammatical gender of the word in any given language. He refers, for example, to the "predominantly male representation of death in Medieval art and literature" which had "little, if anything to do with the grammatical gender of the word for death."[10] There's not enough space here to elucidate the complex historical and cultural reasons why Mexico's personifications of death have tended to favor the female gender, but what is clear is that Bolaños'

[9] *In it, Death is portrayed as a man who successfully convinces Macario, the main character, to share a turkey with him, after God and the devil have failed in their attempts to convince him of the same thing. The tale was adapted into a film in Mexico. It is relevant to note that Bruno Traven was not Mexican—his country of origin is still a matter of debate.*

[10] *Karl Siegfried Guthke,* The Gender Of Death: A Cultural History In Art And Literature *(Cambridge: Cambridge University Press, 1999), 41-42.*

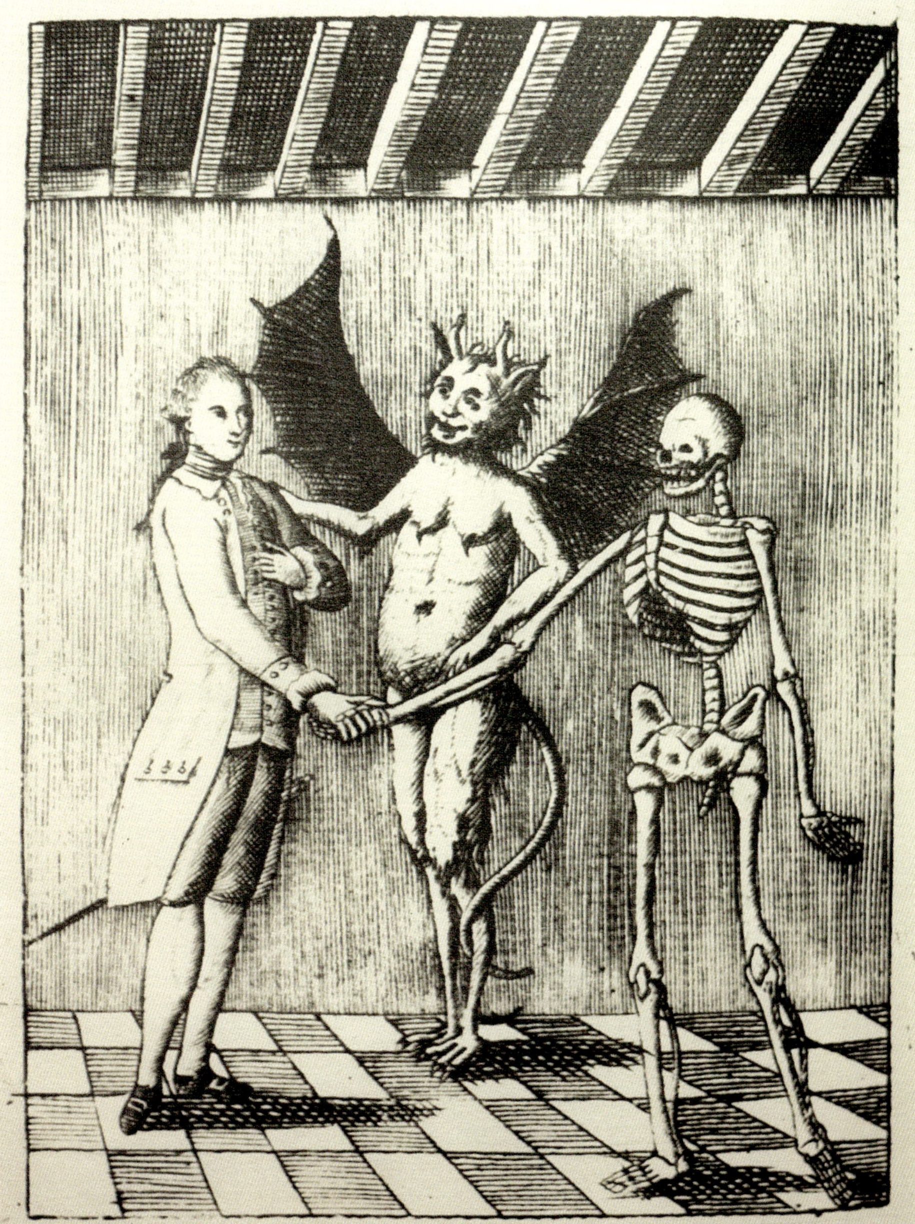

Percussimus foedus cum morte. Isaiae cp. 28.

Image previous page: Death wedding a doctor, from Bolaños, Joaquín. La portentosa vida de la Muerte: emperatriz de los sepulcros, vengadora de los agravios del Altisimo, y muy señora de la humana naturaleza. *México: Impresa en la oficina de los herederos del Lic. D. Joseph de Jauregui, 1792.*

book was one of the first examples of this tendency in the country. His character is not like the monstrous deities from the Aztec underworld, who devoured their adepts. Bolaños' characterization of Death as a clever, passionate and powerful woman was one of the earliest of many future literary and poetic personifications of death in Mexico that would display similar features.

The words Bolaños used to describe Death's physical beauty appear to be echoed by vernacular poems such as a popular folk song from Oaxaca called "La Llorona" (The Weeping Woman). This is a song of love and despair, and it's dedicated to a mysterious lady. Several verses and stanzas as well as a widespread interpretation of the song suggest this lady is none other than death personified—incidentally, "La Llorona" is one of the popular names of Death in Mexico. La Llorona is portrayed as a desired woman or an estranged lover, beautiful and alluring. But the song is melancholic, and often references death and dying while praising this mysterious woman's beauty. In one of the verses of the song we find the following words: "you were wearing such a beautiful *huipil*, Llorona / that I thought you were the Virgin." The song is comparing a lover to the Virgin Mary because she was beautifully dressed, and not because of some moral or spiritual quality, but what's interesting to notice is the suggestion that Death can look as beautiful as the Virgin, which is a way of interconnecting death and the divine that echoes Bolaños' text.

A comparison between Death and the Virgin Mary also takes place in the form of certain figurines used for the veneration of La Santa Muerte. Revering Death for her beauty is a common practice among followers of La Santa Muerte. Santa Muerte adepts call her "mi niña blanca" (my white little girl), and dress her up in beautiful garments. Words of affection are commonly used in prayers to Santa Muerte, who is seen as a powerful yet beautiful woman with whom it is possible to bargain. Among other practices, followers of Santa Muerte share alcoholic beverages, cigarettes and other substances with statues and figurines of La Flaquita (the Skinny Lady). These substances and other offerings must not be absent from her altars, because she is known to enjoy drinking and smoking. In fact, followers are urged to drink and smoke with her, to treat her with familiarity, because she is a dame who enjoys partying.

Mexican representations of the beautiful Death tend to display a baroque sensibility. This baroque sensibility has deep roots in the colonial period. Bolaños never idealizes his main character: he portrays Death as a changing, capricious figure, full of contrasts. "She is as sad as death, and on the other hand, she's as happy as Easter," he writes. And also: "She deceives us all, and she makes us all see the truth. Her thoughts are so delicate and fine that they make some people go mad, and others come back to their senses... She disrupts every order and, at the same time, she puts all things back in order... She's as dark as night, but also as clear as the light of disillusionment. She toys with mortals and nobody toys with her." She is as deceiving as she is beautiful. She's a treacherous lover who enjoys an uncanny proximity with the divine.[11]

[11] *This depiction of Death as a treacherous lover is also echoed by twentieth-century poet José Gorostiza. In his long poem* Muerte Sin Fin *(Death Without End) he teases death and calls her "putilla del rubor helado" ("little whore with frozen blush"), before asking her to go to the devil with him. See José Gorostiza,* Muerte Sin Fin y Otros Poemas *(México, D.F.: Fondo de Cultura Económica, 1983).*

Conclusion

According to Claudio Lomnitz, in *La Portentosa Vida de la Muerte* Fray Joaquín Bolaños teeters "between a fire-and-brimstone moralism and truculent entertainment."[12] Bolaños does get serious in some parts of the book, but the passages where he is moralizing must be taken with a grain of salt. The overall tone invites readers to always keep a healthy sense of humor, and not to take their own mortality too seriously. This doesn't mean *La Portentosa Vida de la Muerte* is not a real attempt to

[12] *Lomnitz, 288.*

entice its readers to meditate about mortality; it just treats the whole subject with humoristic ambivalence. This ambivalence also permeates Agüera's illustrations, and it can be found across the spectrum of Mexico's representations of death even today.

Take, for example, Mexican ranchera music, a genre known for its exaltation of love and passion as well as its blatant machismo. First created during the 1930s, right after the Mexican Revolution, ranchera music cemented a stereotype of Mexico's culture that is still around, and which involves sombreros, fiestas and cockfights. Like in many other cultural expressions in the country, death is an important theme of ranchera; defying death, laughing in the face of death, or fearlessly seeking refuge in death after a love affair that ended badly. Interestingly, many of the elements enlisted by Octavio Paz as being the core of Mexican views on death in *The Labyrinth of Solitude* can actually be traced back to some of the most famous ranchera songs. One of these songs, called "La Muerte," shows that even ranchera falls under the spell of the ambivalent, baroque character that Bolaños' book first drafted back in the eighteenth century. At the beginning of the song, Death comes into the scene wearing colorful garments. The singer asks her to give him a kiss (ven dame un beso, Pelona, or "come give me a kiss, Baldy"). At the end of the song, however, Death leaves him alone and goes away singing, walking by the cacti. The singer replies, in a final stand that is also a proof of Death's indifference: "So what's the deal, Baldy? Will you take me or not?" (*¿En qué quedamos, Pelona? ¿Me llevas o no me llevas?*). Ranchera music stresses again the ambivalent spirit of Mexican representations of death.

Photo of Santa Muerte figurine, from a Los Angeles Santa Muerte botanica. Photo by Joanna Ebenstein.

Even the most stereotypical representations of death in Mexico can present various layers of subtlety. Death seems to bring tension and ambivalence into any formula. Joaquín Bolaños' *La Portentosa Vida de la Muerte*, an almost forgotten, long-lost seminal

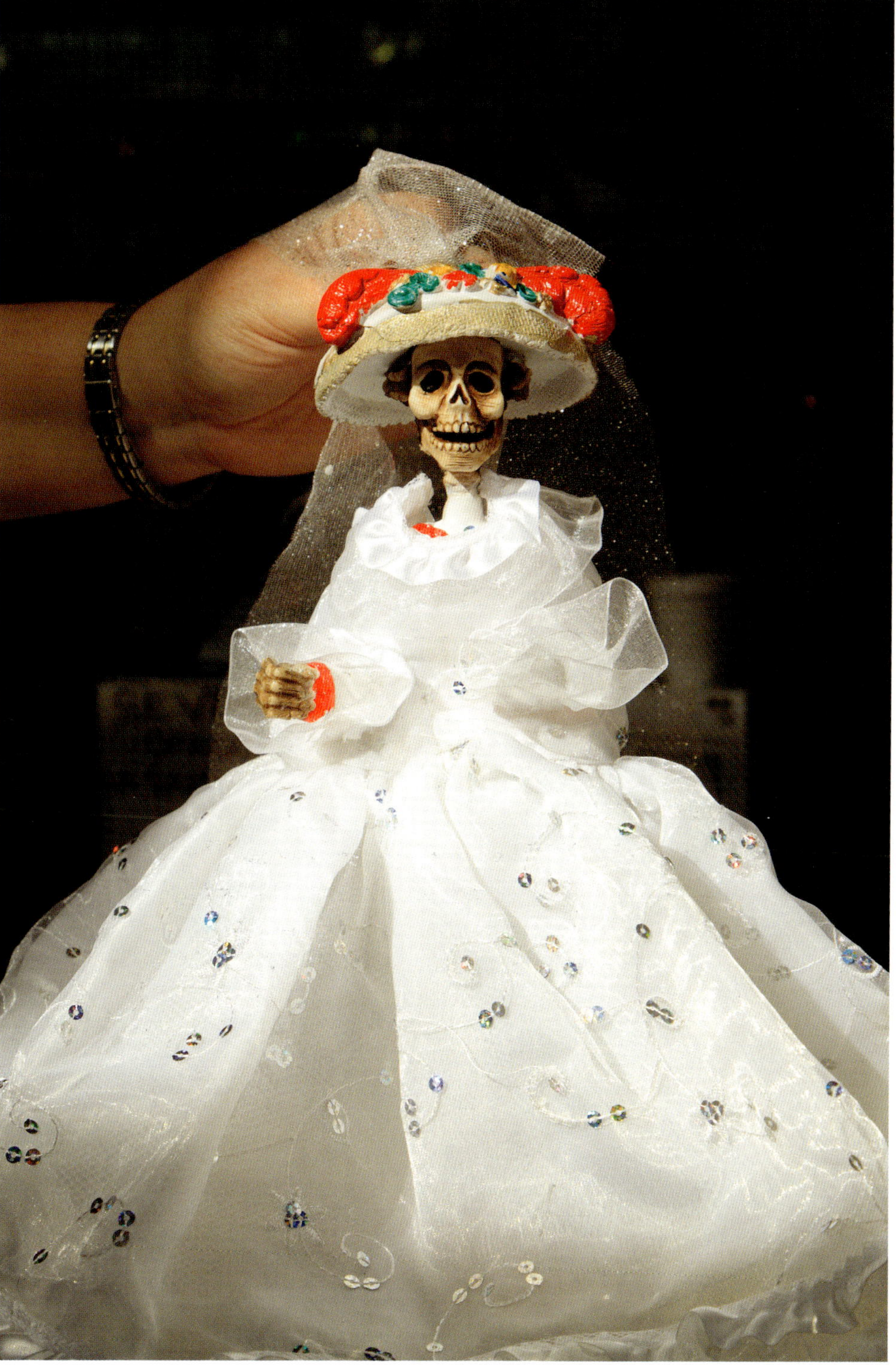

book, has a lot to tell us today about the origins of Mexico's most iconic personifications of death. Its humorous approach and ambivalent spirit make it a remarkable piece within a set of death-related cultural objects scattered worldwide, which project a human face on mortality, something often overlooked by more orthodox points of view.

[BIBLIOGRAPHY]

Bolaños, Joaquín. *La Portentosa Vida de la Muerte, Emperatriz de los Sepulcros, Vengadora de los Agravios del Altísimo, y Muy Señora de la Humana Naturaleza.* 1st ed. Mexico: Impresa en la oficina de los herederos del Lic D Joseph de Jauregui, 1792.

Bolaños, Joaquín. *La Portentosa Vida De La Muerte, Emperatriz De Los Sepulcros, Vengadora De Los Agravios Del Altísimo Y Muy Señora De La Humana Naturaleza.* [Edited by Blanca López de Mariscal.] México, D.F. : El Colegio de México, Centro de Estudios Lingüísticos y Literarios, 1992.

Bolaños, Joaquín. *La Portentosa Vida De La Muerte.* México, D.F.: INBA, Premia Ediciones, 1983.

Bramón, Francisco, Agustín Yáñez, and Joaquín Bolaños. *Los Sirgueros De La Virgen.* México: Universidad Nacional Autónoma, 1944.

Caso, Alfonso, Lowell Dunham, and Miguel Covarrubias. *The Aztecs: People Of The Sun.* Norman: University Of Oklahoma Press, 1970, c1958.

Gorostiza, José. *Muerte Sin Fin y Otros Poemas.* México, D.F.: Fondo de Cultura Económica, 1983, c1964.

Guthke, Karl Siegfried. *The Gender Of Death: A Cultural History In Art And Literature. Cambridge*, U.K.: Cambridge

University Press, 1999.

Lomnitz-Adler, Claudio. *Death And The Idea Of Mexico.* Brooklyn, N.Y.: Zone Books , 2005.

López Casillas, Mercurio and Gregory Dechant. La Muerte *En El Impreso Mexicano: Images Of Death In Mexican Prints.* México: Editorial RM, 2008.

Paz, Octavio. *El Laberinto de la Soledad.* Madrid: Cátedra, 1997.

Traven, B. *Macario.* Mexico: Compañía General De Ediciones, 1978, c1960.

MORBID CURIOSITY *MEETS* MORBID ANATOMY

RICHARD HARRIS

WHEN I FIRST APPROACHED GREG KNIGHT, THE HEAD CURATOR OF the Chicago Cultural Center, about an exhibition based on my art collection, he was very enthusiastic. The fact that the theme of the collection was "death" didn't seem to bother him. However, when he finally found a time slot in his exhibition schedule for my collection to be exhibited, he was not certain that the selection committee would okay a show about death. Fortunately for Greg and I, we both were pleasantly surprised by the committee's acceptance of the exhibition, which ran from January 28 through July 8, 2012. The exhibition, "Morbid Curiosity: The Richard Harris Collection," became the most successful exhibition in the thirty-three year history of the Cultural Center, with a total attendance of well over a hundred thousand visitors.

How did I come to this thematic subject for my collection? I have long had an interest in the art history of the human body and had begun buying antique human anatomy books and prints. I was selling my print collection of Picasso, Matisse and Rembrandt at Maastricht, the world famous art fair in the Netherlands in 2000 and 2001, when I found a dealer who was exhibiting and selling

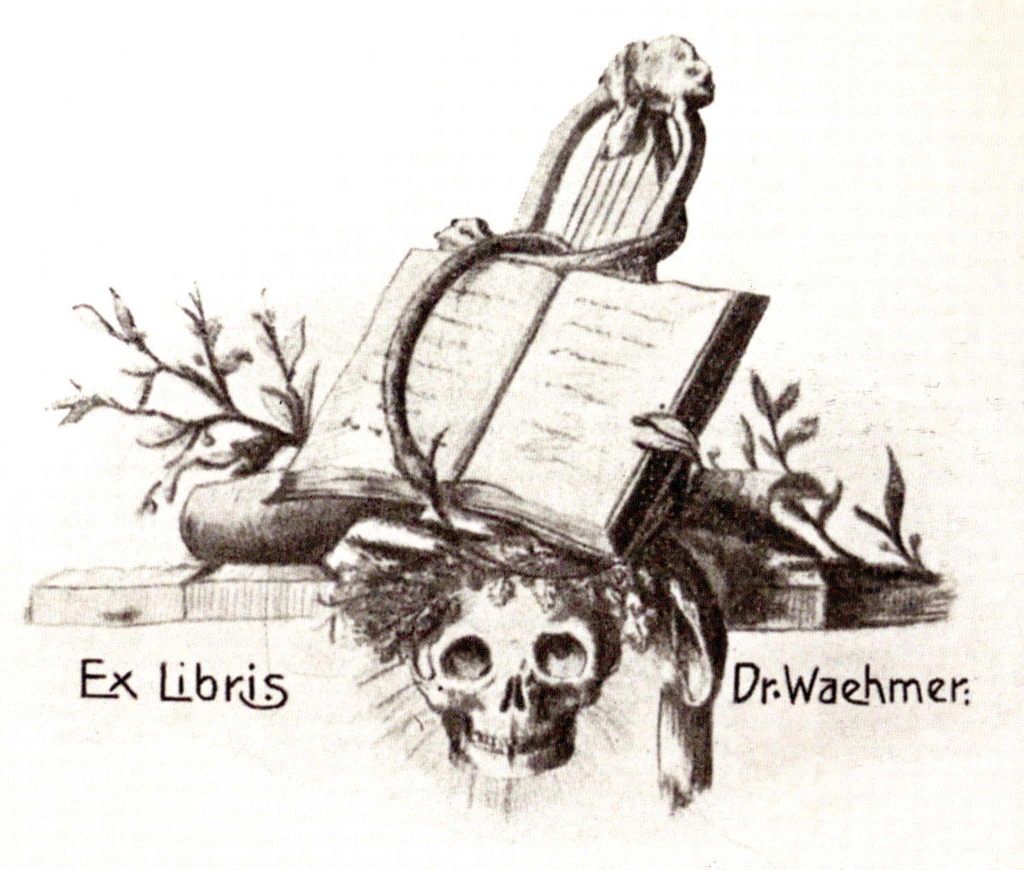

his collection of paintings, prints, photographs and sculptural pieces of human skulls and skeletons under the title *memento mori* (remember we will all die).

It was then that I decided to create a much broader collection of objects that I felt would tell a fuller and more inclusive visual story of death than a collection of only masterpieces. The collection would be a very personal one through my own eyes and aesthetic. My art interests include outsider and ethnographic art, along with ephemera and vernacular photographs. With almost two thousand pieces in this collection, I believe that I have fairly well accomplished my objectives.

Artist Unknown, Ex Libris from a book belonging to Dr. Waehmer. Courtesy of the Richard Harris Collection.

A brief overview of some of the images from my collection is in order. Spanning a broad time frame, from 2000 BC to today, these objects also illustrate the differences and similarities of cultures around the world in their practices of the rituals of "death."

A well-known example of this is the "day of the dead" ceremony of the Mexican community, a celebration that seeks to reunite the living with their deceased loved ones. The grave site is decorated with beautiful flowers, food, and mementos that the deceased enjoyed during their lifetime. One of the two works of art that illustrates this attitude toward death is the wonderful altarpiece by Roberto Hernandez in honor of Miguel Hidalgo, a great Mexican patriot. The altar features a large papier-mâché figure of Hidalgo standing atop a wedding cake-like layered structure holding the Mexican flag; on the lower layers are other figures, as well as food, flowers and candles. Another work on a similar theme is the twenty-four piece ceramic installation by Zenaida Raphael, a young Mexican woman who represents the height of the Mexican folk art tradition. *El Panteon* (*The Cemetery*) is made up of many skeletal figures dancing, singing and carousing at a cemetery site.

Over the years, the collection has grown to inlcude a number of important works of art. Among the more noteworthy prints are *Tod und Frau* by Kathe Kollwitz, *My Portrait as a Skeleton* by James Ensor, *The Coat of Arms with the Skull* and *Four Horsemen of the Apocalypse* by Albrecht Dürer, and *Death Appearing to a Wedded Couple from an Open Grave*, by Rembrandt van Rijn. A few of the special drawings, watercolors, and gouaches are the *Triumph of Death* by Maerten van Heemskerck, *The Death Room / The Last Rites*, a late fifteenth-century page from a book of hours, *Old Fears Are Still Valid*, by Marlene Dumas, and *The Living Shell*, by Pavel Tchelitchew. Some of the wonderful paintings include

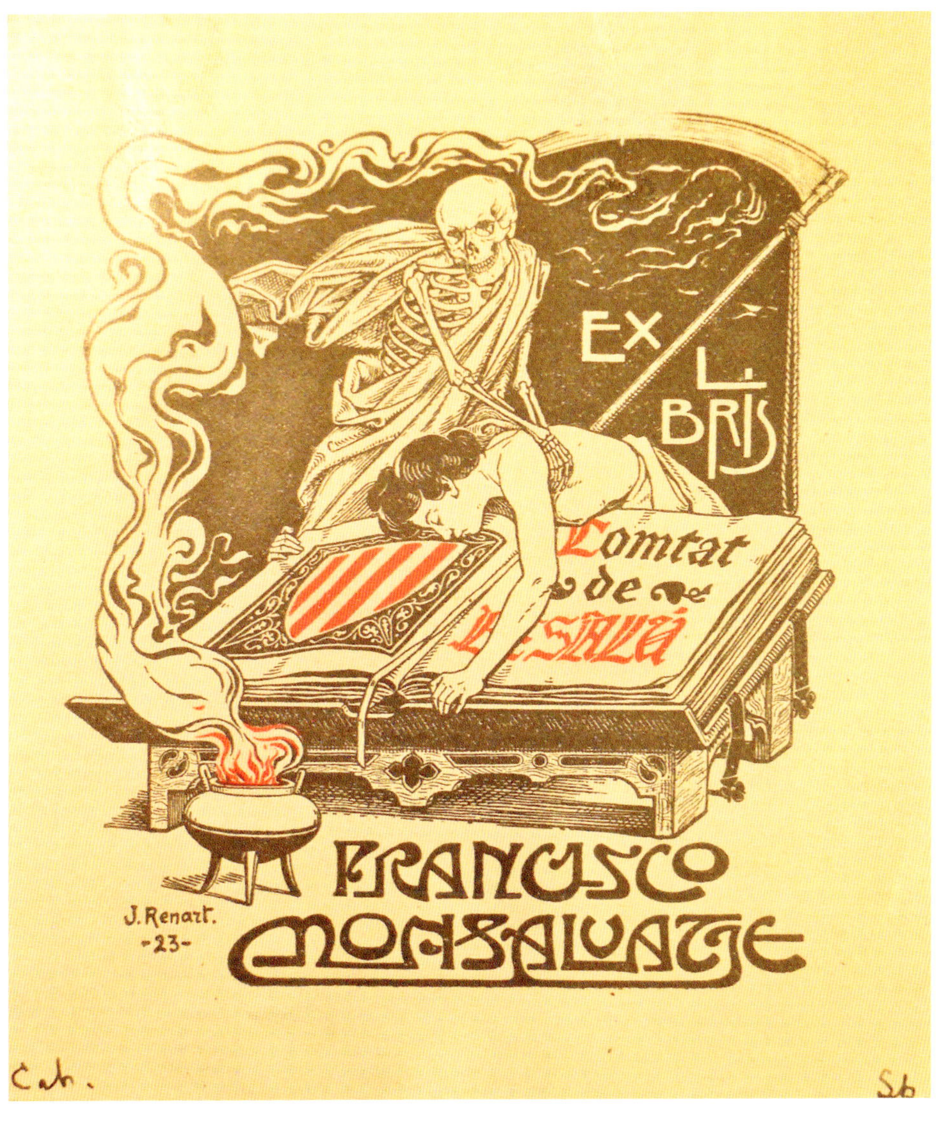

Joaquim Renart Garcia, Ex Libris, 1923, from a book belonging to Francisco Monsalvatge. Courtesy of the Richard Harris Collection.

the northern European masters Adrian van Utrecht, *Vanitas Still Life with a Bouquet and a Skull*; Barthel Bruyn's *Portrait of a Man/A Skull in a Niche*; Marinus van Reymerswaete's *St. Jerome in His Study*; and an unknown lower-German master's *Fall and*

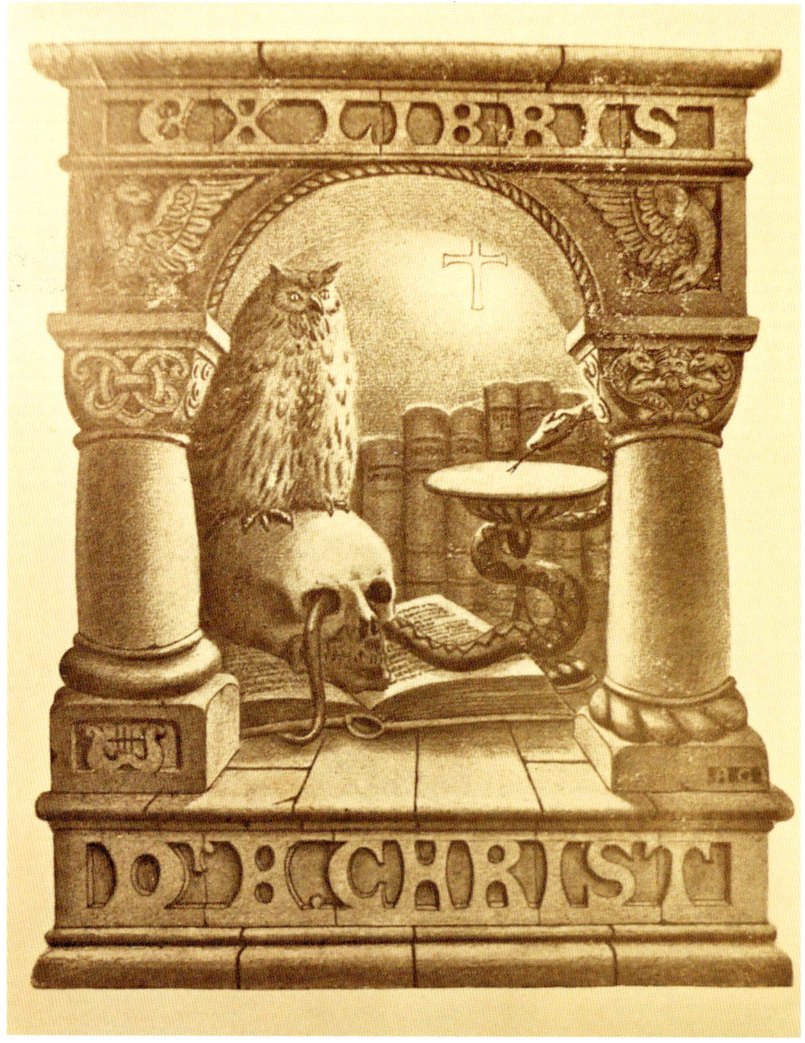

A.G. , Ex Libris from a book belonging to Dr. H. Christ. Courtesy of the Richard Harris Collection.

Redemption of Man. A contemporary painting, *The Face in the Rage of Red*, by Jim Dine, matches these old master paintings in its scale, intensity and power. And then there are the contemporary photographic gems, including *Skull Walking Cane*, by Robert

Mapplethorpe, *Vanitas*, by Vic Muniz, Graciela Iturbide's *Procession*, and Andre Serrano's *The Morgue*. A large collection of vernacular photographs also capture the contemporary world view of death created by amateur photographers.

From my early interest in book collecting I have added a number of bound books and print series based on the "dance of death" theme. The earliest example is a copy of the first Latin edition of Hans Holbein's *Totentanz*, which set the standard for all "dance of death" works of art.

Some of my favorite three-dimensional objects include the late eighteenth-century, elephant-ivory tusk decorated with scenes from Dürer's great print *Knight, Death and the Devil*, John Isaac's grotesque wax sculpture *Are You Still Mad at Me*, the elegant okimono wood carving of a skull and snake by the Japanese artist Sukeyuki, June Leaf's simple *Gentleman on Green Table*, and finally Jodie Carey's great three-chandelier installation, *In the Eyes of Others*. (Each chandelier is created from three thousand plaster bones. It is spectacular!)

Possibly the most unique part of the entire collection is the six great *war/anti-war* print series. The earliest set is the seventeenth-century *Les Grandes Misères de la Guerre*, by Jacques Callot, followed by Francisco Goya's nineteenth-century masterpiece *Disasters of War*. The early twentieth century is represented by the powerful *Der Krieg*, by Otto Dix, and the late twentieth century by the Chapman brothers' *Disasters of War*. In the twenty-first century, the American artist Sandow Birk created fifteen huge woodcuts, *Depravities of War;* his depictions of the Iraq war are the final pieces to this extraordinary war collection. I don't believe that these six extraordinary war series exist together in any collection in the world.

In a collection this large there are unusual specialty groupings that might get lost if not for their sheer numbers. One example is the pop-culture collection of 150 T-shirts of rock groups with their skull/skeleton imagery. Another is the group of 155 *ex-libris* prints all having a definite *memento mori* theme, with skull/skeleton references each representing a disparate view of death iconography. The theme of *memento mori* represents another major portion of the collection, including the themes of *vanitas* and the "dance of death." In the pages that follow are some examples of this tradition: in addition to the *ex libris* plates, there are metamorphic postcards (*Tête de Mort*) of the early twentieth century. These images are meant to fool the eye: from a distance the image on the card appears to be a skull, but on closer inspection you see that the skull image has been created from a grouping of figures and objects placed together to give the appearance of a skull. The collection of these postcards as well as other inexpensive pieces of ephemera give the entire collection its uniqueness and quirkiness, which I love. The balance of the collection amplifies and gives more depth to all the themes and subthemes that make my personal journey through the art world of "death" so important.

Upon completing the collection and after its very successful exhibition run at the Chicago Cultural Center, I realized that the art collection could serve and has already begun to serve another purpose. On my frequent visits to the Chicago exhibition I would often overhear visitors talking about their own personal experiences with the death of loved ones. It is my hope that this exhibition or iterations of it will travel around the world and act as a catalyst for a wider more open discussion and conversation about death.

[FOLLOWING IMAGES]

Page 358: Artist Unknown, "La Vie la Mort, Leben und Tod": *Tête de Mort*, c. 1900s postcard. Courtesy of the Richard Harris Collection.

Page 359: Artist Unknown, "Tête de Mort, Depose Dans Tous Les Pays": *Tête de Mort*, c. 1900s postcard. Courtesy of the Richard Harris Collection.

Page 360-361: Favei Bnichlm (illegible) *Ex Libris* from a book belonging to Karl Andres. Courtesy of the Richard Harris Collection.

Page 362: Artist Unknown "Homo Perit Liber Manet": *Ex Libris*, 1902; From a book belonging to Ramon Peres. Courtesy of the Richard Harris Collection.

Page 363: Artist Unknown, Ex Libris. Courtesy of the Richard Harris Collection.

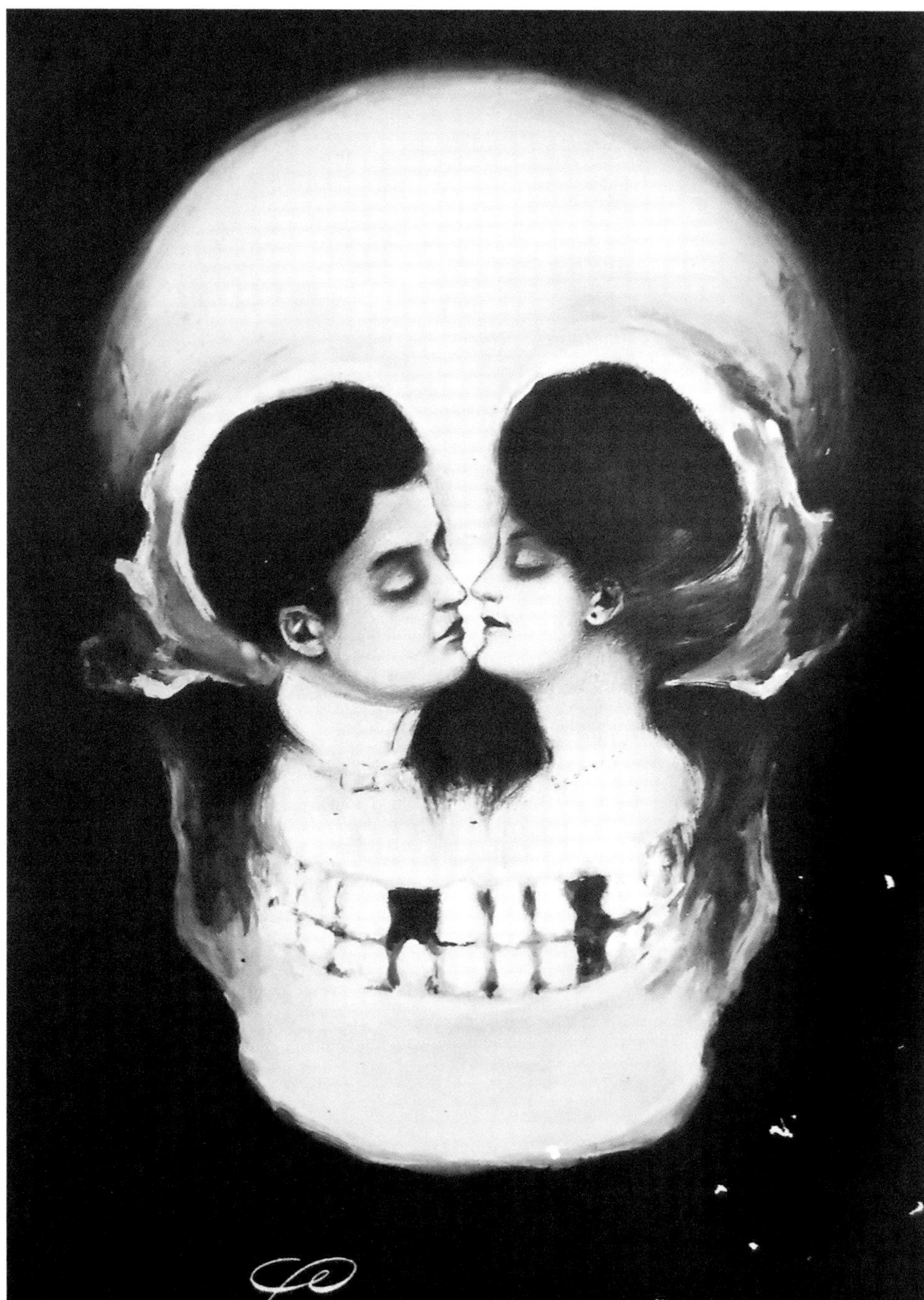
„La vie et la mort"
„Leben und Tod"
A.R.& C.i.B.3969.

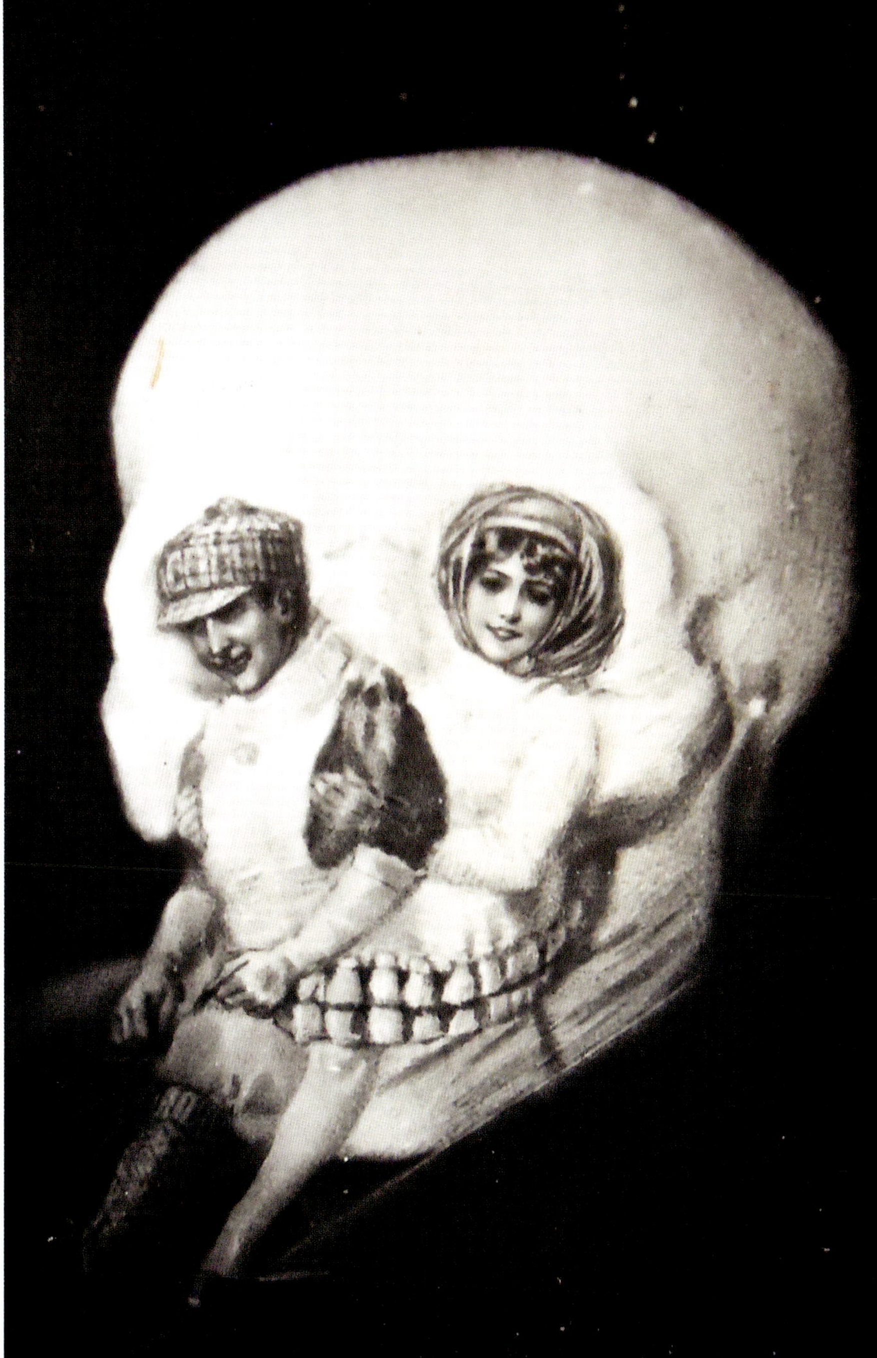
Tête de mort.
DEPOSÉ DANS TOUS LES PAYS

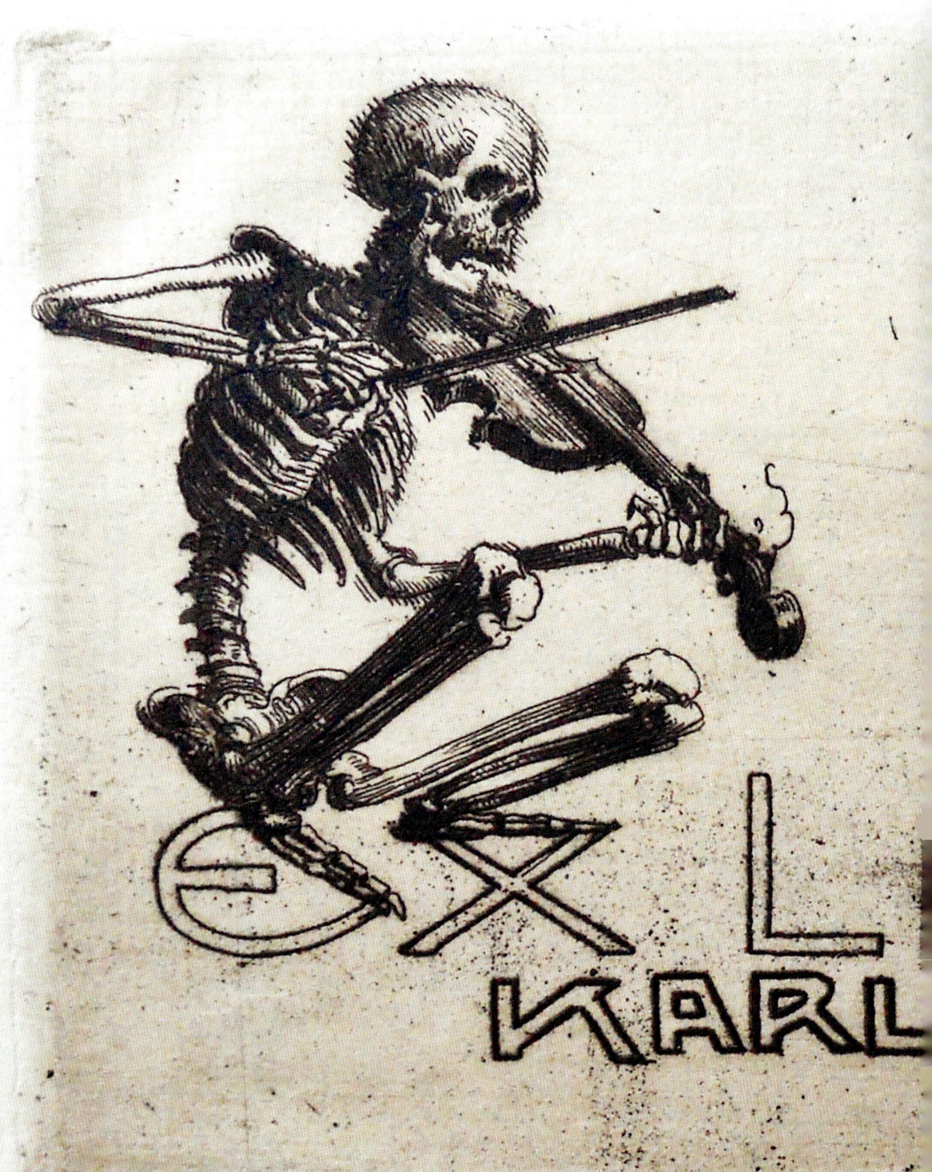
ex L
KARL

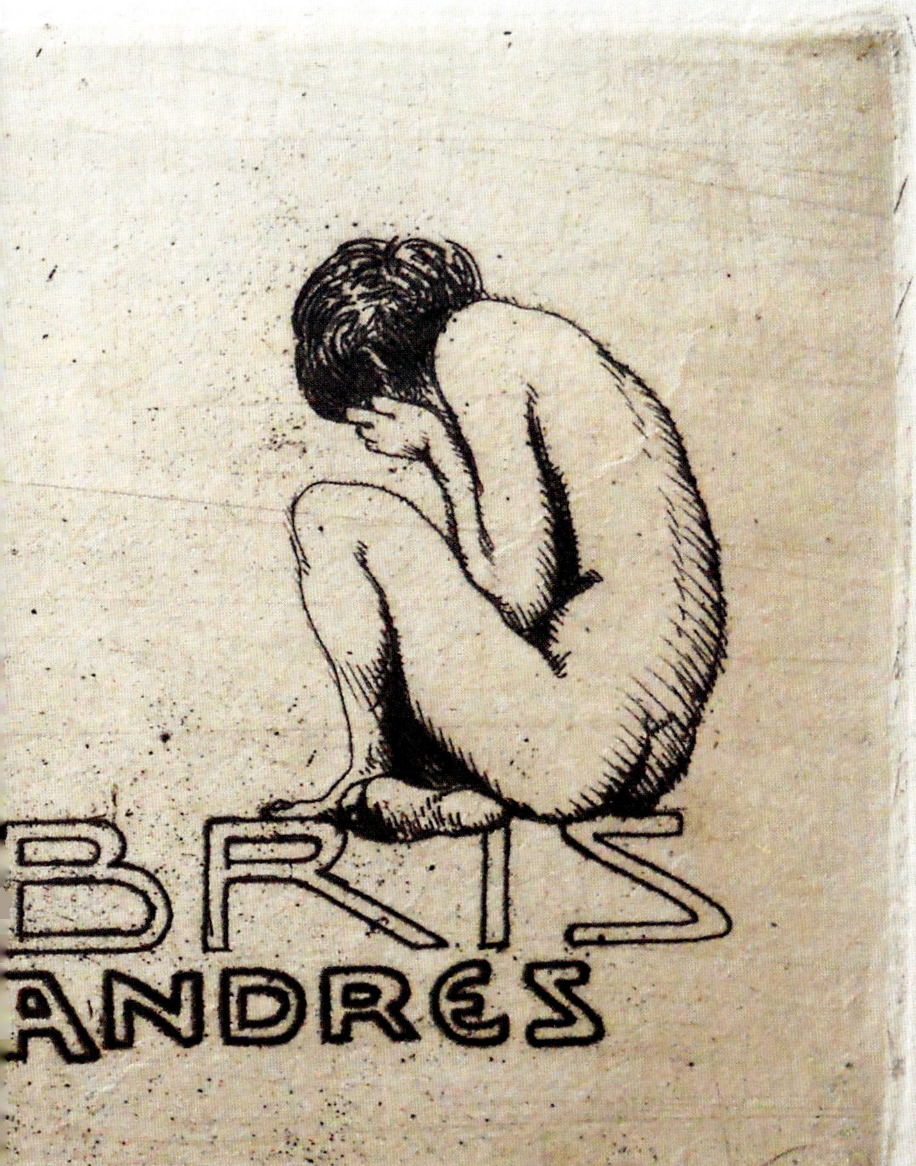
BRIS
ANDRES

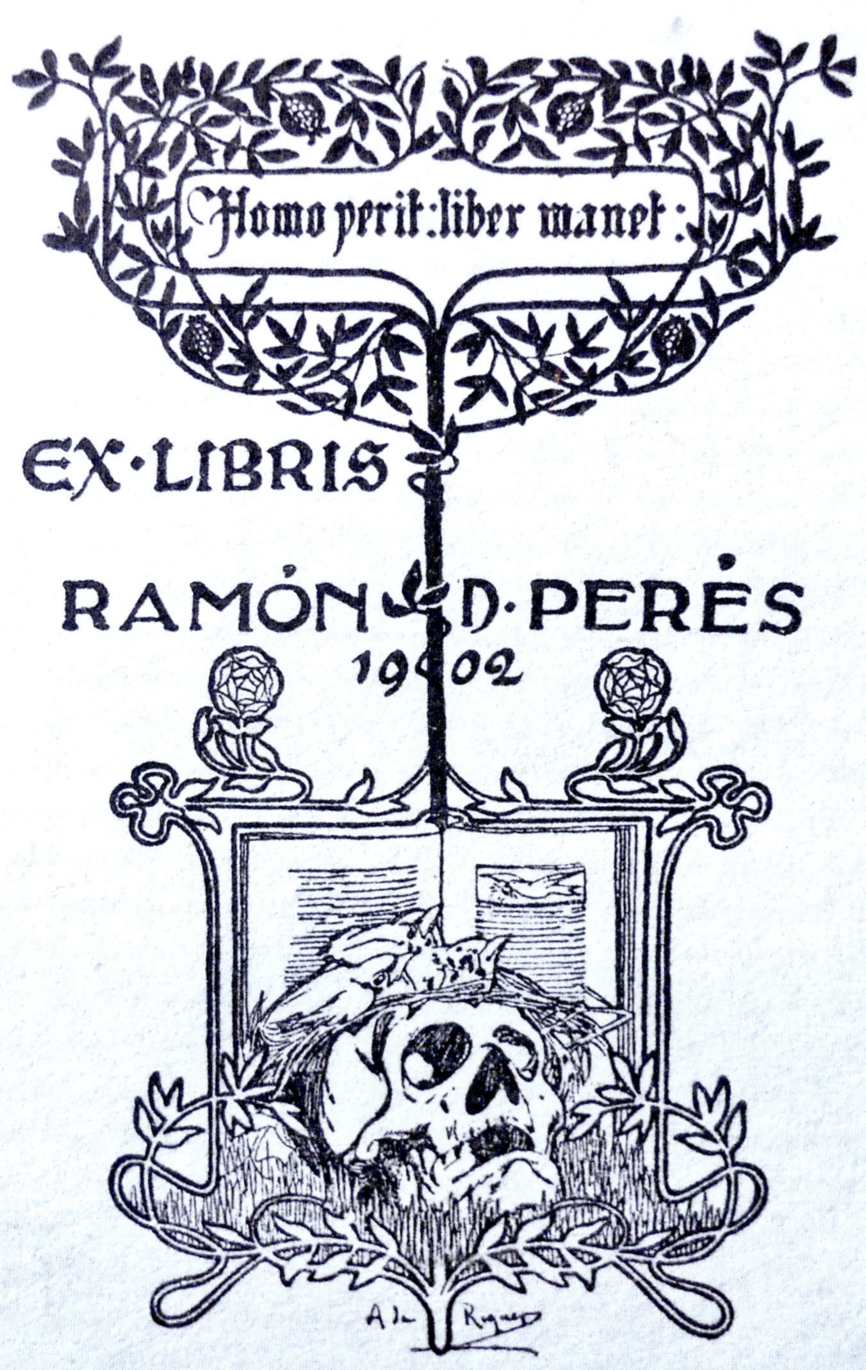
Homo perit: liber manet:
EX·LIBRIS
RAMÓN D·PERÉS
1902

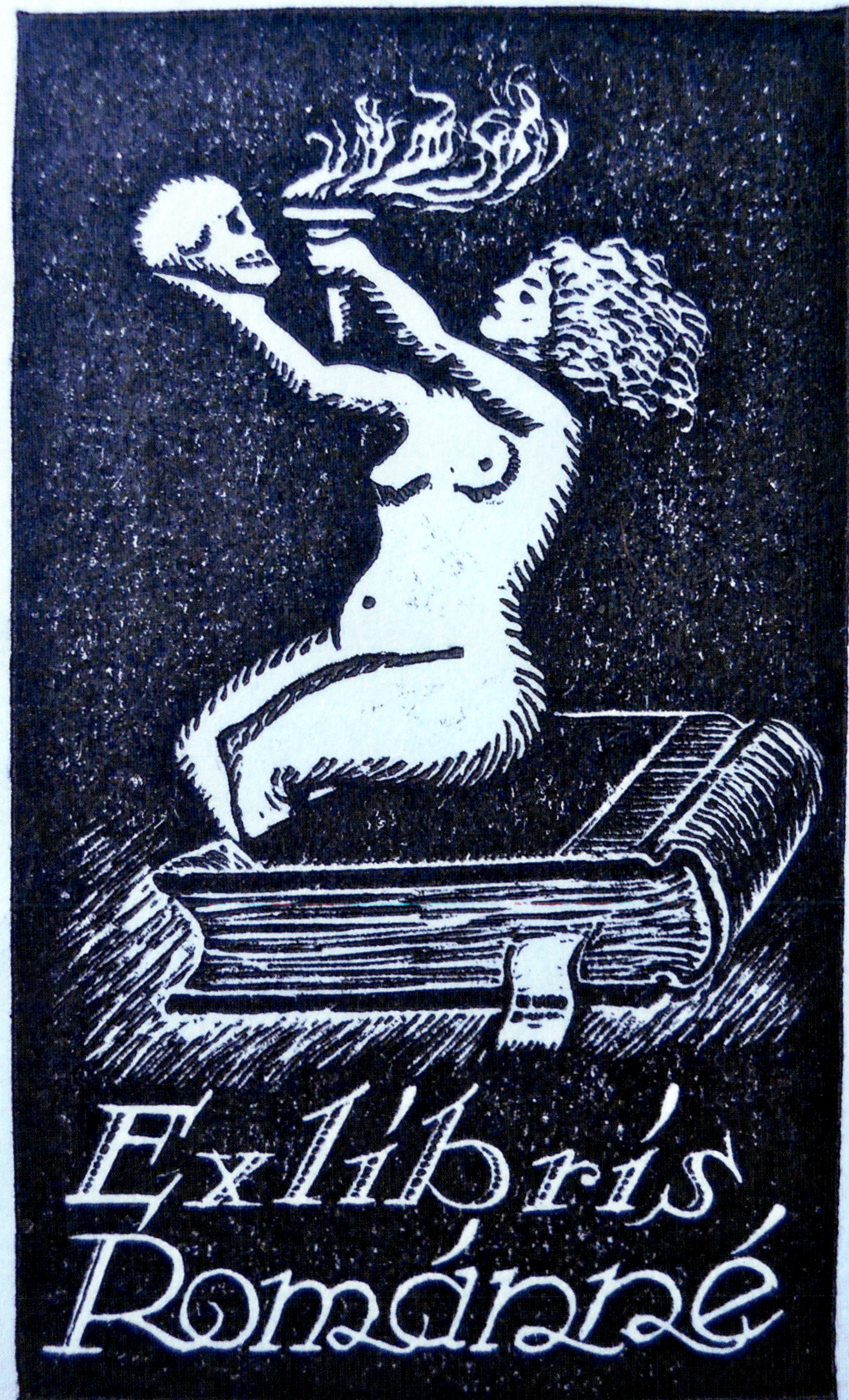

930

DEATH
AND
DOCTOR BUCHAN

ROSS MACFARLANE

OPENED TO WIDESPREAD ACCLAIM IN NOVEMBER 2012, WELLCOME Collection's "Death: A Self-Portrait," brought to London a selection of items from the collection of Richard Harris, a former antique print dealer based in Chicago. Press attention for the show understandably focused on the works by some of the more famous names exhibited: Otto Dix, Goya and Dürer. However, one of the smaller pieces also caught the attention of many of the visitors.

Dating from the turn of the twenty-first century, American artist June Leaf's *Gentleman on Green Table* is a spindly affair: a small, skeletal figure constructed from rusted tin. Harris has mentioned how it's one of his favorite works in his collection, and it's a figure easy to invest emotions onto. Given the particulars of the surrounding exhibition, perhaps the bowed head of Leaf's gentleman is filled with thoughts of others who have passed away before him or of the inevitability of death. Or, is he pausing out of tiredness or fatigue, arms at his side resting as he exhales out of sheer weariness or in a last mortal breath? The hunched figure looks frail, worn out—the shoulders about to sink out of the sheer desperation of it all.

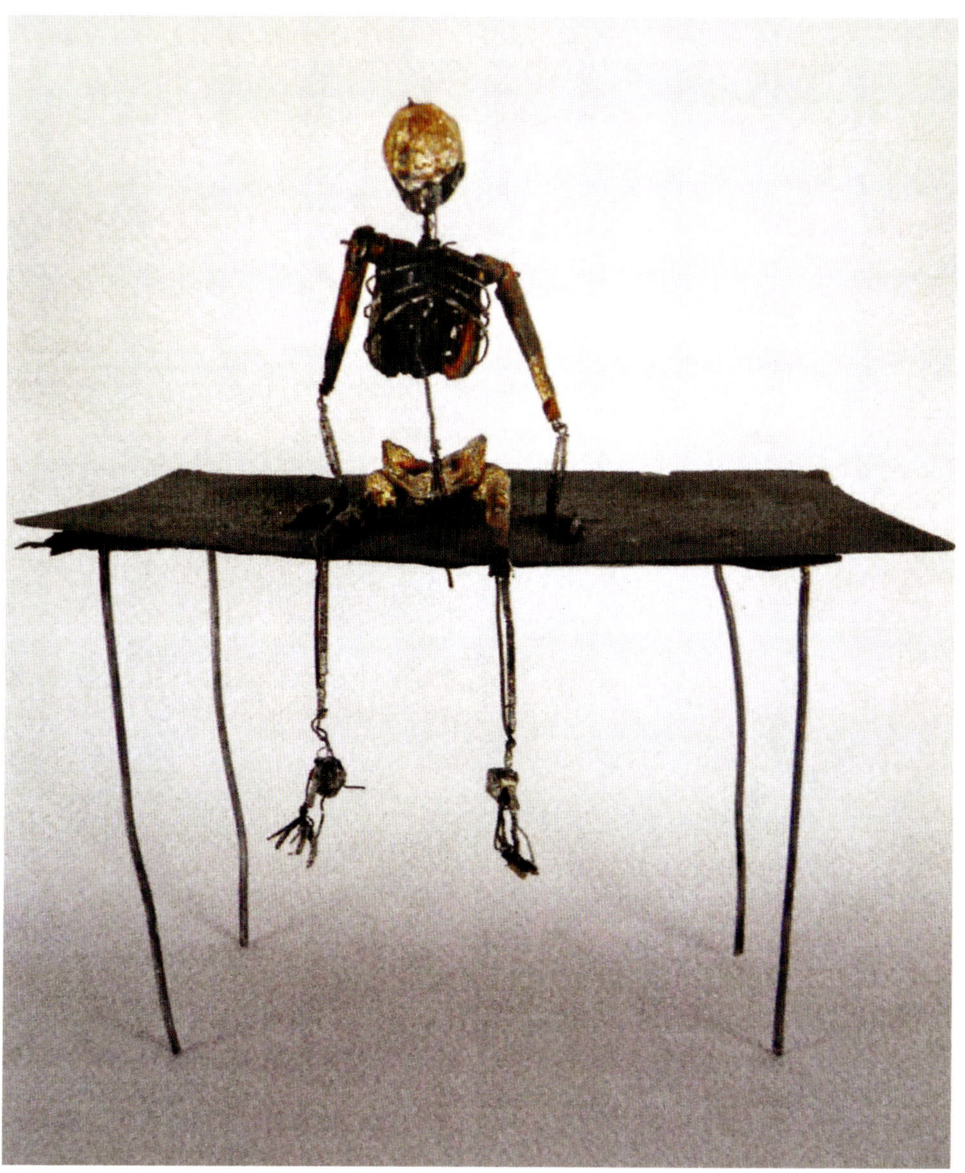

June Leaf, Gentleman on Green Table, *tin and wire, 1999-2000.*
Courtesy of the Collection of Richard Harris.

There's a great Scots word to describe how this chap looks—*drumoid*, or "dull, dejected, woe-begone." But as I pondered this Scottish word another thought struck me. What if our gentleman on his green table wasn't a dejected mortal pondering death, but actually a dejected Death himself? Then more Scots words were recalled, arranged in a poetical form known as the "Habbie Stanza." The poem I was (half) remembering featured just such a character—not only that, its satirical premise was built around one of the most popular medical books ever written.

The poem that was brought to mind was "Death and Doctor Hornbook," by Robert Burns (1759–1796). Although published in Burns' *Poems, Chiefly in the Scottish Dialect* (1786), and so sharing space with many of his best-known poems, "Death and Doctor Hornbook" is a lesser-known part of the Burns canon. It doesn't—like "Address to a Haggis"—form part of the template for the celebratory world of a Burns supper, nor, like "Auld Lang Syne," is it sung across the world on New Year's Eve. It does, though, share a number of features with more familiar titles. Like "Tam O'Shanter," it locates the supernatural in the everyday, and like "Holy Willie's Prayer" it satirizes the actions of Burns' local community.

With more statues erected in his honor than any other poet, and more than two thousand editions of his works existing in more than fifty languages (to say nothing of more than a thousand societies and clubs worldwide honoring him), Burns is clearly one of the most popular and remembered poets. There's also a fair amount of misremembering going on: Burns' radical edges were smoothed down over the centuries by many of his supporters (though recent revisionist scholarship has helped go some way to bring this aspect of his personality and poetry back out into the open). Also, Burns is very much not the "Heaven-taught ploughman" he has long been hailed as: he may have been self-taught, but he was an extremely well-read man, highly political and very much a product of the Enlightenment. Burns' most recent biographer surmised his powers and popularity through the facility of being able to speak for and to anyone, that the voices he captured extended through "muse, mouse and louse."

In "Death and Doctor Hornbook," he brings humanity even to the Grim Reaper himself. The poem begins with its narrator returning home from the alehouse (an opening gambit the poem shares with Burns' later masterpiece "Tam O'Shanter"). Somewhat the worse for wear with drink, our narrator meets a spindly figure sat by the roadside—the image that brought *Gentleman on Green Table* to my mind—who our narrator quickly realizes is Death himself (his accoutrements being all present and correct, including "An awfu' scythe, out-owre ae shouther, / Clear-dangling, hang").

Our narrator is understandably nervous. However, Death assures him that their meeting will not prelude his demise. Becoming more relaxed, our drunken narrator (no doubt sobering up) and Death enter into a chummy conversation. Death confesses that his powers are waning—no longer a figure of fear, he's now being laughed at by children. Why so? Well, Death now has a rival. Even with an outbreak of an unnamed epidemic disease, Death is being undone by the local 'doctor' (the Doctor Hornbook of the poem's title).

Death's scythe and dart—his traditional tools in ending life—have proved ineffective against Hornbook's doctoring:

But Doctor Hornbook, wi' his art
An' cursed skill,
Has made them baith no worth a fart,
Damn'd haet they'll kill!

The narrator takes this as evidence of Hornbook's success as a doctor. Death quickly corrects him: Hornbook isn't curing, he's killing. The death portrayed in the poem is a despondent figure, unhappy that his work has been taken from him. Doctor Hornbook's ill-informed actions—which are revealed to be self-taught—are doing Death's job for him.

As the poem continues, Death describes the range of fatalities Hornbook has inadvertently caused, ranging from the high to the low in society. For instance, these range from the local gentry:

A country Laird had ta'en the batts
Or some curmuring in his guts
His only son for Hornbook sets
An' pays him well:
The lad, for twa guid gimmer-pets,
Was Laird himsel'.

To a local girl:

A bonnie lass—ye kend her name—
Some ill-brewn drink had hov'd her wame;
She trusts hersel', to hide the shame,
In Hornbook's care;
Horn sent her aff to her lang hame,
To hide it there.

The poem gives a sense of the medicines at Hornbook's disposal:

Calces o' fossils, earths and trees;
True sal-marinum o' the seas;

> The farina of beans an' pease,
> He has't in plenty;
> Aqua-fontis, what you please,
> He can content ye.

And also his method of diagnosis:

> Ev'n them he canna get attended,
> Altho' their face he ne'er had kend it,
> Just shit in a kail-blade, an' sent it,
> As soon's he smells 't,
> Baith their disease, and what will mend it,
> At one he tells 't.

"Death and Doctor Hornbook" can be traced to an acquaintance of Burns': John Wilson, parish schoolmaster at Tarbolton in Ayrshire (a "Hornbook" was a simple teaching primer of the age, hence the use of the term in the poem). Wilson also ran a small grocery shop, selling "simple medicaments" and "offering advice" on common disorders. At a meeting of the same Freemason's Lodge of which Burns was a member, Wilson's expression of his medical knowledge was the provocation for Burns to write this poem, which aimed to prick the pomposity of the self-taught doctor.

At one level then, the poem can be read as merely a satire on pretension. To the medical historian Malcolm Nicholson, however, when contextualized in eighteenth-century understandings of medicine, the poem "reveals itself to be more subtle and much more morally ambiguous." Burns has a wider target in mind than just a fellow Freemason.

Nicholson argues that the poem is not merely a satire on unqualified, incompetent physicians but "a satire on the reputation and status of medicine in 18th century society more broadly." As such, he points out the satirical tone in the poem with which the quality of the remedies and the methods of diagnosis (given above) are described. Indeed, the lampooning of the medical profession was rife in the eighteenth century, in part as "medicine was seen as a necessary defence against illness but also feared both for its limited efficacy and for the unpleasantness and toxicity of many of its remedies."

Nicholson leaves aside another reference that would offer more evidence for his argument. At the heart of a poem satirizing the medical profession, there's a reference to someone who wanted to reform medicine. It comes when Death introduces Hornbook to the narrator:

> 'Ye kem Jock Hornbook i' the clachan,
> Deil mak his king's-hood in a spleuchan!
> He's grown sae weel acquaint wi' Buchan
> An' ither chaps,'

Image right: Title page from William. Buchan's Domestic Medicine, Or, The Family Physician: Being an Attempt to Render the Medical Art More Generally Useful, ... *Edinburgh: Printed by Balfour, Auld, and Smellie, 1769. Courtesy of Wellcome Library, London.*

The "Buchan" that Hornbook had grown so "well acquaint" with was William Buchan. The acquaintance wasn't personal: as contemporary readers of Burns' poem would have known, the allusion is being made with the book Buchan published in 1769, *Domestic Medicine, or, The Family Physician.*

Domestic Medicine is one of the most successful medical books ever published. Between its first publication and the last English-language version (in Philadelphia, over one hundred years later) Buchan's work appeared in at least 142 separate editions. Whilst to some, what captures the attention in the twenty-first century is the bizarre-to-our-eyes remedies (2012 saw a republication of sections of *Domestic Medicine* as *Do Onions Cure Earache?*), this shouldn't distract from the book's radicalism. It

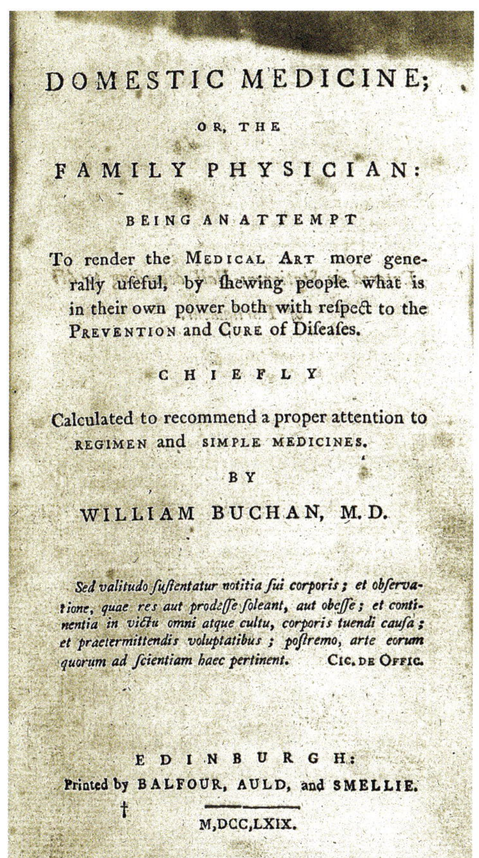

DOMESTIC MEDICINE;

OR, THE

FAMILY PHYSICIAN:

BEING AN ATTEMPT

To render the MEDICAL ART more generally ufeful, by fhewing people what is in their own power both with refpect to the PREVENTION and CURE of Difeafes.

CHIEFLY

Calculated to recommend a proper attention to REGIMEN and SIMPLE MEDICINES.

BY

WILLIAM BUCHAN, M.D.

Sed valitudo fuftentatur notitia fui corporis; et obfervatione, quae res aut prodeffe foleant, aut obeffe; et continentia in victu omni atque cultu, corporis tuendi caufa; et praetermittendis voluptatibus; poftremo, arte eorum quorum ad fcientiam haec pertinent. CIC. DE OFFIC.

EDINBURGH:
Printed by BALFOUR, AULD, and SMELLIE.

M,DCC,LXIX.

was a new kind of medical text: Written by a trained member of the medical profession, it directly questioned medical authority, challenging perceived notions as to who had the authority and legitimacy to tend the sick. It's an immensely political work—and an immensely successful one.

Highly influential across the Atlantic Ocean (there was an American reprint as early as 1772, and in 1795 a Philadelphia publisher issued an edition "revised and adapted to the diseases and climate of the United States of America"), there were also

French, Spanish, Portuguese, Italian, German, Russian, and Swedish translations. Buchan was even the recipient of a gold medal and a commendatory letter from Catherine the Great of Russia. *Domestic Medicine's* contents were even deemed applicable in the South Seas: the National Maritime Museum in Greenwich holds a copy of the book from HMS Bounty that the ship's mutineers took with them to their retreat on Pitcairn Island.

By the time of the publication of *Domestic Medicine,* Buchan had already enjoyed a successful career in medicine. Born in 1729, he spent his childhood on his father's small estate in Roxburghshire in the Scottish Borders. He spent nine years at Edinburgh University, eventually finishing his education in medicine. Most of his working career had been spent in England, particularly as the first surgeon and apothecary at the Foundling Hospital in Ackworth in Yorkshire, founded in 1759 (this was one of the first institutions to be built after the creation of the Foundling Hospital in London, which was founded in 1741 for the "education and maintenance of exposed and deserted young children").

Buchan's experiences treating children in Ackworth fed into his medical dissertation, "On the Preservation of Infant Life" which he submitted to Edinburgh University in 1761. In 1762—when the Government removed a grant to fund the Ackworth Hospital—Buchan moved his family to Sheffield to begin a private medical practice. By 1766 he was back in Edinburgh, writing what would become *Domestic Medicine.*

Following the publication of the work, Buchan appears to have fallen foul of the Edinburgh medical establishment. By the late 1770s he had moved to London, where he enjoyed a successful career, updating *Domestic Medicine,* publishing on gonorrhea and maternal health, and treating many of the eminent members of London society. So successful was his career that, upon his death in 1806, Buchan was buried in Westminster Abbey.

Domestic Medicine was published in 1769 by Buchan's friend, the Edinburgh printer William Smellie. Five thousand copies—each at six shillings—quickly sold. A second edition, with further material, was published three years later. (An argument exists that Smellie was more than just the printer. Evidence—most closely examined by Christopher Lawrence—suggests he had a hand in the re-writing of the second edition).

Why was the book so successful? As summarized by the American historian of medicine Charles Rosenberg, *Domestic Medicine* was a "book to use and a book to be read"—though not by the medical profession. Its readers could take from it advice as to how to preserve their health, maintain a healthy lifestyle, and also how to both identify diseases and prescribe remedies for them. With regards to content, around the first third of the first edition was focused on the former and the rest of the text to the latter.

Whilst many manuscript collections concerning medicine in the domestic realm existed prior to this book's publication, very few similar works had ever come from the presses. Buchan rightly acknowledged Samuel Auguste Tissot's *Avis au people sur sa santé* (which had appeared in 1761), but the aims of Buchan's work went further.

These aims are expressed in the introductions to the first and second editions. Buchan sees medicine in need of reform due to its secretive nature: "the medical art" has become "an object of ridicule" due to physicians "...concealing their pretended virtues from the rest of mankind." Buchan argues that medicine needs openness to improve and innovate itself. However, he claims, some members of the medical profession will fight this—"the interested views of a trade will always obstruct the progress of a science."

Promoting medical knowledge would also have a deleterious effect on quack healers: "Had physicians never affected mystery, quacks and quackery could never have existed. Now that they have over-run all Europe... there is no other method of discrediting them with the people, but a total reverse of behaviour in the Faculty. Let us therefore act with candor [sic], openness and ingenuity, and mankind will soon learn to dread everything in medicine that has the smallest appearance of secrecy or disguise," Or as he elsewhere put it more succinctly (in the context of knowledge of venereal disease): "while people are kept in the dark and told not to use their understanding in matters concerning their health, they will be the dupes of designing knaves."

But Buchan drew boundaries: the lay public couldn't do everything, and there would still be a role for trained medical men. "Nothing is farther from the design of the following pages," he writes, "than to induce ignorant persons to tamper with dangerous medicines, or trust to their own skill, where better assistance can be obtained. But where something must be done, and no medical assistance can be had, it is certainly better to direct people what they ought to do than to leave them to blunder on in the dark." Buchan appears to be suggesting that it's better the public have some medical knowledge rather than no medical knowledge. "We do not mean that all men are to be made physicians. We only mean that they should be taught the importance of due care for the preservation of health, and of a proper regimen in diseases."

To Buchan, changes in how medical knowledge would be disseminated would lead to changes in society, and the responsibility would lie with the self-improving middle-orders to lead the way:

> We make no doubt but the ladies, gentlemen, and clergy who reside in the country will readily concur with us, in endeavouring to root out pernicious and destructive prejudices. Their example will have great weight with their dependents and inferiors; and their advice will be often listened to with more attention than that of a physician. They will teach the poor the importance of a proper regimen both in health and sickness; the danger of trusting their lives in the hands of quacks and conjurers, and the folly of their own superstitious notions. By this means they may prevent much evil, do some good, and prove real blessings to those among whom they reside.

Whilst they may not have proselytized fully on his behalf, the rising middle classes are seen by Charles Rosenberg as key to the success of *Domestic Medicine.* Its purchasers, Rosenberg writes, "represented a cross-section of the literate, servant-employing and self-consciously improving middle-orders—men and women who would think twice before spending hard-earned shillings and pounds on a physician, and who sought a rational guide both to prudent domestic practice and to a moral and health-ensuring regimen. The growth in numbers and self-consciousness of this new class may well explain both the enormous success of Buchan's guide and the specific shape of the genre it created."

As such then, Burns' satirical target in "Death and Doctor Hornbrook," John Wilson, perfectly fits the audience to which Buchan aims *Domestic Medicine,* being himself a schoolteacher and not a professional doctor. And whilst Burns' poem sends up the failings of the medical profession, he does share some of

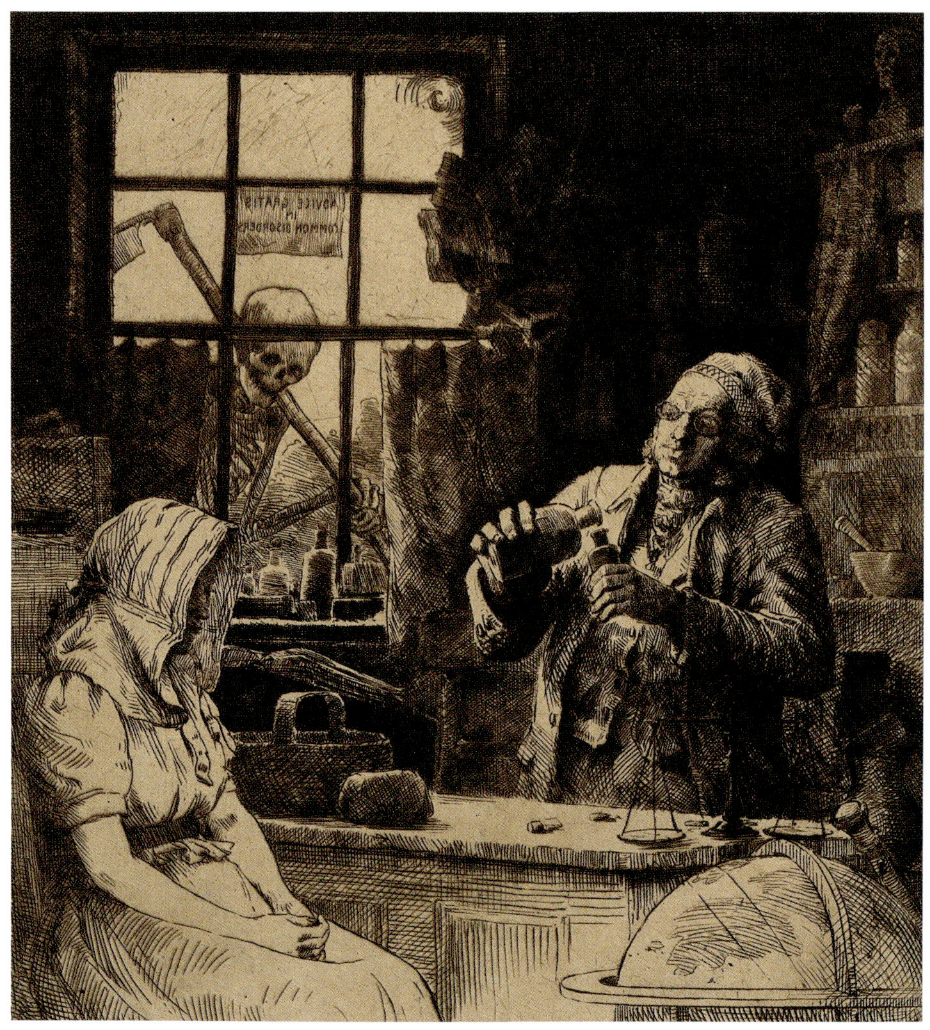

the same concerns of medicine's status and power with Buchan. Indeed, the character Hornbook, carrying out procedures deemed within the layman's knowledge as set out in *Domestic Medicine*, looks even worse when it's realized the character isn't following the advice of the book.

Rosenberg concludes his examination of Buchan by ruminating on his fame following the book's republication and alteration over time. By the end of the nineteenth century, he writes, Buchan "had become a sacred name, invoked to reassure the lowest level of literate consumers of intellectual goods. Buchan had transcended the reality of his own life and become a figure incorporating an almost sacred authority. It is not entirely clear that the enlightened Scotsman would have approved of this particular beatification."

Image left: A woman visits an apothecary; death lurks nearby. Etching, 1895. Courtesy of Wellcome Library, London.

A similar beatification had also fallen upon Burns in the nineteenth century after his early death in 1796. Burns died a landowner and an employee of the state (he had worked in his last years as an exciseman), precisely the educated member of the middle classes Buchan had appealed to. As such, we have to wonder if a copy of *Domestic Medicine* ever found its way on to Burns' bookshelf?

Although "Death and Doctor Hornbook" begins with Death diminished and bemoaning his lot, by the poem's conclusion, Death seems revitalized and ready to wrestle back his authority over Hornbook. Death confides of his plan with the poem's narrator:

"But, hark! I'll tell you of a plot,
Tho' dinna ye be speaking o't;
I'll nail the self-conceited sot
  As dead's a herrin';
Niest time we meet, I'll wad a groat,
  He gets his fairin'!"

But just as he began to tell,
The auld kirk-hammer strak the bell

Some wee short hour ayont the twal',
Which rais'd us baith:
I took the way that pleas'd mysel',
And sae did *Death*.

And so the poem ends with a fortified Death revealing to the narrator his plan of action, but without the all-important detail of when he will set it in motion.

To the reader it's not the most pleasant of conclusions, as it reminds us of not only the inevitability of death, but also its unpredictable timing. Perhaps it's this curiosity over our own mortality that drew so many visitors to see the *Gentleman on Green Table* and the other objects in Richard Harris' collection at "Death: A Self-Portrait." This same morbid curiosity might also be the inspiration for the other artworks in the exhibition.

[BIBLIOGRAPHY]

Buchan, William, *Domestic medicine; or, the family physician; being an attempt to render the medical art more generally useful, by shewing people what is in their own power both with respect to the prevention and cure of diseases. Chiefly calculated to recommend a proper attention to regimen and simple medicines* (Edinburgh: Balfour, Auld and Smellie, 1769).

__________________, *Domestic medicine. Or, A treatise on the prevention and cure of diseases by regimen and simple medicines* (London: W. Strahan, etc., 1772).

__________________, *Observations concerning the prevention and cure of the venereal diseases: with an appendix containing a list of the most approved medicines now used in the cure of this disorder* (London: T. Chapman and Mudie and Sons, Edinburgh, 1796).

Burns, Robert, *Selected Poems* (London: Penguin Classics, 2007).

Crawford, Robert, *Scotland's Books: The Penguin History of Scottish Literature* (London: Penguin, 2007).

___________________, *The Bard: Robert Burns a biography* (London: Jonathan Cape, 2008).

King, Melanie (ed.) *Can Onions Cure Ear-Ache?: Medical Advice from 1769* (Oxford: Bodleian Library, 2012).

Lawrence, Christopher, "William Buchan: Medicine laid open," *Medical History*, vol. 19, 1975; pp. 20-35.

___________________," Buchan, William (1729–1805)," Oxford Dictionary of National Biography (Oxford: Oxford University Press, 2004).

Nicholson, Malcolm, "*Death and Doctor Hornbook* by Robert Burns: a view from medical history," Medical Humanities, vol. 36 (1), 2010, pp. 23-26.

Online Dictionary of the Scottish Language, accessed 2 May 2013. http://www.dsl.ac.uk/

Porter, D. and Porter, R., *Patient's progress: doctors and doctoring in eighteenth century* England (Oxford: Polity, 1989).

Rosenberg, Charles, "The Fielding H Garrison Lecture. Medical text and social context: explaining William Buchan's *Domestic Medicine*," *Bulletin of the History of Medicine*, vol. 57, 1983, pp. 22-42.

BOOKS BOUND IN HUMAN SKIN

A Survey of Examples of Anthropodermic Bibliopegy

DANIEL K. SMITH

THE FIRST REACTION IS ALWAYS, "IS IT REAL?" ONE LEATHER CAN look quite a lot like any other. The book covering has no smell, no tactile sensation or visible clue to suggest a tale greater than a writer's narrative; that is, until you open the covers and read the inscription on the flyleaf—*Bound in Human Skin.* Eventually your eye finds an unevenness of color, a blemish or even a faint tattoo. We know this is the fate of some unfortunate soul and assume there's no volunteering. The question is: How did this come to be?

The Newberry Library in Chicago has a handsome dark-brown book with gold decoration that contains the inscription, "Found in the Palace of the King of Delhi, Sept. 28th 1857, seven days after the assault James Wise MD Bound in human skin." Unfortunately, that's all the doctor tells us.

We get a bit more about one book's history from a seventeenth-century treatise on Spanish law in the Harvard Law Library titled "Practicarum quaestionum circa leges regias hispania." A faint,

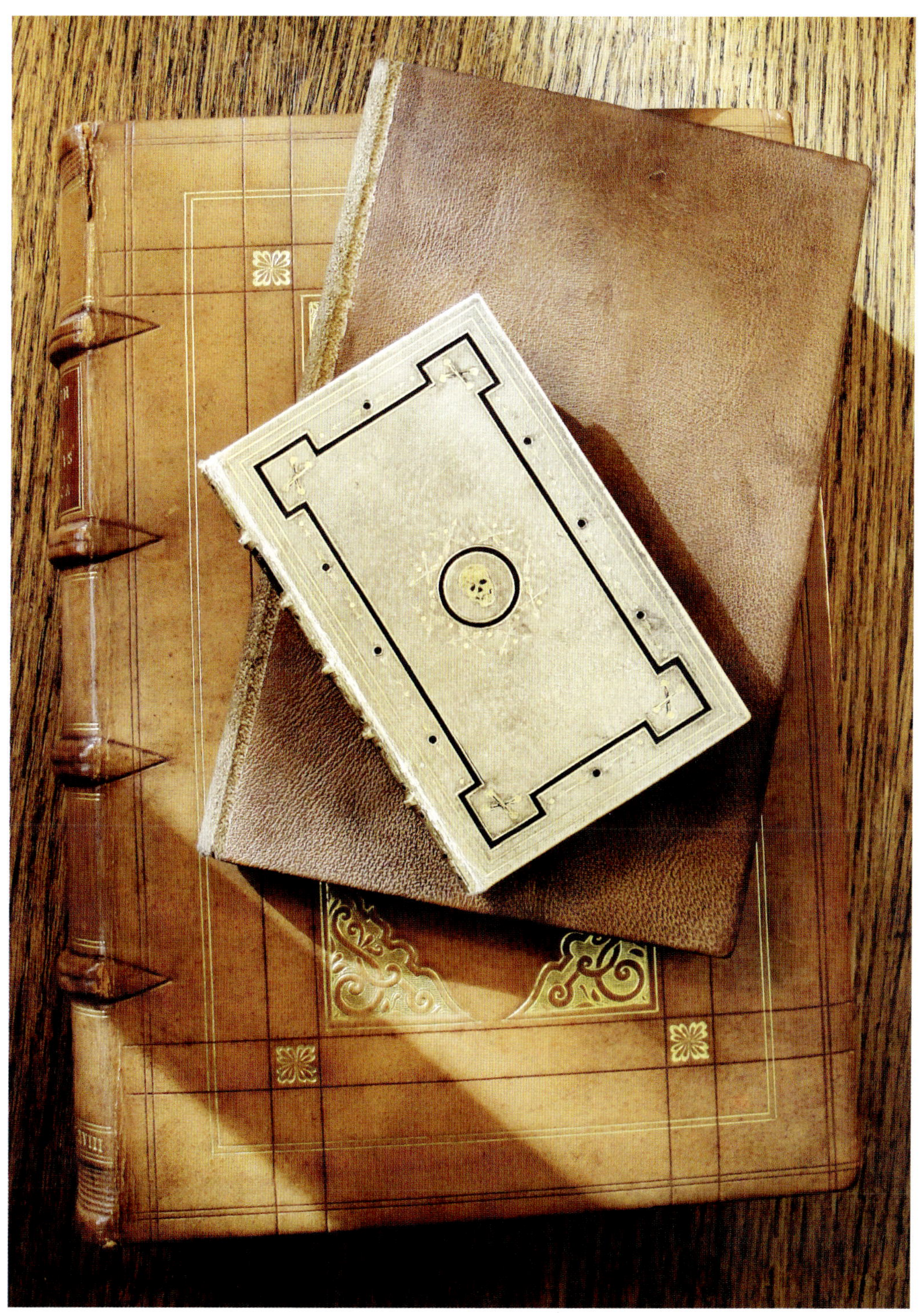

Image previous page: Books bound in human skin from the John Hay Library at Brown University. Bottom: Andreas Versalius' De Humani Corporis Fabrica*, 4th edition, bound by Schavye for the King of Belgium; Middle: Hans Holbein's* Dance of Death*, London 1816, bound by Zaehnsdorf in 1893 with headbands of human hair.; Top: Hans Holbein's* Dance of Death*, London & New York, George Bell and Sons, 1898, bound in Chicago by Cox 1898. Photo by the author.*

handwritten inscription explains that the skin comes from a "dear friend" of the inscriber, Jonas Wright, who was flayed alive by the Wavuma (an African tribe) in 1632. The book was very important to Mr. Wright and was given to him along with "ample of his skin to bynd it." The inscription ends "Requiescat in pace."

In 1992, Harvard had this book tested for human DNA. The test came back inconclusive, killing any hope the library might have had that science would unmask a fraud. Today this book is just a grisly curiosity, off-limits to the public and researchers alike. Like most of these volumes, it lives darkly between authenticity and symbol. Ghoulish prank or *memento mori*?

The practice is primarily a nineteenth-century phenomenon. What was missing prior to this was a reliable supply of human epidermis. That started to change when superstition about human remains began to wane, giving way to a popular interest in science, especially the study of the human body. What follows is a selective list of books bound in human skin. These are old books, some dating back to the fifteenth century—some bound by the skilled craftsmen of the day, some rather crude and hasty productions.

The Executed

The skin of executed criminals was sometimes used to bind the records of their trial. The authorities found execution wasn't enough of a deterrent and hoped to add further terror and infamy by ordering the dissection of the corpse. Surgeons then had free rein of the cadaver. There would be no remains for the family to inter and pray over for a Christian resurrection. In payment for their crimes, not only was their life taken but also their afterlife.

Father Henry Garnet was executed in 1606 for his involvement in the Gunpowder Plot against King James I of England.

He was sentenced to hang and then be drawn and quartered. It's not clear if the last part of his sentence ever happened; contemporary accounts say sympathizers seized his legs while he was hanging to end his suffering, and then beheaded him. But Father Garnet continued to annoy the English church after his execution: a straw husk that was stained with his blood and taken from the site of his beheading was preserved as a religious relic, and sometime afterward, a face revealed itself on the husk. It became a focus of devotion among England's Catholics, and wound up in the possession of the Society of Jesus, though it disappeared around the time of the French Revolution.

In 2007, a British auction house listed a book of the trial of the Gunpowder Plot participants, "believed to be bound in human skin, possibly that of the aforementioned Jesuit Priest; Father Henry Garnet." This book was printed three years after Garnet's execution by Robert Barker, printer to the King (and several years later, printer of the King James Bible). Video and still images show a very thin, translucent cover and an insubstantial binding similar to a paperback. This book was protected in a box, which probably accounts for the volume still being in one piece. Images of the cover show wear that resembles an old bearded man, and the BBC quickly made the suggestion it was Father Garnet. Pareidolia redux? According to the auctioneer, Sid Wilkinson, the book was sold for 5,400 pounds (about 8,500 dollars) to a private collector.

Eighteenth-century England was faced with ever-increasing crimes against property that was mostly in the hands of the aristocracy. To maintain their wealth and position, such criminals were punished in a very public way: hanging. Before the technique was perfected by adjusting the height of the drop, these well-attended displays couldn't always be counted on to work as intended. Victims had an unexpected way of coming back to life. Sometimes the condemned would simply pass out from lack of oxygen, only to revive while being carted away or worse, while naked on the anatomist's table and being cut open. The most famous instance involved Margaret Dickson who, in 1724, popped up out of her coffin, then lived to a ripe old age and bore many children. At the time there was no legal way to rehang her. While rare, such miscues happened often enough to give the friends and family hope that the person could be, if not revived, given a chance of resurrection with a Christian burial. The problem was getting the body away from the sheriff. Riots were common at these executions, which often attracted over ten thousand people.

The list of capital crimes at this time is incomprehensible to us today. Servants could be hanged for stealing forks or poaching for their dinner—all of which led to a great deal of frustration and anger toward the prosecutors. A trial might end with the condemned promising revenge—if not in this life then in the hereafter (witchery was taken seriously). Combine this with very credible stories about hanging victims popping out of coffins and turning up in America or running away from the surgeon, and it becomes clear why the prosecutors and court personnel couldn't always rest easy. Ghosts can be very hard to handle.

The interest in science and anatomy provided an excuse for judges to add dissection of the corpse to the sentence. This is how a body wound up in the hands of a person capable of removing the skin and then getting it tanned and bound, and without a funeral or burial, the book could now function as a gravestone.

The Murderers

William Burke was one of the most notorious murderers of the nineteenth century and terrorized Edinburgh from Christmas

1827 to October 1828. Burke teamed up with William Hare, who ran a lodging house. When a boarder died owing a debt to Hare, the two men decided to sell the body to Dr. Robert Knox of the Edinburgh Medical College. Demand for cadavers for scientific purposes had already created a rash of grave robbing; it was common knowledge that the Medical College would pay cash for a body, no questions asked. Finding this an easy way to earn money, Burke and Hare started to murder other boarders by getting them drunk, then smothering them, leaving little evidence of violence. Soon, they expanded their enterprise to include prostitutes and others seized on the street. (Robert Louis Stevenson based his short story "The Body Snatchers" on these murders.) Burke was finally arrested when a body was found under his bed. Hare was granted immunity for testifying against Burke, who was executed in January 1829. He was anatomized at Edinburgh Medical College, his skin used to make souvenirs and a small notebook—which, along with his skeleton, is still on display at the Royal College of Surgeons of Edinburgh.

In Bristol, England's Record Office Archive is a volume of bound papers with the inscription "Cutis Vera Johannis Horwood" stamped in gold, which translates to: "Here is the actual skin of John Horwood." Horwood, 18, was convicted for murdering Eliza Balsum with a rock. His sentence read: "John Horwood, convicted of the wilful murder of Eliza Balsum—Let him be hanged by the neck until he shalt be dead, on Friday 13th April [1821] instant, and let his body be delivered to Mr Richard Smith, of the City of Bristol, Surgeon; to be dissected and anatomised." Smith removed enough of Horwood's skin to bind the records of the trial. In 2011, Horwood's great-great-great-grandniece, Mary Halliwell, discovered his mounted skeleton in a cabinet while doing research on the case; the rope that killed him was still around the neck. She had him buried with his father exactly 190 years to the minute after his execution.

In 1827, William Corder had arranged to meet his lover, Maria Marten, with the intention of eloping at Red Barn, a local landmark in Bury St. Edmunds, England. Instead of running away together, Corder shot and killed her, burying her in the barn. He left town, but sent letters to Maria's family so they would think she was still alive. According to legend, Maria's stepmother dreamt that Maria was buried in the barn, and so her father searched the ground, soon enough finding a soft spot. The young woman's body was discovered and Corder was brought back from London, tried and found guilty of murder. The trial generated massive publicity and attracted a huge crowd for his hanging in Bury St. Edmunds. An hour after his hanging, his body was cut down by the hangman, and taken to the courtroom where it was slit open. Corder's skin was tanned by the surgeon George Creed, and used to bind an account of the murder. It is held at Moyse's Hall Museum, Bury St. Edmunds. The inscription on the endpaper reads, "The binding of this book is the skin of the murderer William Corder tanned by myself George Creed." Along with the book, Corder's preserved scalp and death mask are on display.

The Doctors

Medical books are also a common medium for anthropodermic bibliopegy. Most instances come from doctors with enough resources to remove the skin, tan it, and have a bookbinder use it to bind a favored medical textbook. Sometimes the text on a specific ailment was paired with the skin of a patient that suffered from the disease. At the Clendening History of Medicine Library in Kansas City is an early study of the pituitary gland, *Exercitatio anatomica de glandula pituitaria* (1688);

Dr. Charles Humberd, who studied gigantism, had this book bound in the skin of an eight-foot, six-inch Ringling Brothers Circus giant by the name of Perky. The Wellcome Library in London has a collection of gynecological essays by various authors, *De integritatis et corruptionis virginum notis*, published in 1663, that was bound in Paris for Dr. Ludovic Bouland by Marcellin Lortic. A letter from the doctor states that he felt it deserved a binding to match its subject matter; he had secured a piece of a woman's skin when he was a medical student, and had waited many years before he found worthy subject matter.

Dr. John Stockton-Hough was a dedicated collector and his library of medical and bibliographical rarities formed the nucleus of the collection at the College of Physicians of Philadelphia. It contained over 3,200 works on early medicine and bibliography. He had one of his rarest books, a study of anatomy from 1550, bound by the well-known Parisian bookbinder Bruyere. But some books in his collection were done in a far cruder manner by a local binder, bound with the skin of some of his patients and put on display at the Mütter Museum in Philadelphia. In 1869, while performing an autopsy, Dr. Stockton-Hough discovered calcareous points, which he diagnosed as trichinosis. This was the first reported case in Philadelphia, and so, perhaps to celebrate the discovery, he removed a large portion of flesh from the inner thigh of a patient known as "Mary L." He preserved the skin by putting it into a chamber pot filled with tanning fluids, subsequently incorporating the flesh into his library. Also included in the collection is an edition of Leidy's *Human Anatomy* that was bound in the skin of a Civil War soldier—the inscription reads: "The leather with which this book is bound is human skin from a soldier who died during the great southern rebellion."

The John Hay Library at Brown University has a copy of Andreas Vesalius' *De human corporis fabrica* bound in a most

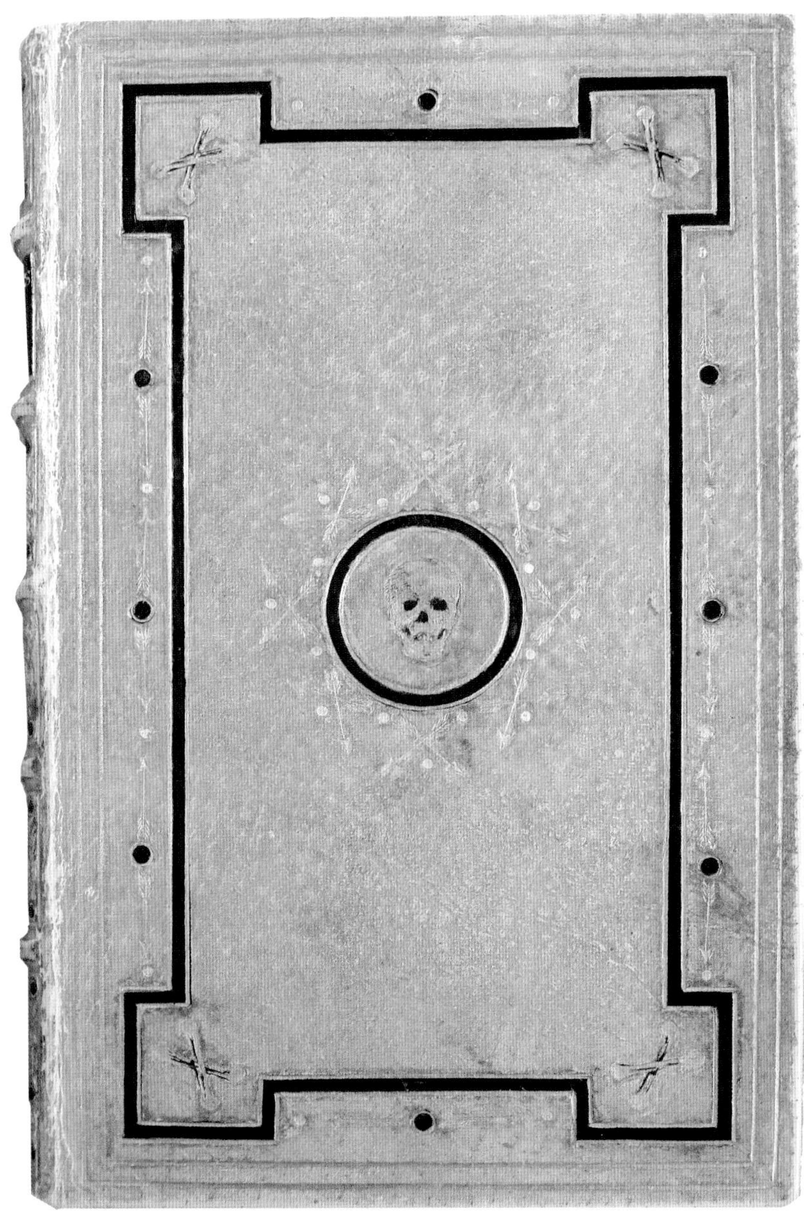

Front cover and spine from Hans Holbein's Dance of Death, London & New York, George Bell and Sons, 1898, ound in Chicago by Cox 1898. Photo by the author.

beautiful manner by Josse-Corneille Eugène Schavye. The illustrations in Vesalius' book, which first appeared in 1543, were based on dissected human subjects and rendered with a level of artistry that had not been seen before. The book became an instant classic and it was quickly pirated and distributed around the world, helping persuade the medical community to establish surgery as its own medical field of study. Brown University's copy is a large volume, about twelve and a half inches high, eight inches wide and several inches thick. As beautiful as it is, with handsomely tanned leather and gold tooling, it's hard to imagine any book that combines the best and worst of humanity more than this particular volume. Using one piece of human leather, Schavye bound it for King Leopold II of Belgium, who was at the time directing the mass murder of millions of Africans in the Congo. Under the guise of stopping the slave trade in the Congo, he sent European adventurers and mercenaries to the unmapped African interior, where they killed, enslaved, tortured, raped, and maimed in the most brutal ways while harvesting ivory and later rubber. Vesalius' bold and daring work had formed the art of surgery out of what was at the time more butchery than treatment—and here it was, gifted to one of the greatest butchers of the nineteenth century.

The Dance of Death

It's not clear when and where the images that we now know as the "Dance of Death" originated: the research points to a wall in a Parisian cemetery or a nunnery in Basel, Switzerland. The arrival of the plague brought home the idea that death comes to anyone, anytime, at every station of life. Some strains would produce fatalities within twenty-four hours from the first sign of illness. Without warning, people living in urban areas could wake up and find themselves surrounded by sickness. The affected suffered a horrible death and the unaffected lived in dread and witnessed the death of their loved ones. In the late nineteenth and early twentieth century, bibliophiles couldn't resist the irony of pairing books on the Dance on Death with human leather: dealers commissioned bindings to add a macabre quality to a collectible and desirable work.

Some of the leading bookbinders of the day produced these books without any hint of squeamishness. In a letter to the book dealer L.W. Bangs from the distinguished British bookbinder Joseph Zaehnsdorf dated 1893, the craftsman confirms he used human skin to bind a collection of Hans Holbein's woodcuts, but claims the piece was too small to cover the copy. To fix this, he writes, "I was obliged to split the leather in two: the result of this is that the skin which is quite smooth is on one side, and the rough unfinished skin is on the other." This binding is plain and unadorned with a remarkable exception: human hair was used as headbands, and a few strands still remain. Another example comes from the binder Cox in Chicago from 1898. Where the European Zaehnsdorf's work features the color and texture of the skin in a natural state, the American Cox's binding is much brighter and highly adorned with gold skulls and crossbones and black-leather inlays.

The famous bookbinding firm of Sangorski & Sutcliffe bound a copy of the Dance of Death in 1914 with a page signed by George Sutcliffe added to certify the covering is indeed human skin. This cover features a medallion with the words "Mortis Saltatio Hans Holbeino" surrounding a human skull with teeth made of ivory. This was commissioned by the Maggs Bros. in 1914, appeared in a book auction in 1935, and reappeared for sale by James Cummins in 2007 at the Boston Book Fair—it remains in private hands.

Image right: Allen, James. Narrative of the Life of James Allen, Alias George Walton, Alias Jonas Pierce, Alias James H. York, Alias Burley Grove, the Highwayman Being His Death-Bed Confession, to the Warden of the Massachusetts State Prison. *Boston: Harrington & Co., 1837. Collection of the Boston Athenaeum.*

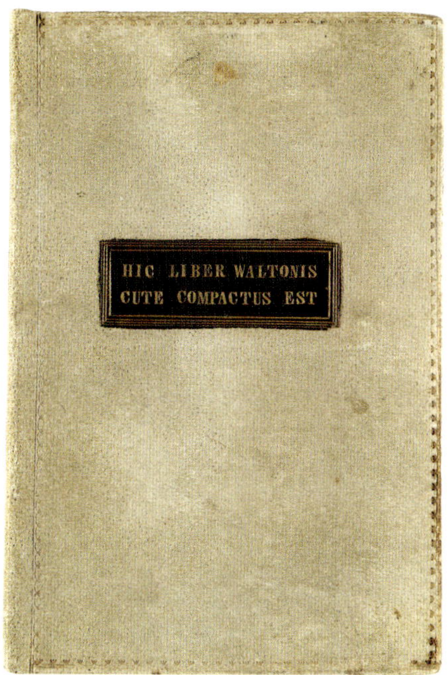

The Volunteer

The Boston Athenaeum contains a unique example of human-skin bookbinding, with a suede-like texture and off-white tone. A gold-stamped label reads "Hic Liber Waltonis Cute Compactus Est." It's the autobiography of James Allen, a famous Boston highwayman of the nineteenth century. The book starts with Allen's birth in 1809, and describes with remarkable candor and frankness the temperament and misfortunes that led to Allen's life of crime. At an early age Mr. Allen became distrustful of his "fellow men" and turned to crimes like bank robbing and breaking into stores. He was imprisoned numerous times starting as a teenager, though he was rather resourceful in obtaining tools to free himself from incarceration. From every jail, he escaped or attempted escape, always ending up under strict watch and bound in irons. Later in life he turned to highway robbery, using a pistol to hold up travelers on deserted stretches of road. Most victims gave up their pocketbooks quickly, but one, John Fenno, stepped down from the wagon and put up a fight. Allen was recognized and a one-hundred dollar reward was offered for his capture. He fled to Canada but returned to the Boston area for a brief visit and was apprehended.

He spent the rest of his life in prison. As he lay dying, the warden spent time with him and was able to write down Allen's account of his life. Allen asked the warden to promise he would publish his words and have two copies bound in his own skin, one presented to the prison doctor and the other to John Fenno, the only victim brave enough to resist a robbery and him. Miraculously, this happened; Fenno's trophy book stayed in his family for several generations, until a descendant tired of the macabre relic and gave it to the Boston Atheneum.

[1] *Émile Zola wrote an introduction shortly after the early editions, arguing it should be placed anywhere in the house so the women could read it as a cautionary tale: "Stop hiding his book; put it on your tables; just as our fathers did with the canes with which they whipped their children."*

The Allegories

At the Grolier Club in New York is a copy of *Le Traicte de Peyne,* an allegorical poem dedicated to Monseigneur and Madame de Lorraine from a sixteenth-century unpublished manuscript. Bound in human skin by Kauffman-Petit, it is a beautiful example of the binder's craft and a treasure that would be a highlight of any collection. The title translates to "A Treatise on Pain and Suffering"; according to the introduction written in 1868, the poem is by three penitents, the Penitent d'Arches, and begins with a dedication to the Lord and Lady who protected them.

But perhaps the example of anthropodermic bibliopegy that has had the most lasting impact on twentieth-century literature is another volume in the John Hay Library: a copy of Adolphe Belot's 1870 novel, *Mademoiselle Giraud, ma femme.* Belot's novel tells the story of a man discovering his wife is gay and the subsequent disintegration of his marriage and mental state. As with most of Adolphe Belot's work, this created quite a stir and was condemned as moral outrage while selling very well.[1] Handwritten on the front flyleaf of the John Hay Library's copy is "Bound in human skin/S.B.L." and on the back "Genuine human skin" in the same hand. The library also holds a letter written by Sam Loveman of Bodley Book Shop further attesting to the binding's authenticity.

Loveman, as it happens, was a good friend of H.P. Lovecraft, and accompanied the horror writer on a visit to the graveyard of Brooklyn's Flatbush Reformed Church. This visit was Lovecraft's inspiration for the short story, "The Hound," which contains the first mention of the Necronomicon, a grimoire bound in human skin—a mythical tome that had its inspiration in a very real book with a very real history.

This survey is more concerned with a book's DNA than human genetics, and as such I've included some volumes that I'm skeptical about. It's not hard to imagine the reaction of some bookbinders on being presented with a roll of freshly harvested skin. Do you suppress your repulsion and fears or substitute it with hide from a less empathic creature? The color and texture of leather can easily be manipulated. It's my belief this happened more than once, but I haven't let a question of authenticity ruin a good story.

PART V

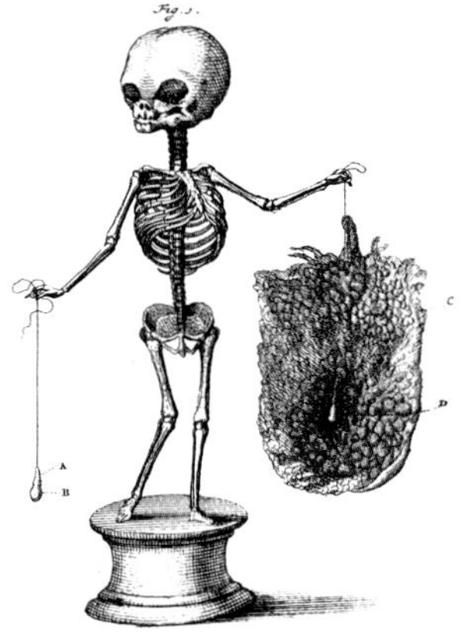

THE DEVIL *IN* THREE DIMENSIONS

RONNI THOMAS

IN 2012, I ATTENDED AN ONLINE AUCTION IN PARIS, FRANCE, with the hopes of securing a nearly complete set of dirty old tissue stereoviews. The auction house estimated that the collection would sell for no more than four hundred euros, and I was confident that I'd be able to secure these stereoviews for my own collection. As it happened, though, the bidding was far more intense—by the time it was over, I had bid what amounted to almost fifteen hundred euros (money I didn't have), only to lose anyway to a French bidder who, in the end, paid twice that for the collection.

But let me back up a bit... For my thirtieth birthday, my wife got me a beautiful stereograph complete with a set of 3D stereoviews from around the world. Having a deep love affair with early technology and art, I was fascinated by how amazing seeing the world in 3D photography might have been for our early ancestors. But of course, it was a fleeting novelty. Until, that is, I decided to see what exactly people nearly two hundred years our senior felt they needed to take 3D pictures of. The strange and unusual has sort of been the one consistent theme in my life, and so I decided to start my search there. Amazingly, I found 3D images of ghosts, dead cats, skin deformities, fat, naked women and a library of just amazing imagery.

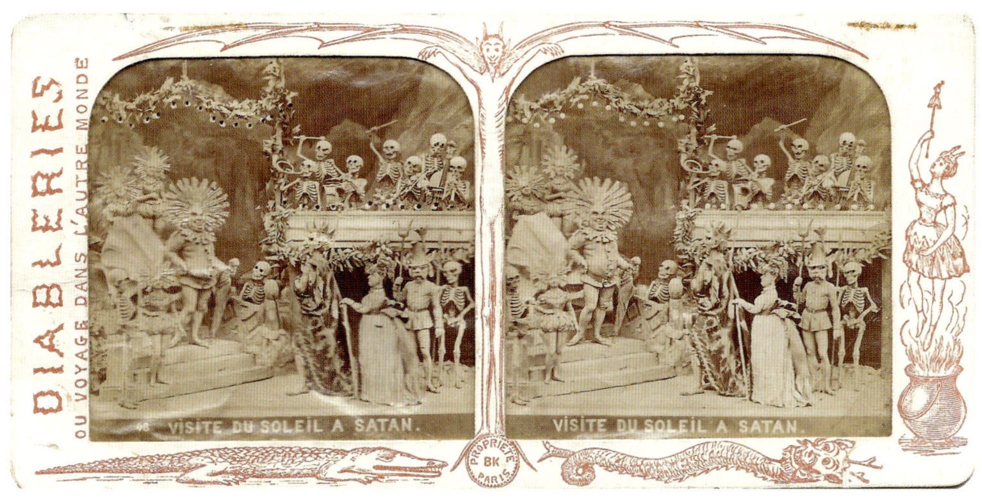

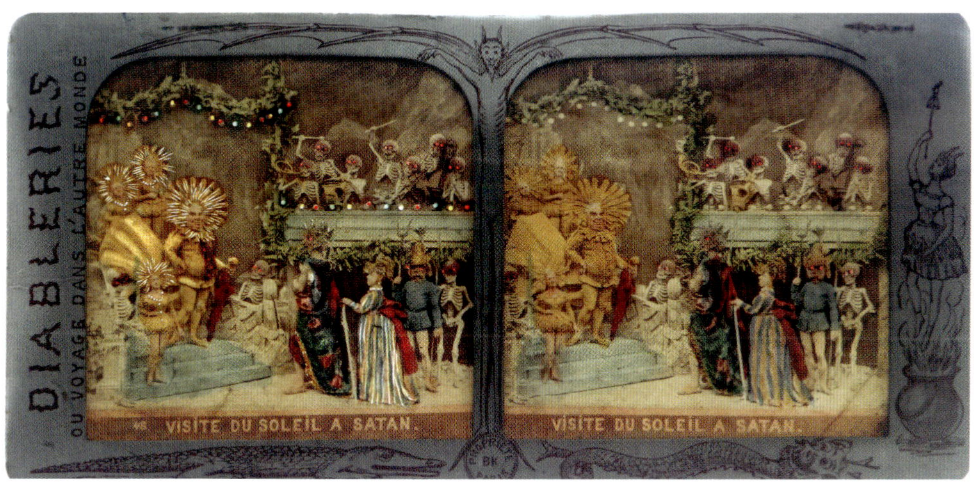

Image above: Front- and backlit Diablerie. Photographed and courtesy of Corey Schjoth, http://www.phantasmagoriaphoto.com.

But nothing prepared me for the slides I would wind up bidding on at that Paris auction...

They are called *Les Diableries*: a series of 3D slides depicting Satan's daily life in hell. Each slide consists of a beautifully sculpted, miniature scene (probably no larger than ten to

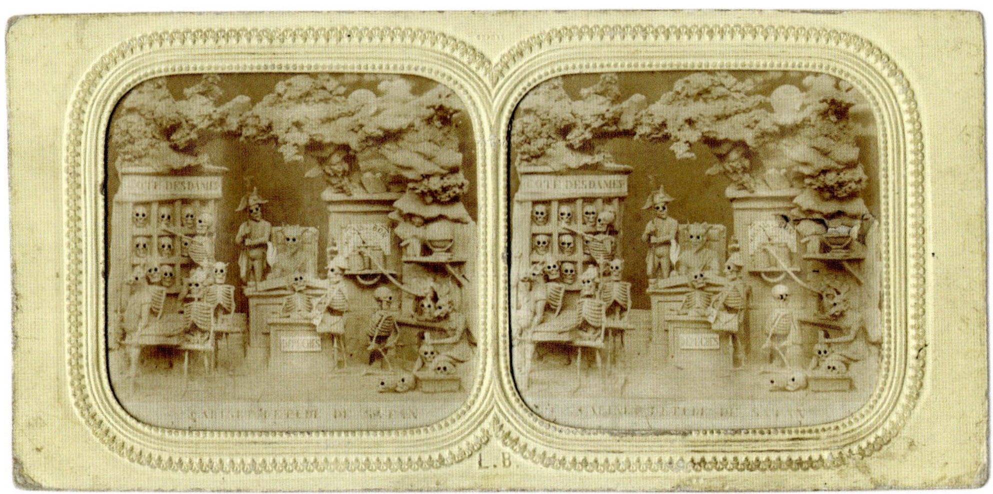

Images on following pages are all Diableries from the author's collection.

twelve inches, total) which was then photographed in 3D and printed onto translucent tissue paper. The series dates back to the 1860s, and only recently, it seems, have they begun to gain attention from the mainstream world. While I lost that online auction in 2012, I've still managed to acquire quite a few of these stereoviews from various sources, occasionally unearthing an overlooked gem in a stack of bargain-bin antiques.

My personal obsessions lay with the content—it's the lighter side of hell. Scenes such as Satan's kitchen and Satan home in bed with a bit of a cold. One of my favorite slides has a group of damned skeletons playing cards outside the gates of paradise. The skeletons seem to be having a grand old time (except of course when they are being playfully tormented by their dark ruler), and express their joy through dancing, playing the double bass, and drinking champagne. They are a testament to the Romantic obsession with excess, decadence, and, of course, my personal favorite theme: rebellion.

The whole idea strikes me as a very forward-thinking concept. That they used the devil as their central figure is no surprise; in the

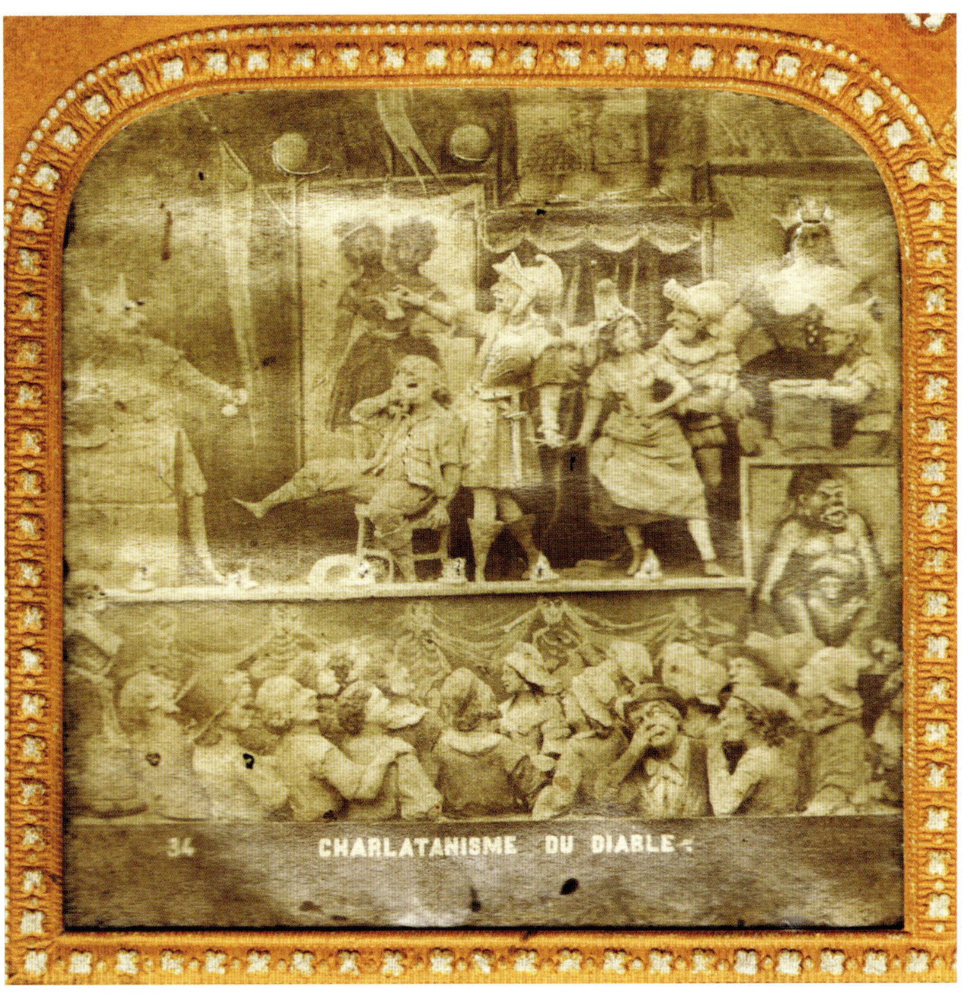

early nineteenth century, even in a very Catholic territory, the devil had become somewhat of a metaphor for quite a few things that would evolve into "modern entertainment": the thrill of fear, the drama of rebellion. No longer was the devil the scary, multiheaded dragon from the early Christian days, or the horned torturer of the Medieval era. By the eighteenth century, our modern devil was the trickster, the affable master, and, of course,

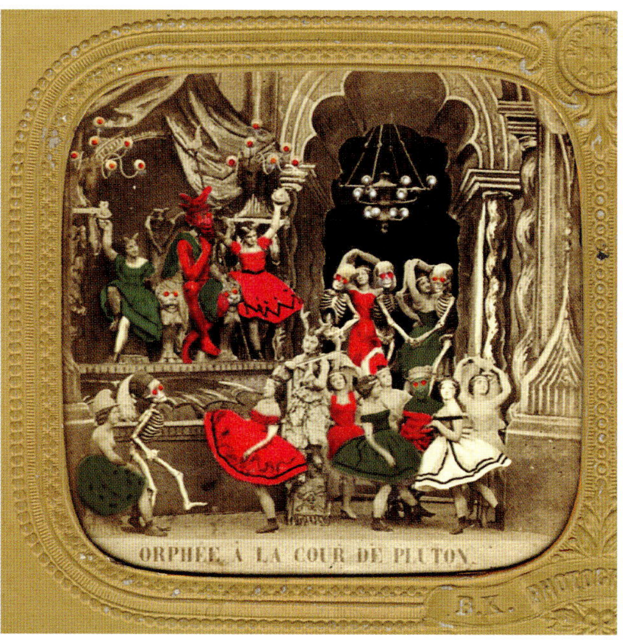

all too human (if not metaphorically the "true savior" for many poets and artists). So having the devil in scenarios that are decadent and human in these slides seems to make perfect sense. Arguably, 1860s France was pretty hellish, at least for the struggling artist, and to choose an almost cartoonish rendering of what daily life in hell would be like seems awfully provocative. Which may be the reason that so many of these stereoviews go uncredited.

Of course, quite a few of the sculptures used to make the slides *do* have a few signatures. The three names associated with sculpting the scenes of *Les Diableries* are Louis Alfred Habert, Pierre Adolph Hennetier, and Louis Edmond Cougny, all documented legitimate artists. In fact, I was proud to discover something very interesting that links Habert to one particular slide. In the slide for "Satan Malade," behind the ailing devil, sitting atop a clock, is a miniature sculpture of a woman. This is

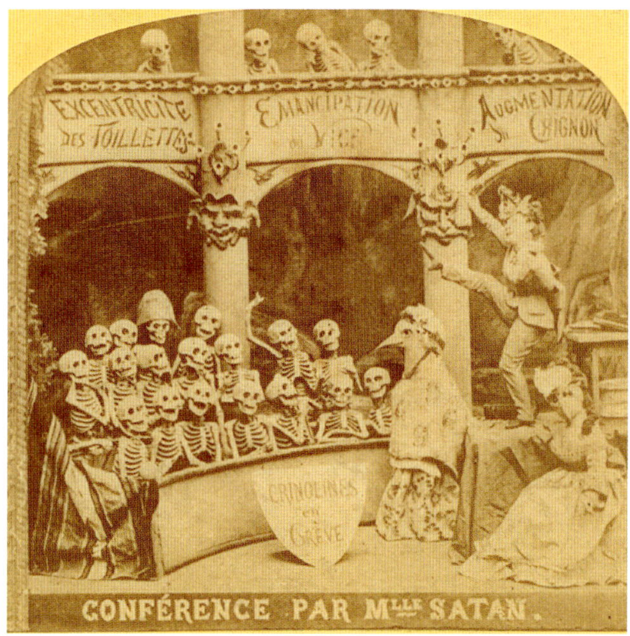

a nod to a very famous sculpture Habert had made in bronze, a subtle signature embedded in the backdrop of hell.

How many actual sets of *Diableries* there are out there is something that comes with a great deal of suspicion, but the most wildly recognized series is referred to as the "A Series": this specific series contained seventy-two individual slides, which were all "tissue" views. The design of these slides is simply fantastic, down to the outer wrapping (sometimes framed in demon wings with devils on each side of the printing). Each of these views would be hand painted in watercolors on the backside of the actual image, so when light would pass through you got an array of color. Another interesting trick the designers of the slides did was to prick tiny pinholes in the eyeballs of the skeletons; with lights shining from behind the slides, it gave the illusion that the skeletons' eyes were flickering.

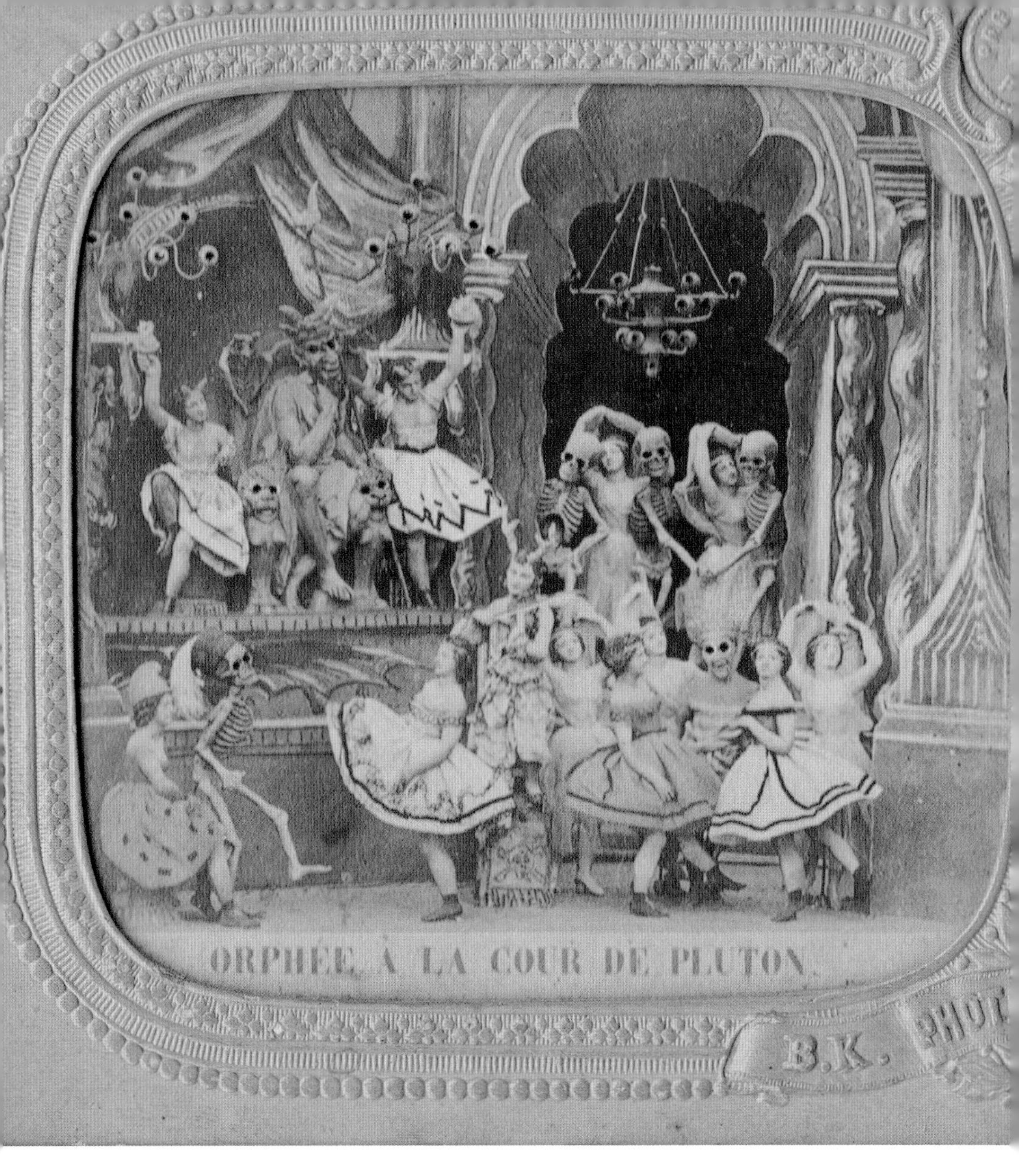

We can safely assume that this specific "A Series" was primarily sculpted by Hennetier and Habert. Assuming, though, that these are the work of just two artists, what's strange about the slides is the variety of styles they depict. Some of the slides are presented to be quite silly and almost look ripped from a Ray

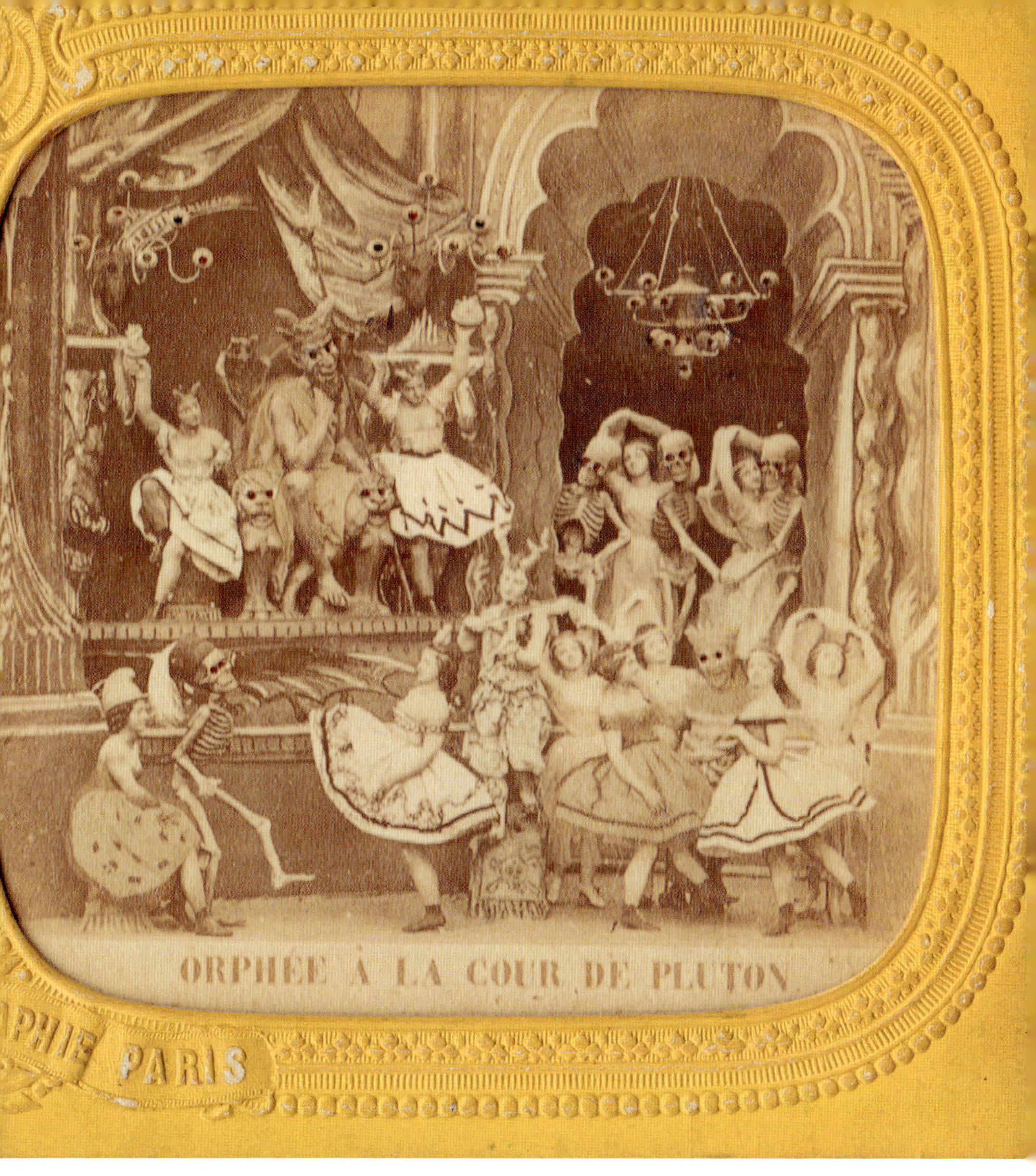

Harryhausen film, as with the slide "Le Bibliothèque infernal," which has a witty scene of a Claymation-like devil in his library. Others maintain a more classical, almost religious view of the underworld such as "La Résurrection," which features the devil locked in battle with heralding angels.

Past the seventy-two most well-documented slides I've come across—in my own collection as well as others—many *Diableries* that time seems to have all but forgotten. A lot of the alternate slides mirror slides from the "A Series." As discovered by Thomas Weynants of the *Early Visual Media* website, there are two versions of "Satan Malade," both similar but of course presented in different styles. It has been suggested that there were possibly "stereo-rivals," competing for "Diabolical Dominance"!

The one consistency that links each of the slides, however, is the apparent satire of the excessive, decadent lifestyle of the upper classes. Many people look at these as some sort of a social or political commentary of Napoleon's tyranny. I have often said that politicizing them takes the fun out of it, and I stand by that; the images themselves speak loudly enough without the glass eye of political history picking them apart. One can look at these images as early entertainment, early cinema, or a very new and exciting way to get lost in the underworld. My specific interest in this series, as a filmmaker and storyteller, is its connection to a wild history of devilish satire, from the Middle Ages to present day. Here—truly—are *our* ancestors. Not only were they using the new technology of the day to explore the world of art, but they were using the devil as their metaphor to get their creative point across. And it's the devil we know and love, far from the scary (though equally entertaining) devil of the Middle Ages. Our *Diableries* devil throws parties and drinks champagne, he sings and dances with his skeleton band, and, he occasionally tortures a dead soul, just for fun.

And so more than just a curious interest in their history and design, I feel as though I am a certain part of these images. If nothing else, the world of *Les Diableries* is certainly the world I'd enjoy spending all eternity.

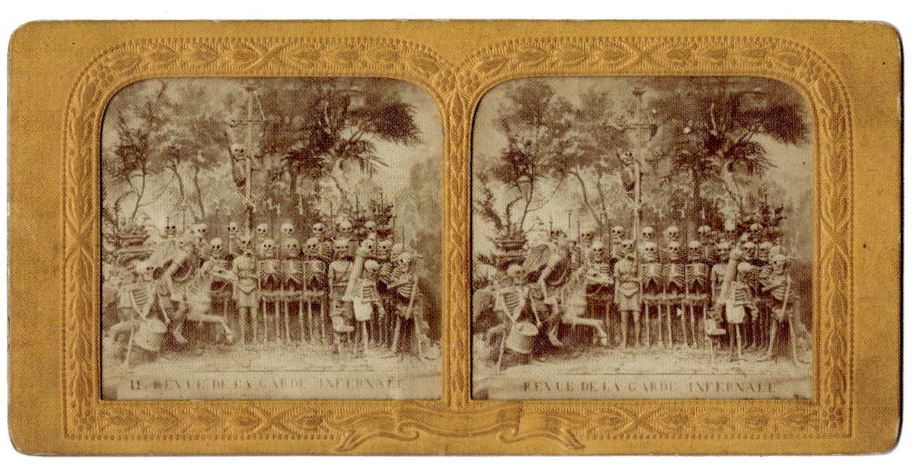

12. REVUE DE LA GARDE INFERNALE
REVUE DE LA GARDE INFERNALE

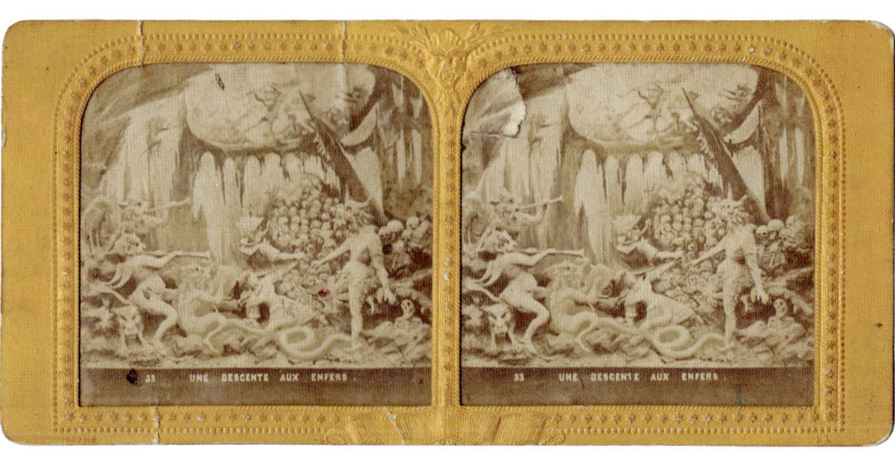

33 UNE DESCENTE AUX ENFERS.
33 UNE DESCENTE AUX ENFERS.

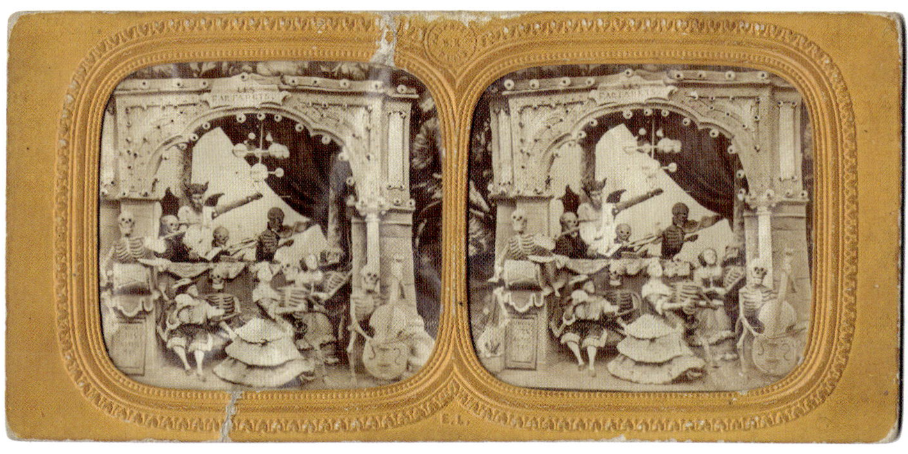

E. L.

ANTHROPOMORPHIC MOUSE TAXIDERMY CLASS

AMBER MAYKUT

Strive to put your mounted animals in easy natural poses unless you are making a grotesque, in which case go the length.
—Albert B. Farnham, *Taxidermy for Pleasure and Profit* (1944)

THE WORD "TAXIDERMY" IS DERIVED FROM THE GREEK: "TAXI" means arrangement and "derm" refers to skin. A deer head on a wall, a hunting trophy preserved and mounted for display, may be the first or most familiar image that comes to mind when the average person thinks of taxidermy. This stylized preservation, in itself, is a scientific art form that requires much time, patience, and skill, as one must carefully prepare and stuff, or mount (in the taxidermy community, the term "mounting" is the preferred term and has come to replace the term "stuffing"), a once-living thing in a fashion that renders it true to life. Traditionally, a taxidermist's goal is to re-create or reproduce the animal so that it looks realistic. But long before hunters were hanging their kills over fireplaces in cabins in backwoods America, taxidermy—and its predecessors—had a long and varied history. The first preserved animals can be traced as

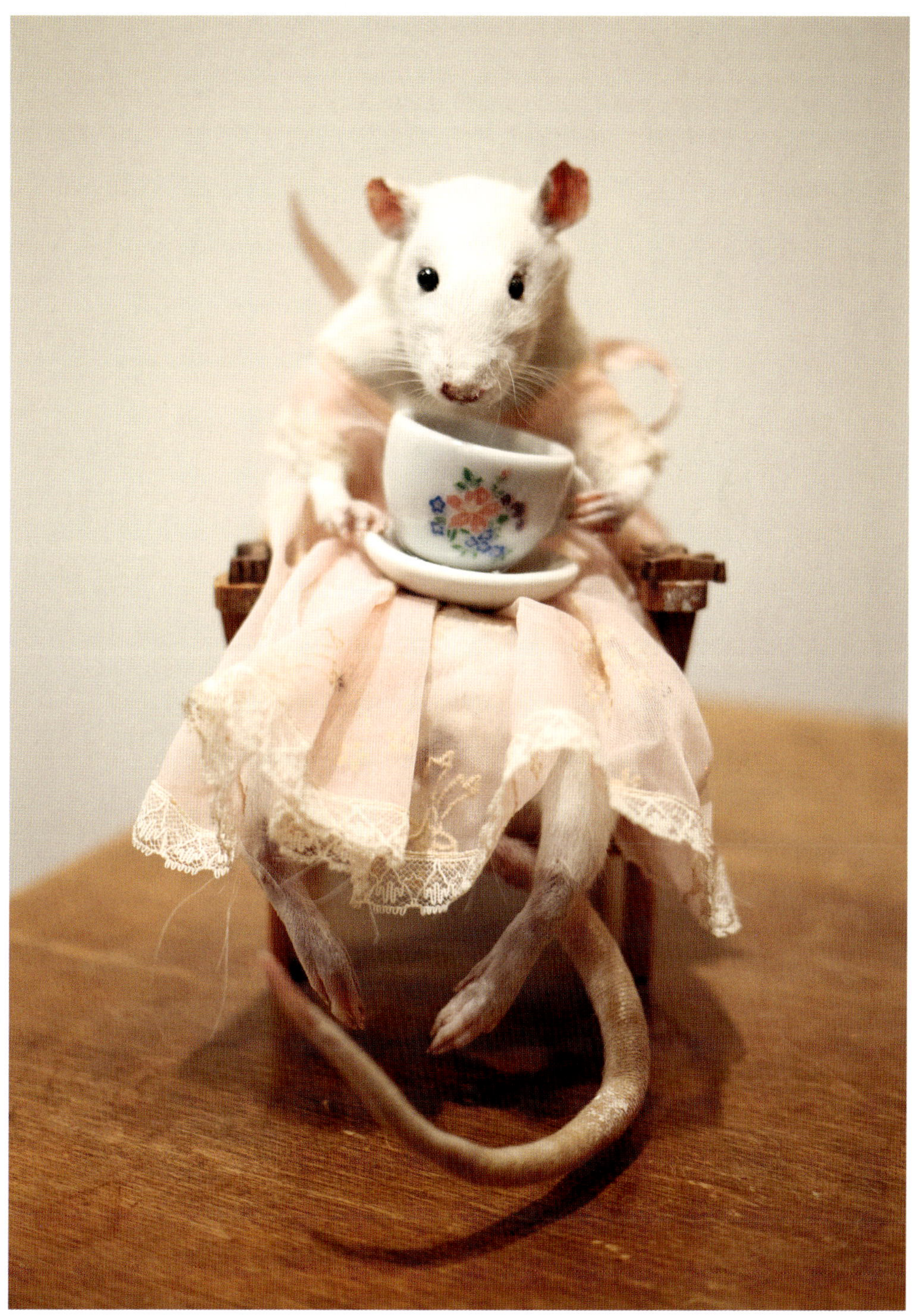

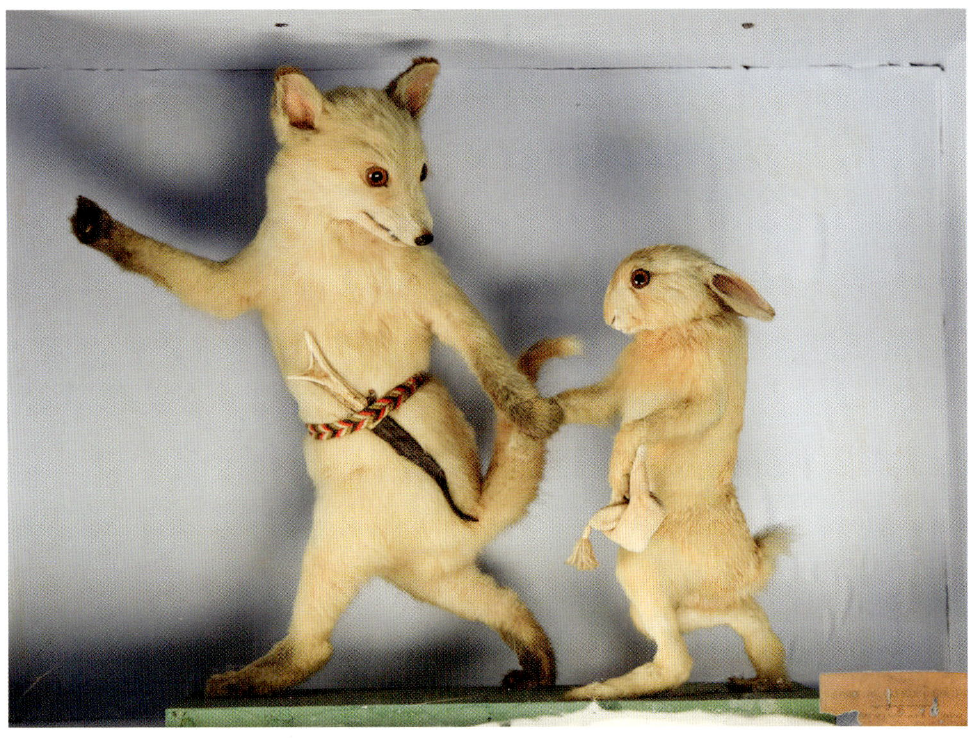

All photos by Joanna Ebenstein.

far back as their appearances alongside mummies in Ancient Egypt, where animals like cats were embalmed, mummified, and buried with their presumable owner. To many, this type of preservation is not considered true taxidermy, but more of an evolutionary step leading to it. Taxidermy as we know it today found its humble beginnings in the nineteenth century, as the demand for leather and quality skins was growing. Most every town at the time had its own tannery business, and a busy, successful one at that. Hunters started bringing their kills into upholstery shops requesting the skins be stuffed with cotton and rags and sewn shut. From there, it wasn't long until taxidermy stepped away from realistic representations found in nature and crept into caricature.

Anthropomorphic taxidermy consists of taking a taxidermied animal and personifying it, or dressing it up and posing it to make it appear to be involved in a human activity. A mouse wearing a suit, sitting at a table, drinking a cup of tea, is an example of such. This style of taxidermy was popularized in the Edwardian and Victorian eras, where taxidermists like Herman Ploucquet exhibited his fantastic work to the British for the first time with his Great Exhibition of 1851. Edward Hart was another early practitioner of the genre, whose portrayal of two red squirrels competing in a boxing match against each other is quite striking. Likewise, British taxidermist Walter Potter is probably the most well-known anthropomorphic taxidermist you'll find. Potter lived from 1835 to 1918 in Sussex, England. For decades, taxidermying dead animals was considered a suitable hobby for young boys all over the world. The book, *The American Boys Handy Book*, published as late as 1963 and a predecessor of sorts to the *Dangerous Book for Boys* that was oft-displayed in Barnes and Noble storefronts in this century's early aughts, contained step-by-step information about how to tie knots, train a dog, build animal traps, confiscate and preserve bird eggs and nests, and (gasp!) taxidermy dead animals like owls (which is now highly illegal in the U.S.). Thus, it is not surprising that Potter was more or less self-taught as a boy, using only attained manuals and books for guidance. Having also read his sister's books of English nursery rhymes, which depicted animals as the main characters of fictional stories, Potter thought of using nursery rhymes as a basis for many of his anthropomorphic works. At the age of 19, he started working on one of his most famous works, *The Death and Burial of Cock Robin*, based on the nursery rhyme of a similar name. The piece took him seven years to complete. The diorama, or tableau, was an elaborate depiction of the events in the story: an owl digging

Image left One of Hermann Ploucquet's tableaux telling the story of Reynard the Fox. Courtesy of Pat Morris.

a grave for the robin, a dove leading a funeral procession, a parson rook holding a sacred text. Potter gained attention by displaying his works in his father's inn, located in Bramber, a small village. As his works grew in number, so did attention for his work. Eventually, his works were moved onto their own premises, a museum of sorts, next door to the inn, where patrons and visitors were welcomed.

It is in the very spirit of Walter Potter that the Anthropomorphic Mouse Taxidermy Class began at Observatory, a gallery and event space hidden off the beaten path near the Gowanus Canal in Brooklyn, New York. The class is conducted by Sue Jeiven, whose taxidermy skills are largely self-taught. Exploring the annals and anals of dead mice with an inquisitive nature and beginner's results, Jeiven concluded that skinning an animal, no matter the size, is no simple task; it seemed a natural solution to cover up a blood stained, shredded pelt with props and clothing. Why should a perfectly imperfect, taxidermied mouse go to waste? Each creation, with its own imperfections, misgivings and teachable moments felt exponentially endearing when it came to life with the right dollhouse accoutrements. Roadkill and whatever vermin her pet cats could scrape up from her dilapidated Brooklyn apartment seemed like shady, yet fair game. A dead mouse diva was born.

In preparation for the class, Jeiven and her assistant, Emily Hexe, would collect whatever appropriately sized props they could come up with, including modified doll clothes and dollhouse furniture, bizarre thrift store finds, and an assortment of fabrics, ribbons, and makeshift material from craft stores. Going to thrift stores and dollar stores would never seem the

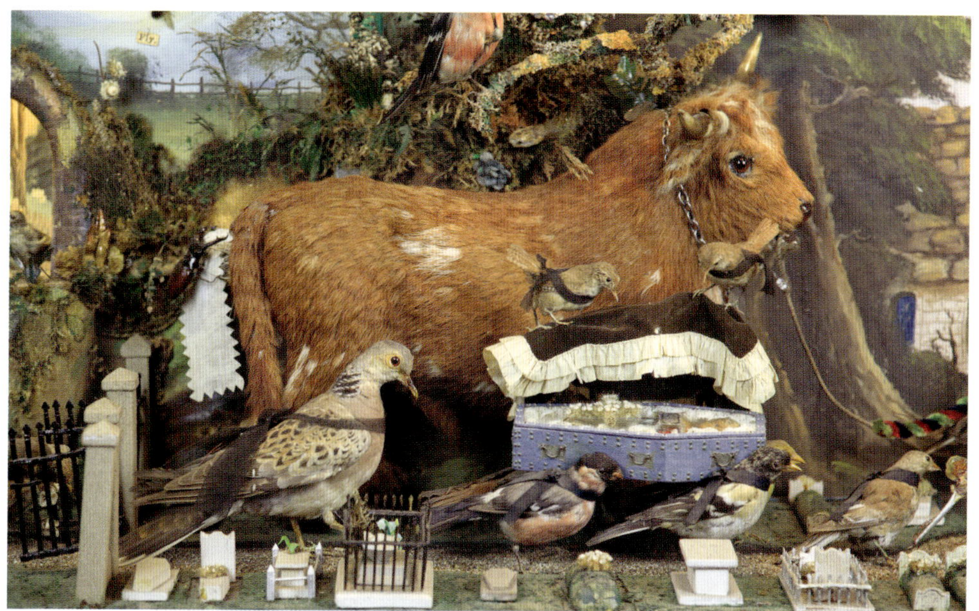

The Death & Burial of Cock Robin by Walter Potter, 1861. Courtesy of Pat Morris.

same to those constantly on the hunt for whatever miniature items could be dug up or ripped off a doll or stuffed animal. Reusable tools and instruments were cleaned and prepared, new boxes of gloves and scalpels were purchased. The feeder mice were collected and kept in the freezer until about an hour before class, which is about how long they took to thaw. The assistants maintained the setting up and breaking down of the four-hour class, and helped students along. Tablecloths would go on the tables, and placemats would lie on the tables in front of each folding chair to delineate individual workstations. Bowls of borax, a natural, powdered laundry detergent, disinfectant, and all-purpose preserver (not to be confused with powdered boric acid, which is highly toxic and used to poison and kill pests, vermin, and other small animals) would abound. A collection of wire, wire cutters, needles, thread, scissors, and modeling clay were shared among the group. Since 2011, eager students

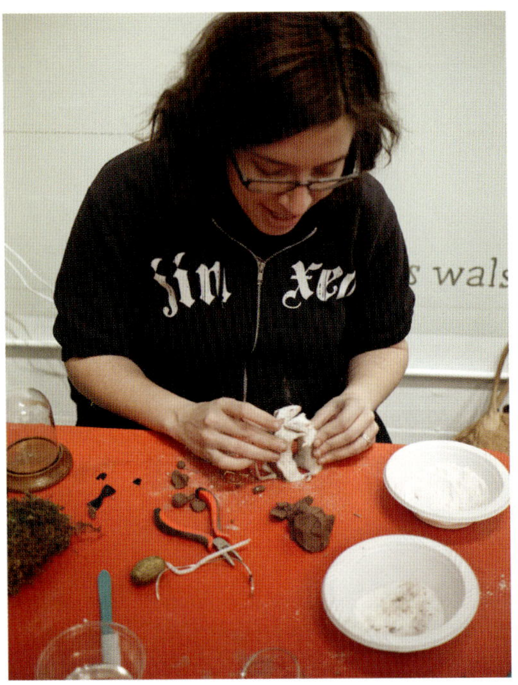

Student Elizabeth New putting the finishing touches on her taxidermied mice.

have shown up to the one-day class empty handed, having walked in with no previous knowledge, and left with their very own taxidermy mouse creation, fully fashioned to their own likings.† Students would gather around the teacher and assistants to watch and learn what to do in the following step-by-step fashion:

---

† *It is worth noting that those making up the class also often seemed to be animal lovers who shared a deep belief that their taxidermy should be ethically sourced. Many were collectors only of vintage taxidermy pieces or were concerned with how a newly taxidermied animal was acquired. Many taking the class wouldn't dream of eating crappy fast food, or, surprisingly, were vegetarians or vegans. If ethically procured, and if the craft maintains an air of mischief and classicism, making taxidermy in the present day and age can be a fantastic throwback to an ancient art that stirs modern morbid curiosity. By using animals that have died of natural causes or by accident (road kill), or unused animal remains that would otherwise go to waste, it felt much easier to find humor and beauty in a piece than if that animal was hunted, trapped, and killed for the sake of taxidermy alone.*

Lay your mouse down on its stomach, spreading out its arms and legs to the sides. Using a scalpel, cut one, straight, initial incision down the back of the mouse from the base of the neck to above the base of the tail, along the spine. Seeing the difference between skin and muscle tissue is easy. Use the scalpel and your hands to gently push and pull the flesh, separating it from the carcass. Use borax to deter the look and smell, as well as disinfect and toughen the skin along the way. Free the entire mouse torso from the skin, being careful of the mouse's abdominal wall; opening the digestive area can lead to some foul sights and smells.

Once the torso is fully separated from the skin, the front and hind legs are then severed from the skin and meat, and detached at the joints using the scalpel. The four leg bones, from the paws to the knee joints, are left attached and inside the skin. The inside of the tail is then carefully but firmly removed, sliding the skin off almost like a sock. The legs and tail will later be wired into place. The next step is fully detaching the rest of the carcass from the pelt, which is only attached at the head. Pull the skin up over the neck of the mouse and behead the mouse, slicing at the base of the neck until the carcass is fully separated from the head. The skull is left inside the pelt and stays attached.

You may next want to pull the skin up over the neck as high up as the eyes and pluck out the eyes with a needle. If not, the eyes can be detached externally later. Remove any remaining flesh from around the skull, including the brain from the base of the mouse head. With the carcass fully detached and pelt inside out, the mouse is then fully submerged in borax for a period of time to dry out a bit.

Meanwhile, grab some clay and model it into the approximate size and shape of your carcass. Remove your pelt from the borax and place your clay inside it. Mold the clay, adding or removing clay until the pelt seals perfectly around the clay, leaving no clay exposed. Then, using five pieces of cut wire (four pieces if you choose to use pipe cleaner for the tail), run a wire inside each leg, down alongside each leg bone until the end of the wire goes into the paw pad. Position the other end of each wire into the clay body to maintain the position you want each limb to stay in.

Sew your mouse closed using double thread and a surgical-style stitch down the initial incision, then use a toothbrush to brush the fur in a fashion that camouflages the white thread into the white mouse fur. The mouse is then posed into the position of choice, easiest usually being that of sitting upright, using the hind legs and tail for balance. Remove the eyes using a fine needle, if not previously removed, and insert ball head sewing needles, cut short, in the color of choice. Traditional black was most popular, but devil-red, angel-white, and little-boy-blue mouse eyes would make their appearances in each class. One student, after trying various eye colors, removed her small cubic zirconium stud earrings from her ears, and used them as sparkling eyeballs.

With needle and thread, a hot glue gun, and some trial and error, attach your desired clothing, props, and base to your mounted mouse until you are happy with the finished product. Voila! You have successfully channeled Walter Potter and have made a one-of-a-kind piece to add to your cabinet of curiosities/*wunderkammer.* Or, what a splendid ornament he will make for a mantelpiece. How appropriate that rascally little face will be peering out from behind some books in a NYC tenement apartment.

Image right: student project from Sue Jeiven's anthropomorphic taxidermy class.

It is important to note that one should not think that after reading a taxidermy essay or book, or taking a class, that without any other experience, you would be able to taxidermy an

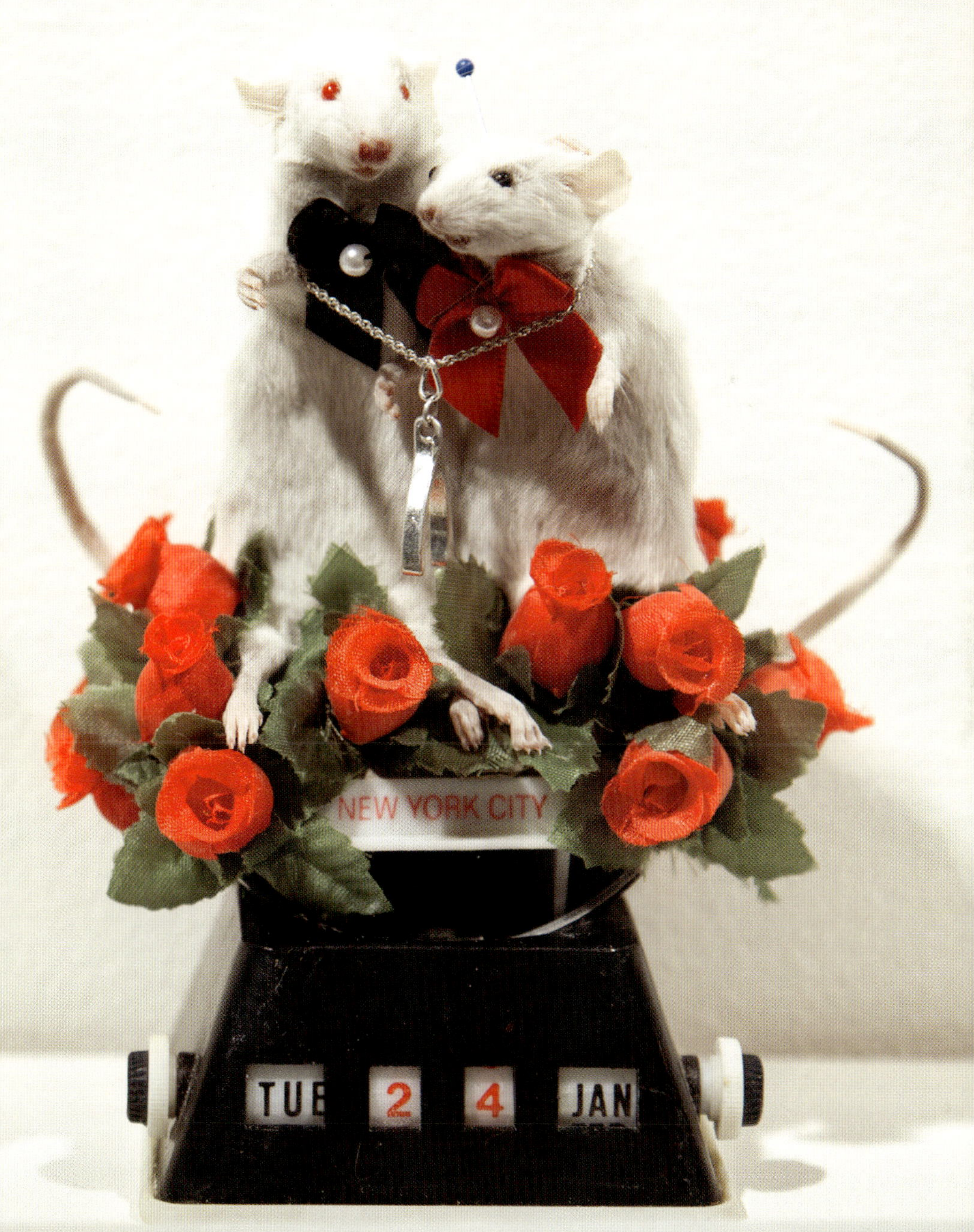
NEW YORK CITY
TUE
2
4
JAN

animal as neatly and perfectly as those you see in the natural history museums of the world, or even in the junk shop storefront windows of the world. On the contrary, the self-taught, amateur taxidermist must expect to make some pretty dismal failures. But each failure can teach you what to avoid during your next attempt. This is where the anthropomorphic aspect of the class played a big role: clothing and props were forgiving as Band-Aids, happily covering soon-forgotten hack jobs. As each student left class, their dressed up creation was photographed for posterity.

It is not overestimating to say that the class had a lasting impact on many of those who were lucky enough to take it—some students used this introductory course as a precursor to their own studies, going on to make taxidermy creations to sell, use in art pieces, or just grow their personal collections. The Anthropomorphic Mouse Taxidermy Class was often made up of a group that demonstrated that there exists a resurging interest in bizarre cultural relics, including the classical naturalist collections and studies of the likes of Charles Darwin.

For Darwin, a traditional naturalist, gaining knowledge of taxidermy wasn't just an interesting, amusing accomplishment. It was also a necessity that was more than a supplementary part of his profession. In the same way that a hunter would take pride in displaying his trophies or successes, a naturalist uses his/her taxidermy to show that he/she has gained experience and obtained a hands-on understanding of the natural makings and anatomy of their trophy.

In the past, these naturalists' works, collected in natural history museums, were considered beautiful re-creations, offering people a way to see realistic representations of wildlife that otherwise may have not been available to be examined and admired in person. As museums modernize themselves, their taxidermy items are often the first pieces to go. In the age of technology, where one has almost unlimited access to exploring the realities of wildlife and animals by just turning on the computer or television, taxidermy is argued to be needless, gratuitous, or perverse. Today, taxidermy feels like more of a cultural relic than nature. These animal representations are immortal, and as these antiquated living dead things have survived through the years, their original use and culture has become obsolete. They are now often seen as unusual timepieces or memorials rather than up-close opportunities to study science and nature. In the similar fashion that many modern young people may not subscribe to a religion but are intrigued by its relics and imagery, an old taxidermy piece is not just an antique—it can hold an almost mystical power as a timepiece from another era of thought and human consciousness.

THE

SPIRITUALISTS

SHANNON TAGGART

> *I asked these spirit figures if I was seeing them or if I was seeing what was in my own brain. They answered "both."*
> —Eileen Garrett, twentieth century medium
> (via Barbara Weisberg)

SPIRITUALISM IS A RELIGION BASED ON COMMUNICATING WITH spirits of the dead. Hugely popular in the nineteenth century, it radically impacted scientific inquiry and popular culture before fading into obscurity. I became aware of Spiritualism as a teenager when my cousin received a reading from a medium—the woman revealed a secret about my grandfather's death that proved to be true. Since then I have been deeply curious about how someone could know such a thing.

In 2001 I began photographing the place where that message was received: Lily Dale, New York, the world's largest Spiritualist community. I quickly immersed myself in the philosophy of Spiritualism; I had readings, experienced healings, joined in séances, attended a psychic college and sat in a medium's cabinet, all with my camera. I expected to spend one summer figuring out the tricks of the Spiritualist trade. Instead I peered into something truly mysterious. I stumbled upon a hidden world, an abandoned system with a storied history that became a resource and an inspiration for my own photographic theory and practice.

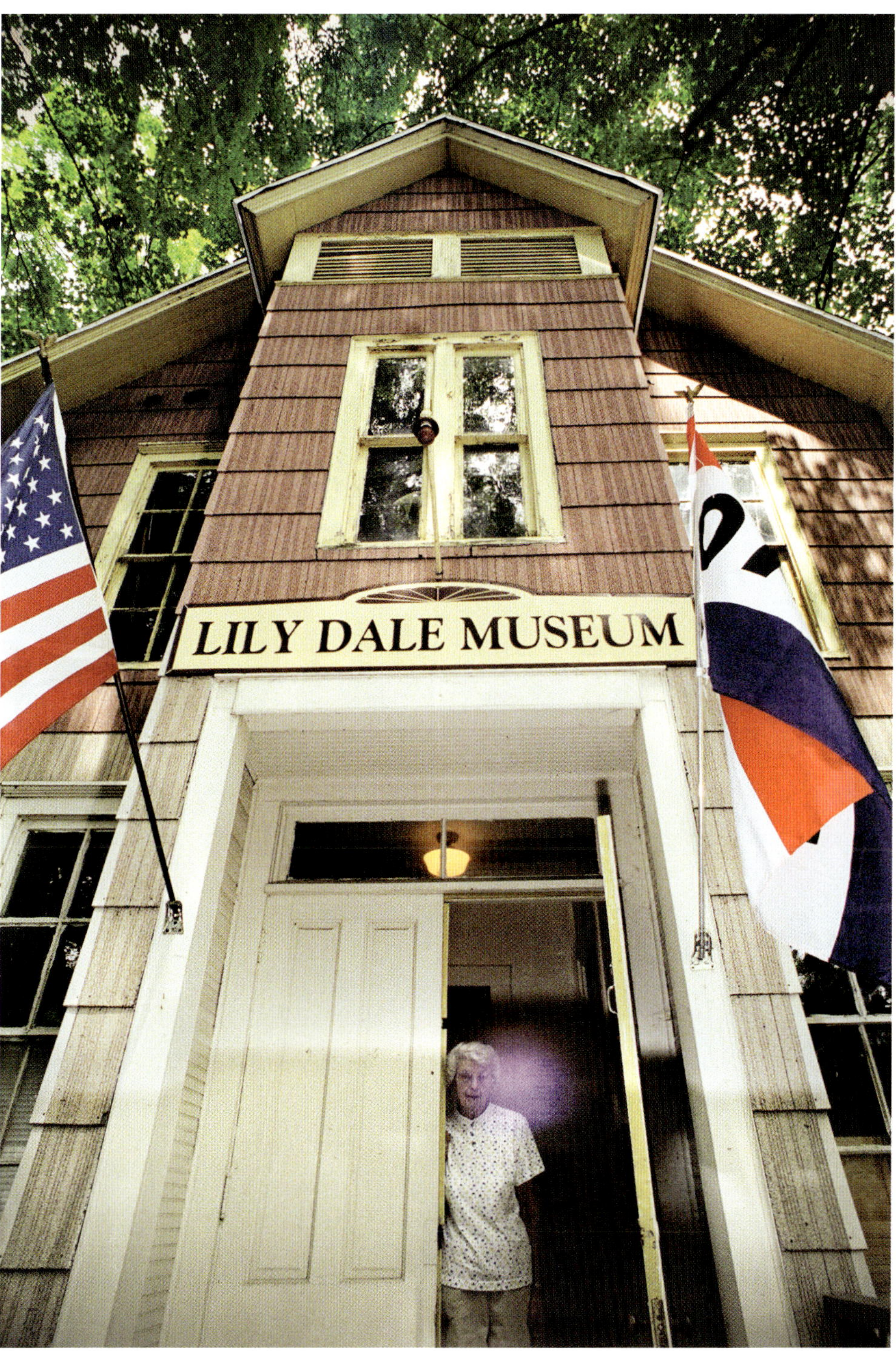
LILY DALE MUSEUM

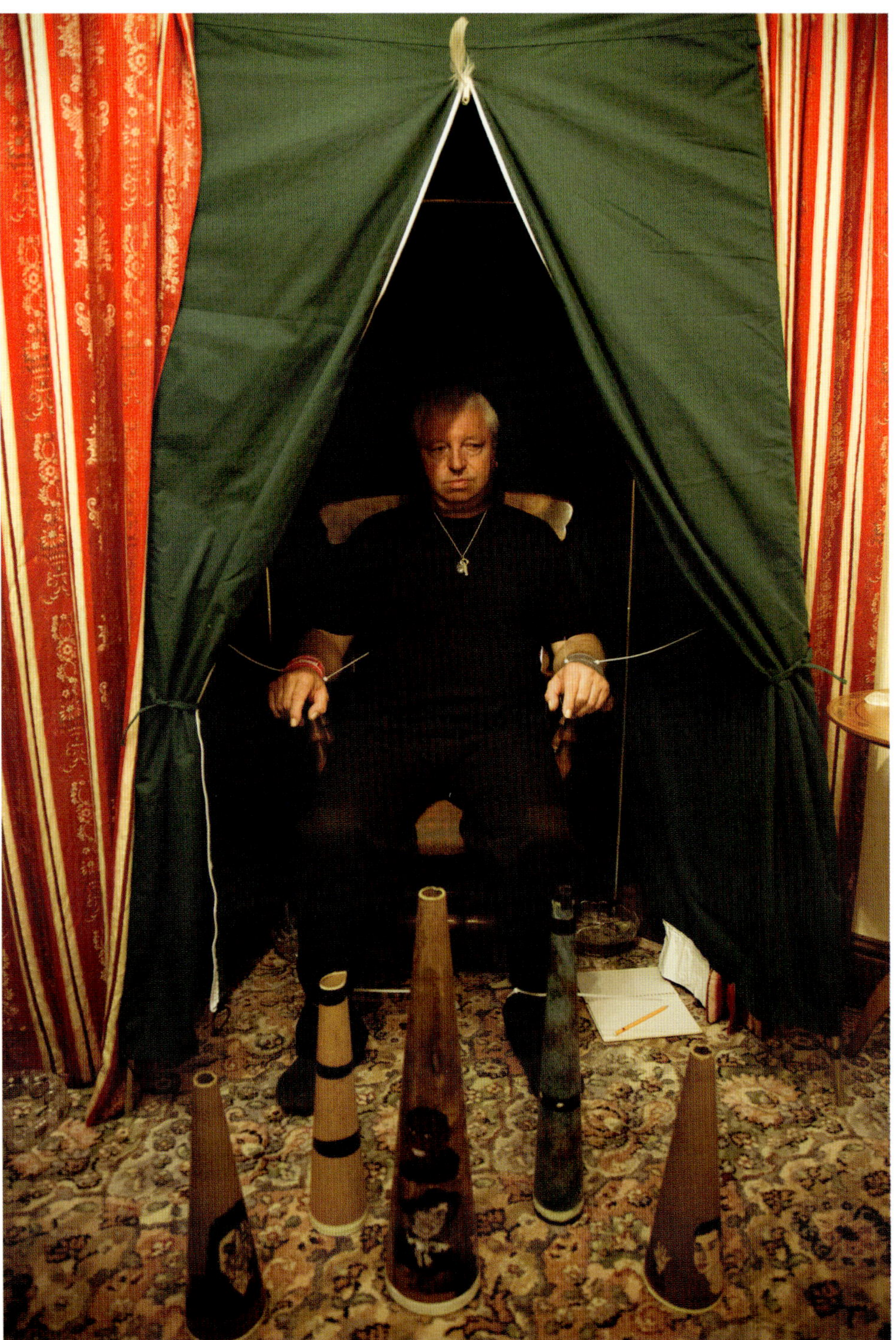

All photos by the author.

How do you photograph the invisible? Spiritualists communicate with the unseen and have always employed technology (however rudimentary) to amplify their connections. Trumpets, tables, talking boards, slates, canvases, cabinets, radios, cameras and audio recorders are used and misused in order to assist engagement with the spirit world. Even the body of the medium becomes an instrument for reception and transmission. Like a camera or a womb, the séance room is a dark chamber for origination and development. Sitting in these charged atmospheres, my thoughts focused on how to photograph these latent proceedings.

The answer came when I pushed my camera to the edge of its functionality and crossed the boundary of what is considered bad, wrong or unprofessional. Chance elements and the inherent imperfections of the photographic process (blur, abstraction, motion, flare) offer an agent for the immaterial, and the long exposures necessary to document séances are a catalyst, rendering time capsules from the exchange between a veiled presence and a visible body. The resulting photographs are records that seem to confirm these invisible correspondences.

Photography and Spiritualism have an intrinsic relationship. Photography's ability to trace the reflection and preserve time directly links it to mortality, Spiritualism's main concern. Both originated in the mid-nineteenth century and were popularized in the same city, Rochester, NY. Each has used the other as a tool to understand its own objective limitations and subjective complications. Photography itself is a paradox, both art and science, it serves each without the ability to leave the other untainted.

The intersection between Spiritualism and photography is a place where many opposites meet—mind and matter, heaven and earth, art and science, life and death. My pictures are meant as meditations on this riddle of liminality, the alchemy of ritual and the magic of the photographic process.

[FOLLOWING IMAGES]

Page 419: Dorothy with Bob's orb, Lily Dale, New York.

Page 420: Physical medium Chris Howarth before a séance, North Yorkshire, England.

Page 424 –425: Parade, Lily Dale, New York.

Page 426 –427: Ron with the Fox Sisters, Lily Dale, New York.

Page 428, top left: Student medium's cabinet, Stansted, England.

Page 428, top right: Sharon Harvey's medium's cabinet, Cheshunt, England.

Page 428, bottom left: Kai Muegge's medium's cabinet, Cassadga, New York.

Page 428, bottom right: Gordon Garforth's séance set up, Stansted, England.

Page 429, top: Vintage mold of ectoplasm, Stansted, England.

Page 429, bottom: The utensils Willa bent with her mind, Lily Dale, New York.

Page 430: Physical medium Gordon Garforth in trance, Harrogate, England.

Page 431: Physical medium Kai Muegge with ectoplasm, Cassadaga, New York.

Page 432: Gordon Garforth in trance, Stansted, England.

Page 433: Gordon Garforth with elongated hand, Stansted, England.

Page 434: Written message from Elvis Presley by physical medium Myra Basey, England.

Page 435: Apported penny in my tea cup, Stansted, England.

Page 436–437: Reverend Jean heals Jennifer, Lily Dale, New York.

Page 438: Sylvia Howarth working with her parallel world, North Yorkshire, England.

Page 439: Physical medium Sharon Harvey's spirit guide asks to show his mask, Cheshunt, England.

Page 440–441: After Sylvia Howarth's spirit art demonstration, North Yorkshire, England.

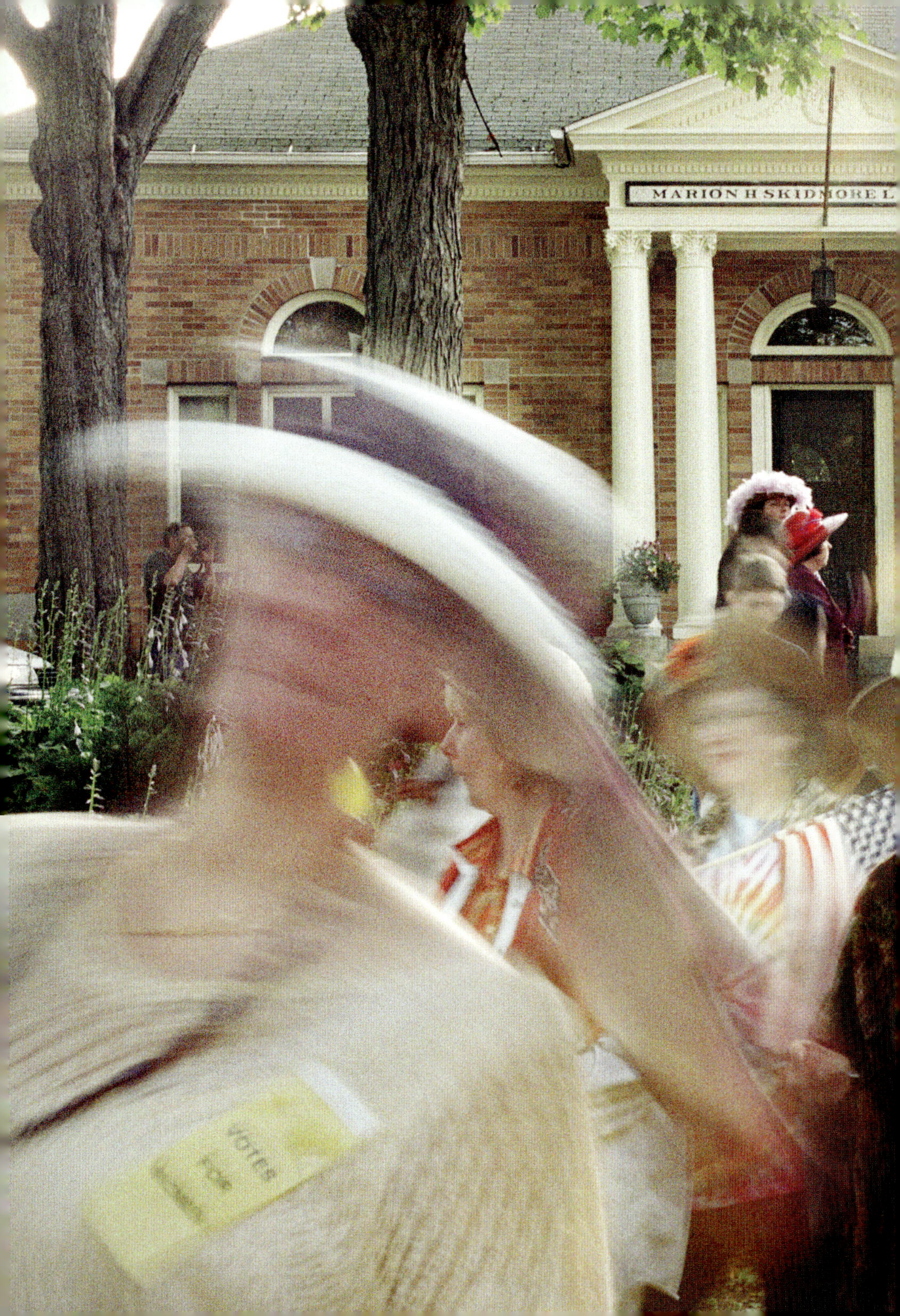
MARION H SKIDMORE L
VOTES FOR

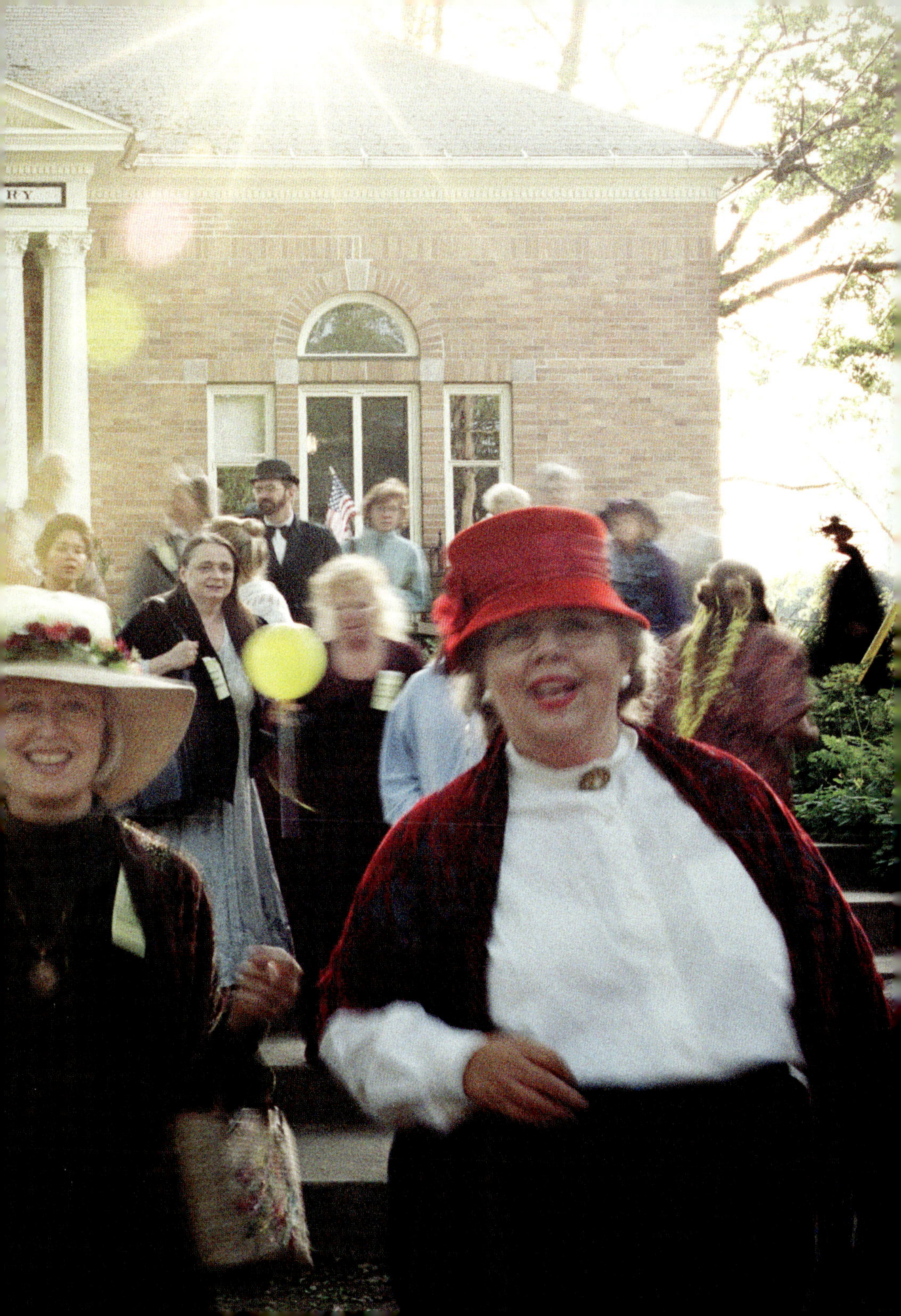

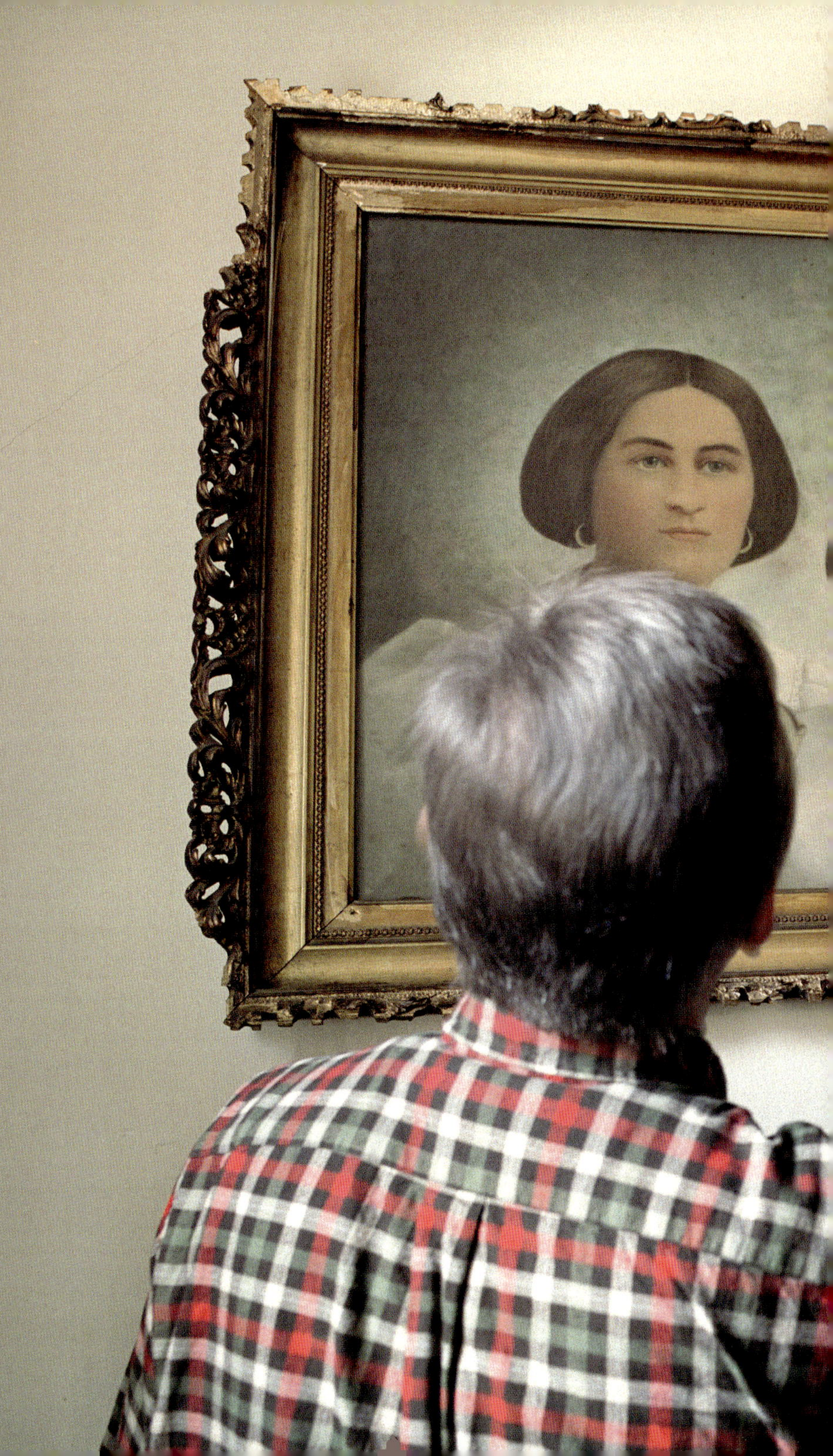

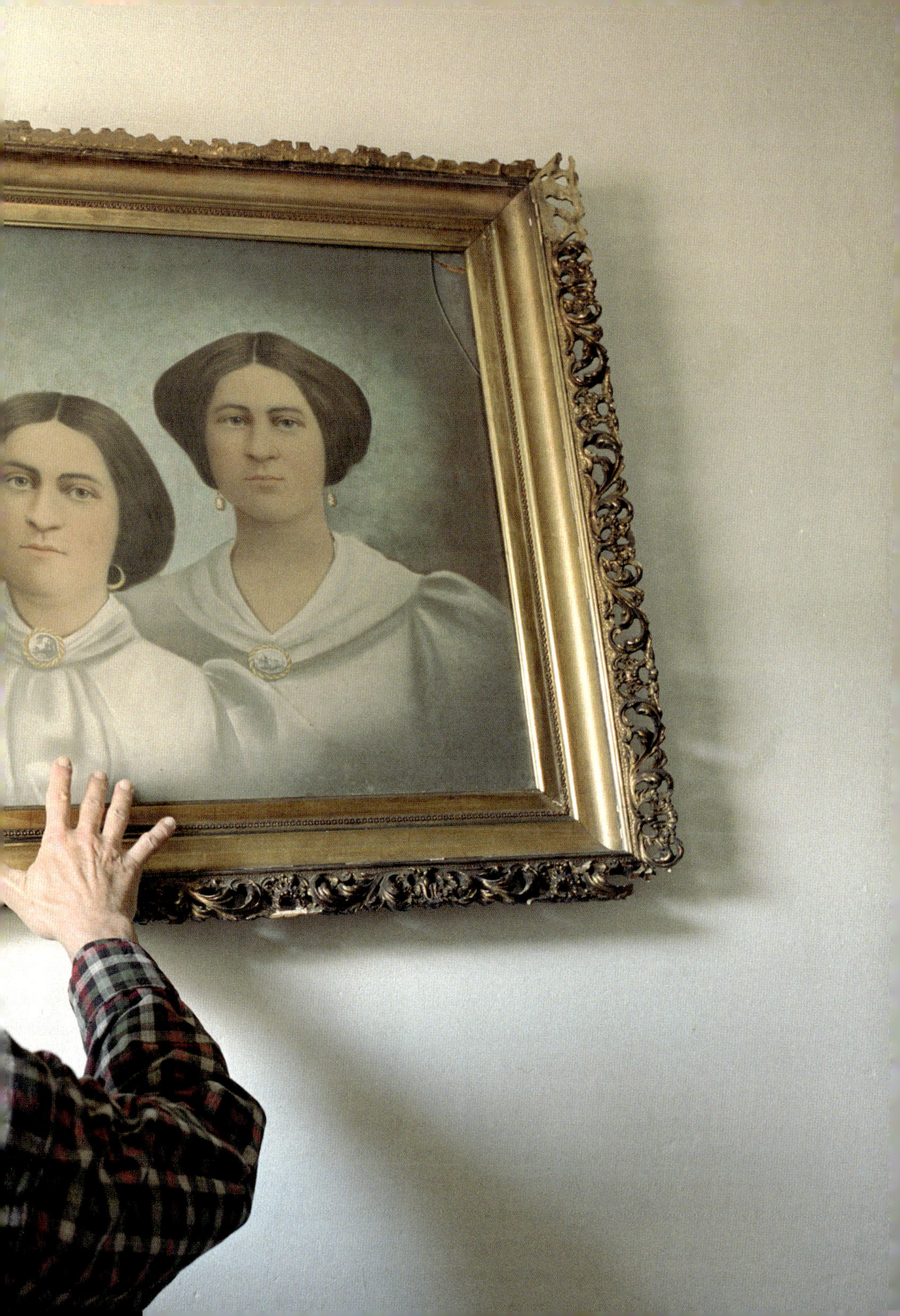

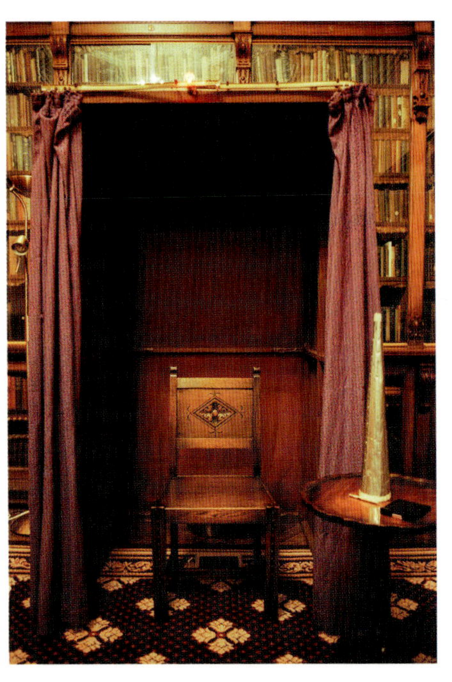
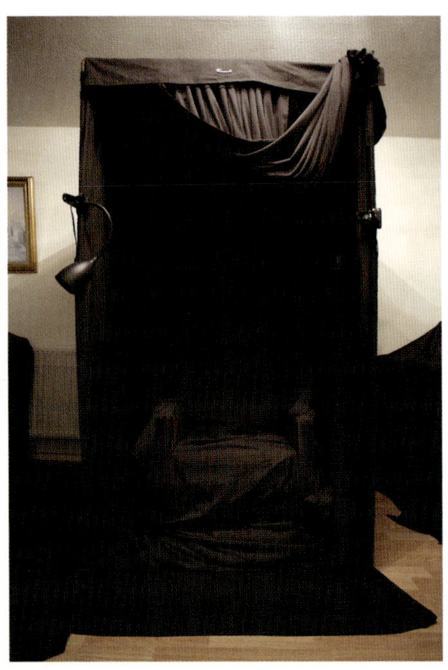
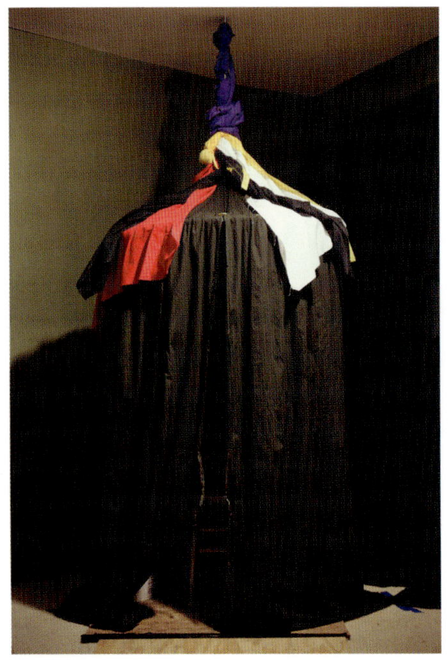
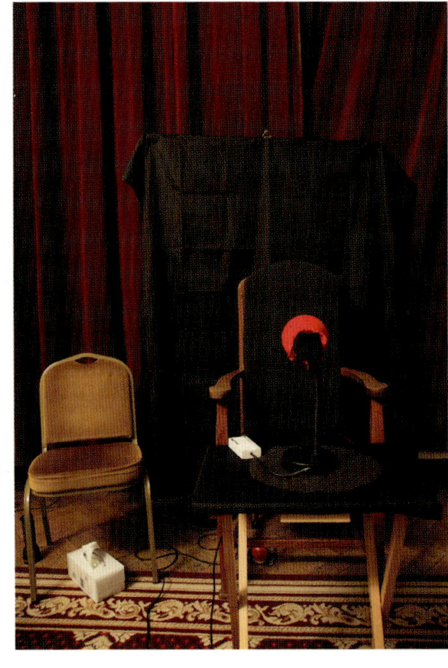

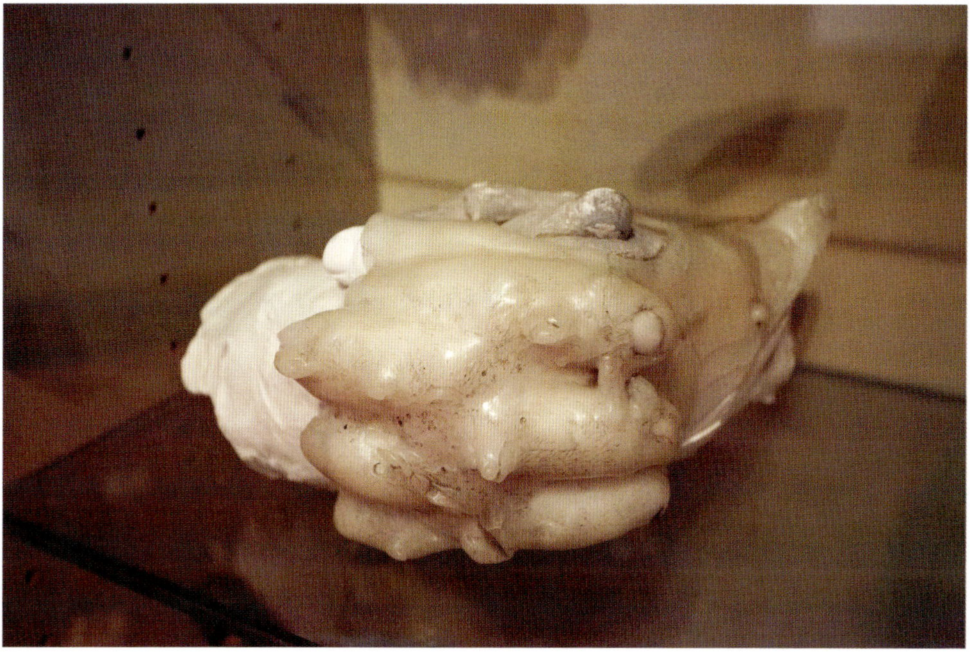

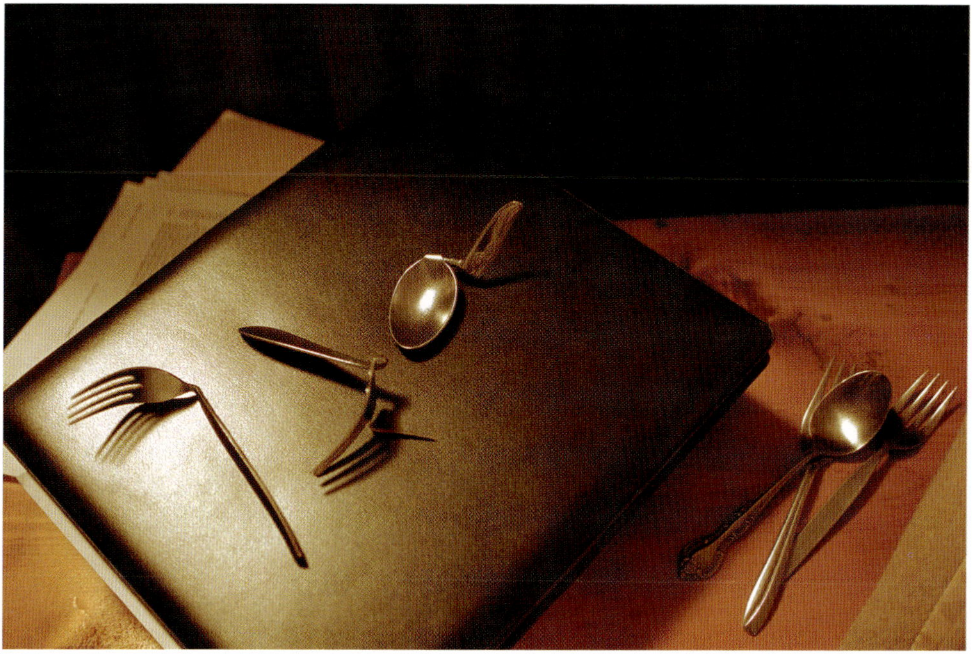

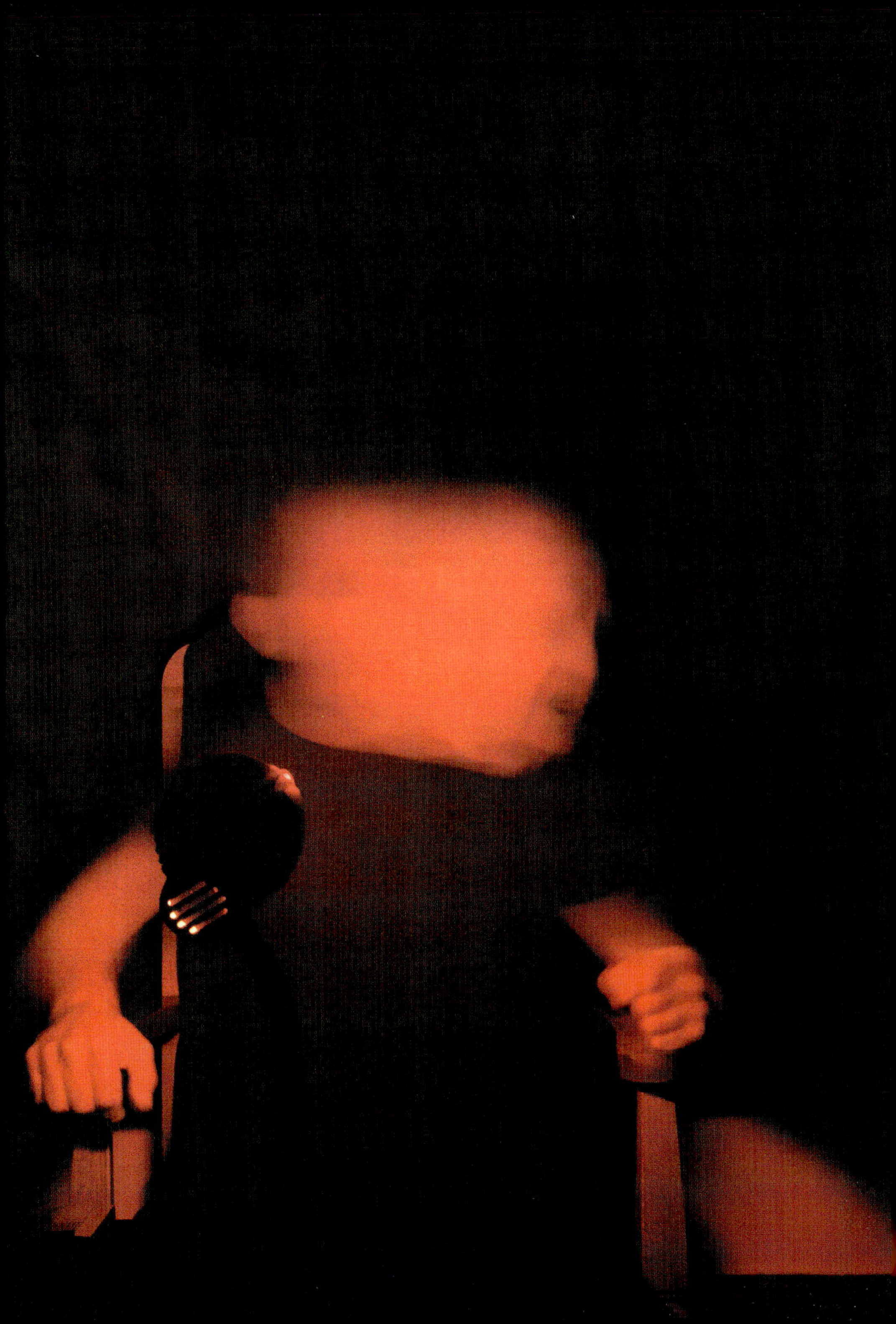

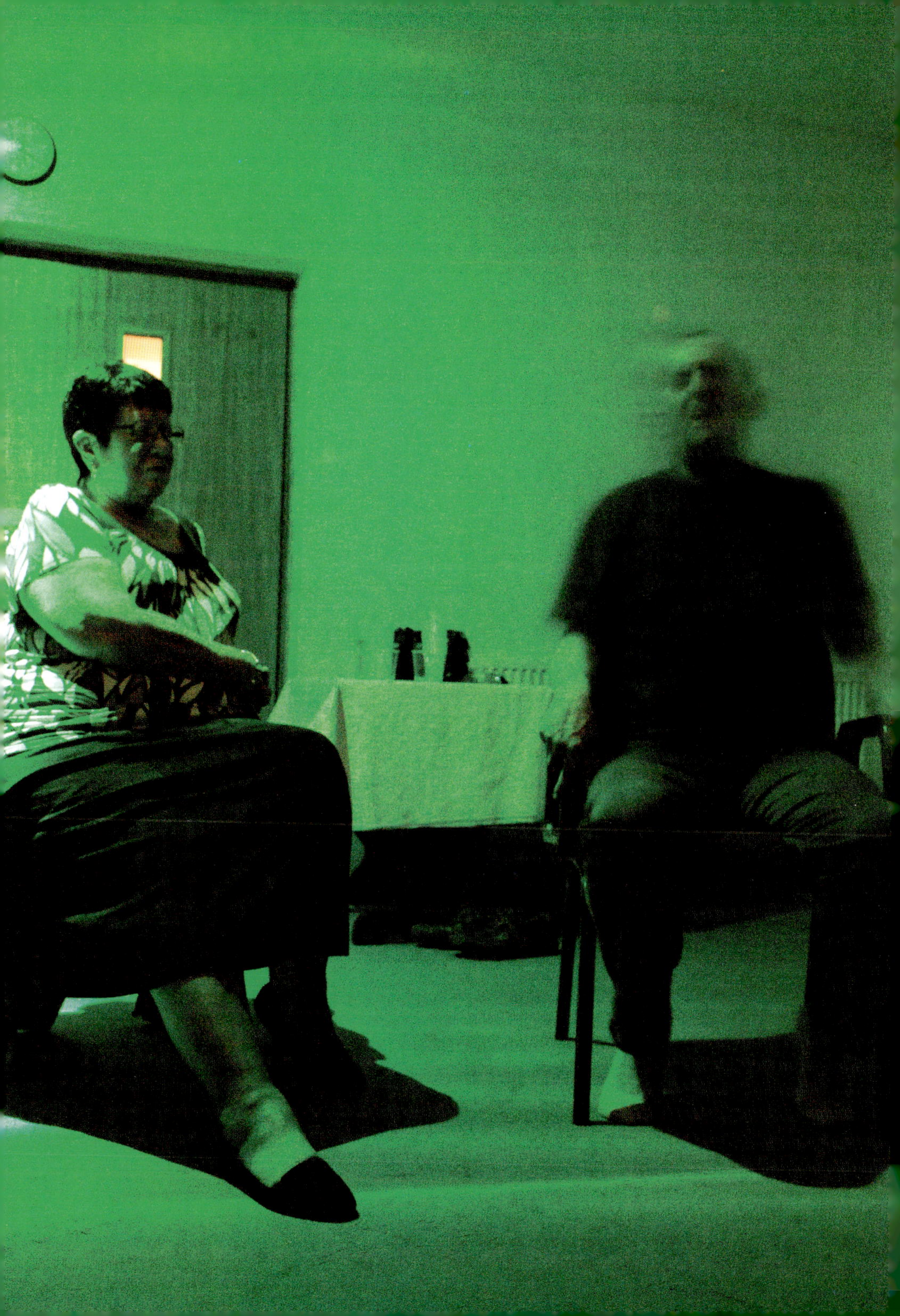

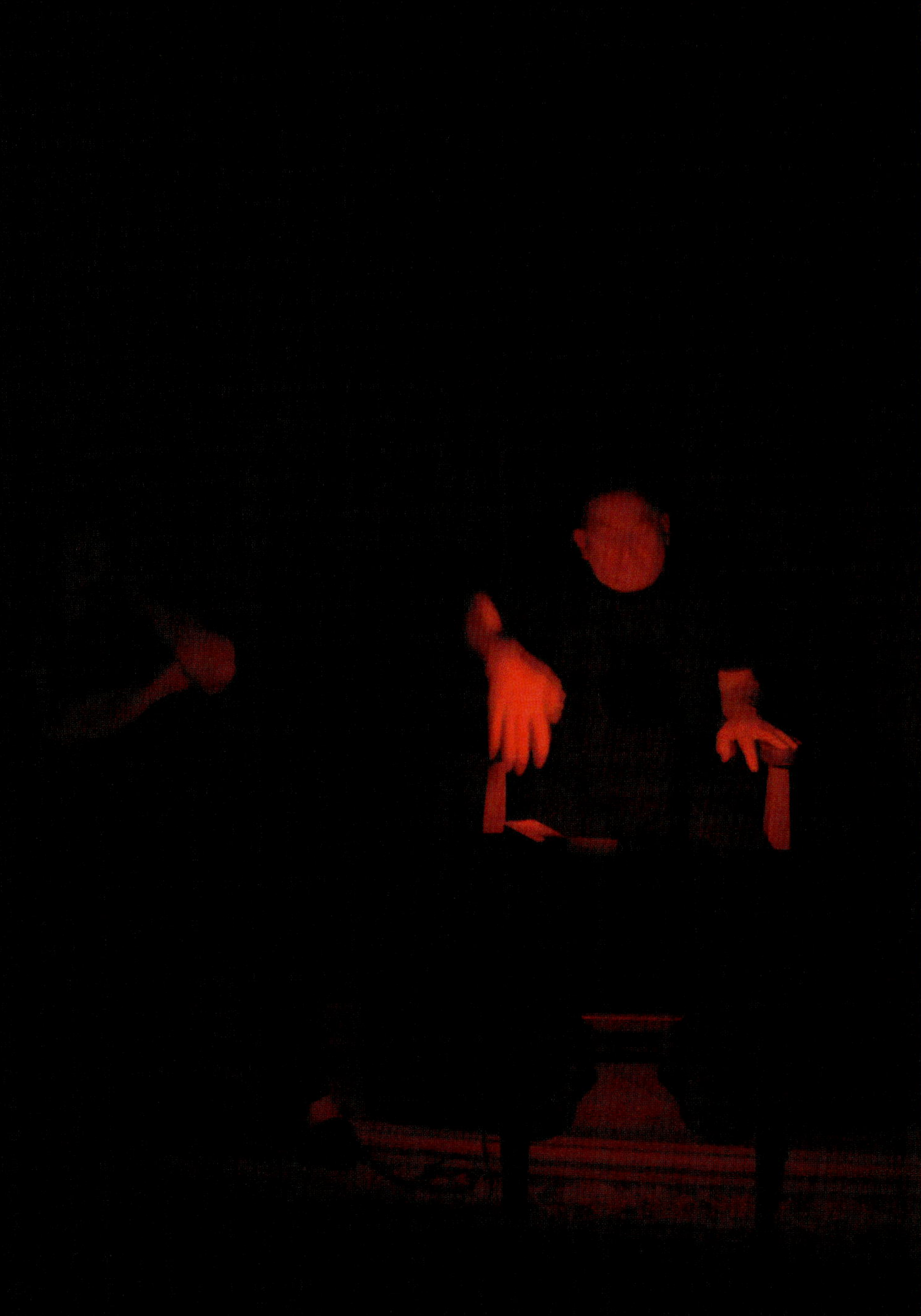

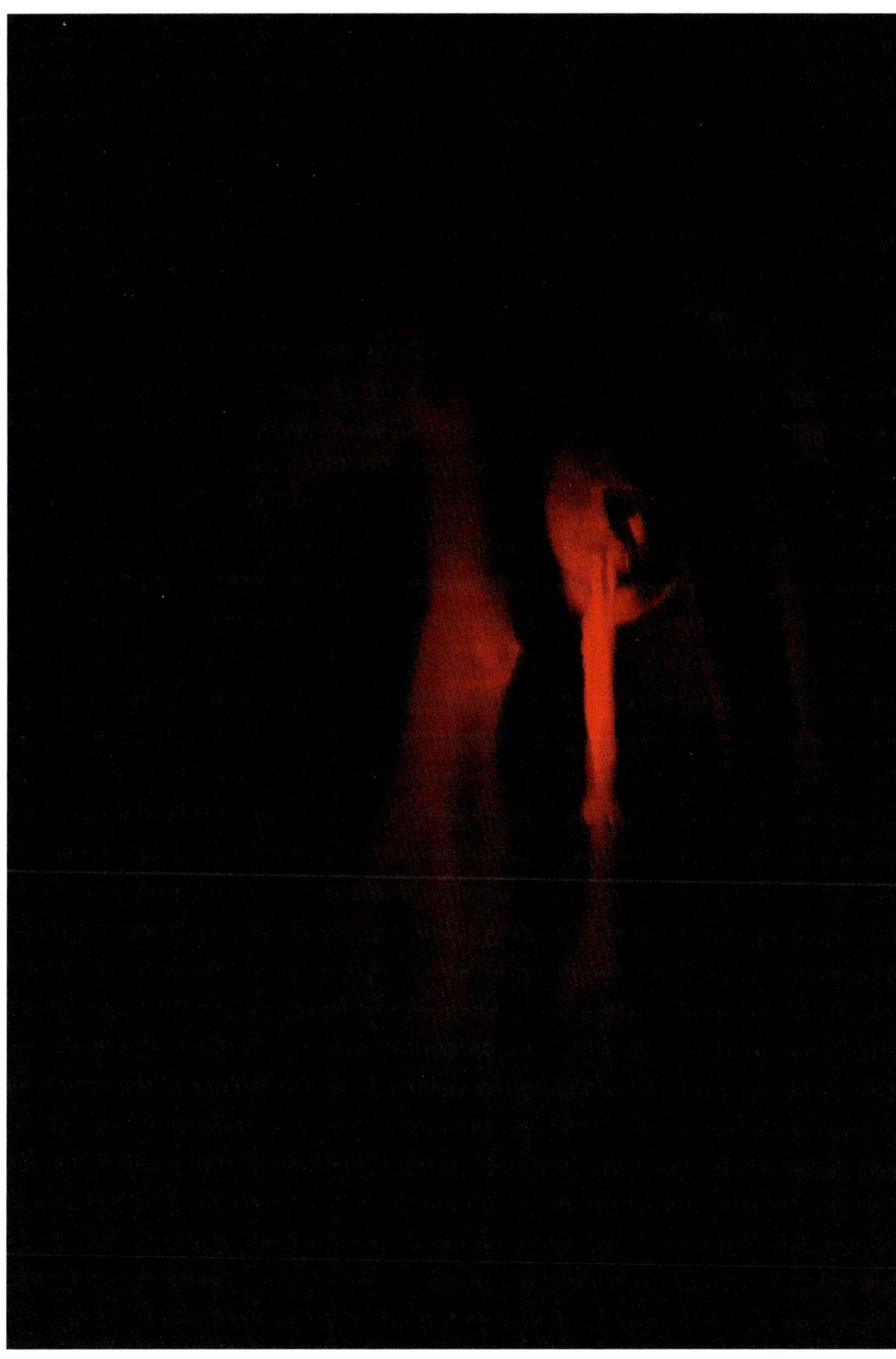

Saturday 3/30/13

Hi

I sure am glad to ~~be~~ have the chance to work & show how I am still able to rite! We ALL survive human death — No Matter what color, race, or creed we are.

I used to sing — I still do!

The Earth plane is a "school" for learning & everyone should make the most of time.

Bye

Elvis Presley

Elvis Presley

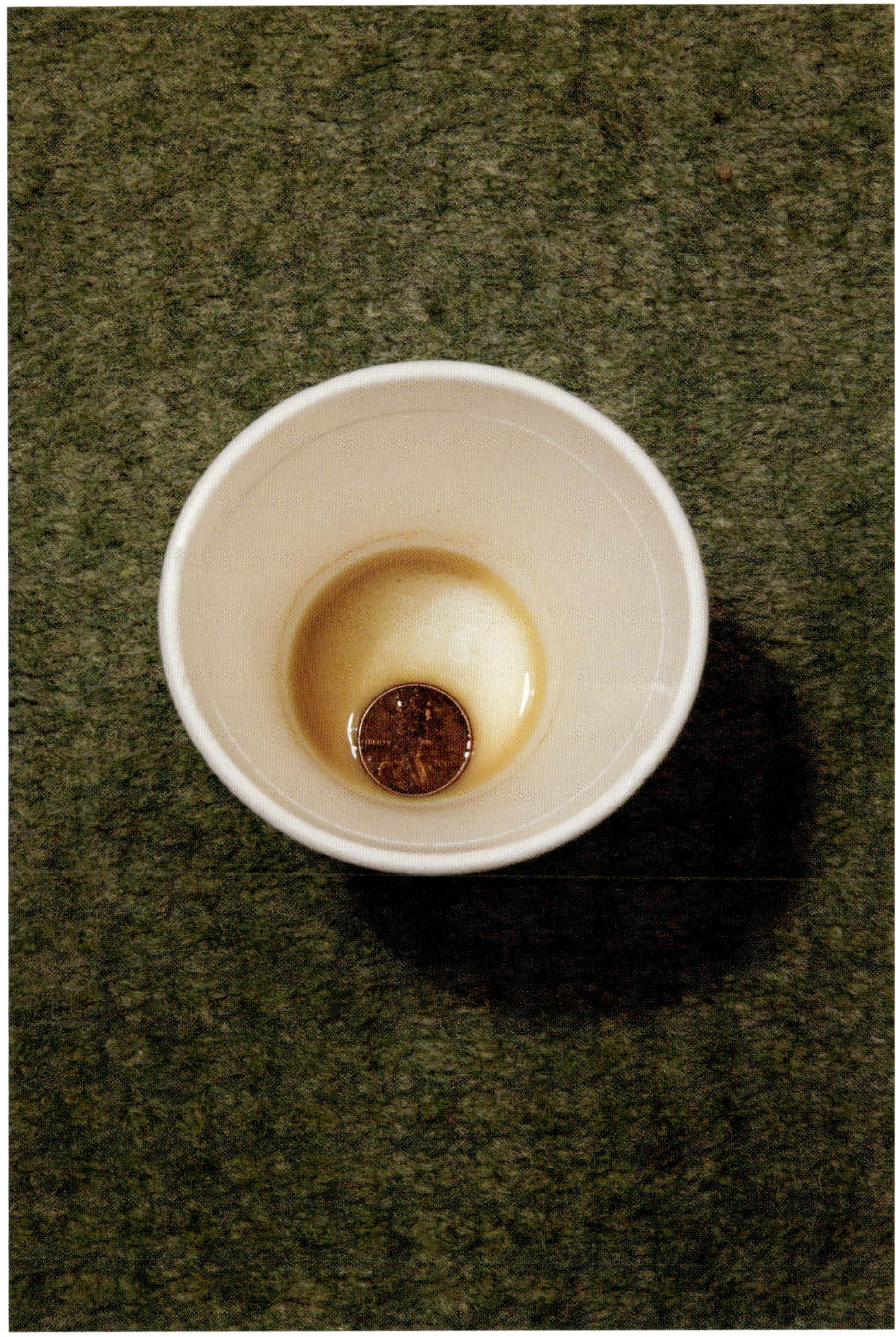

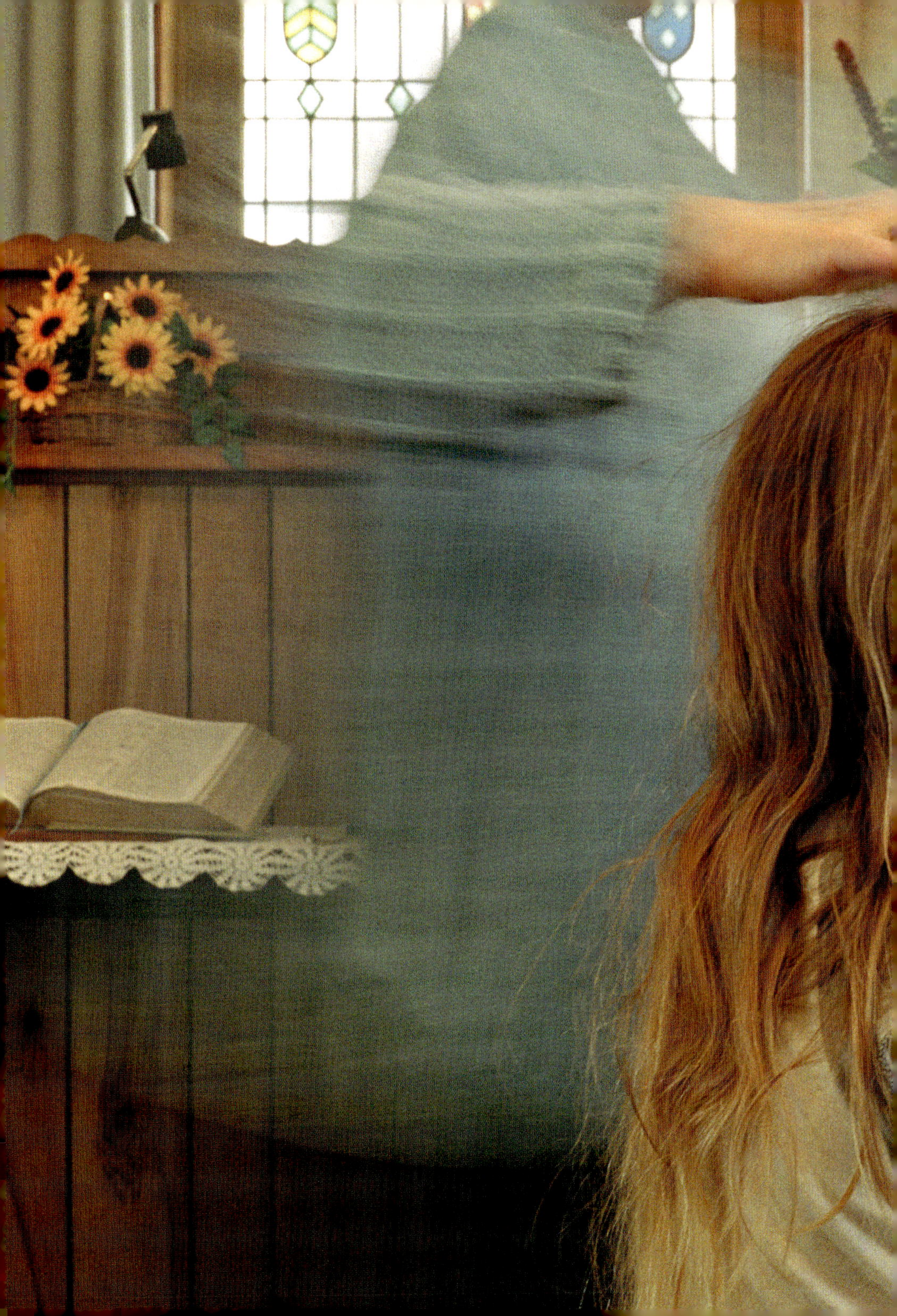

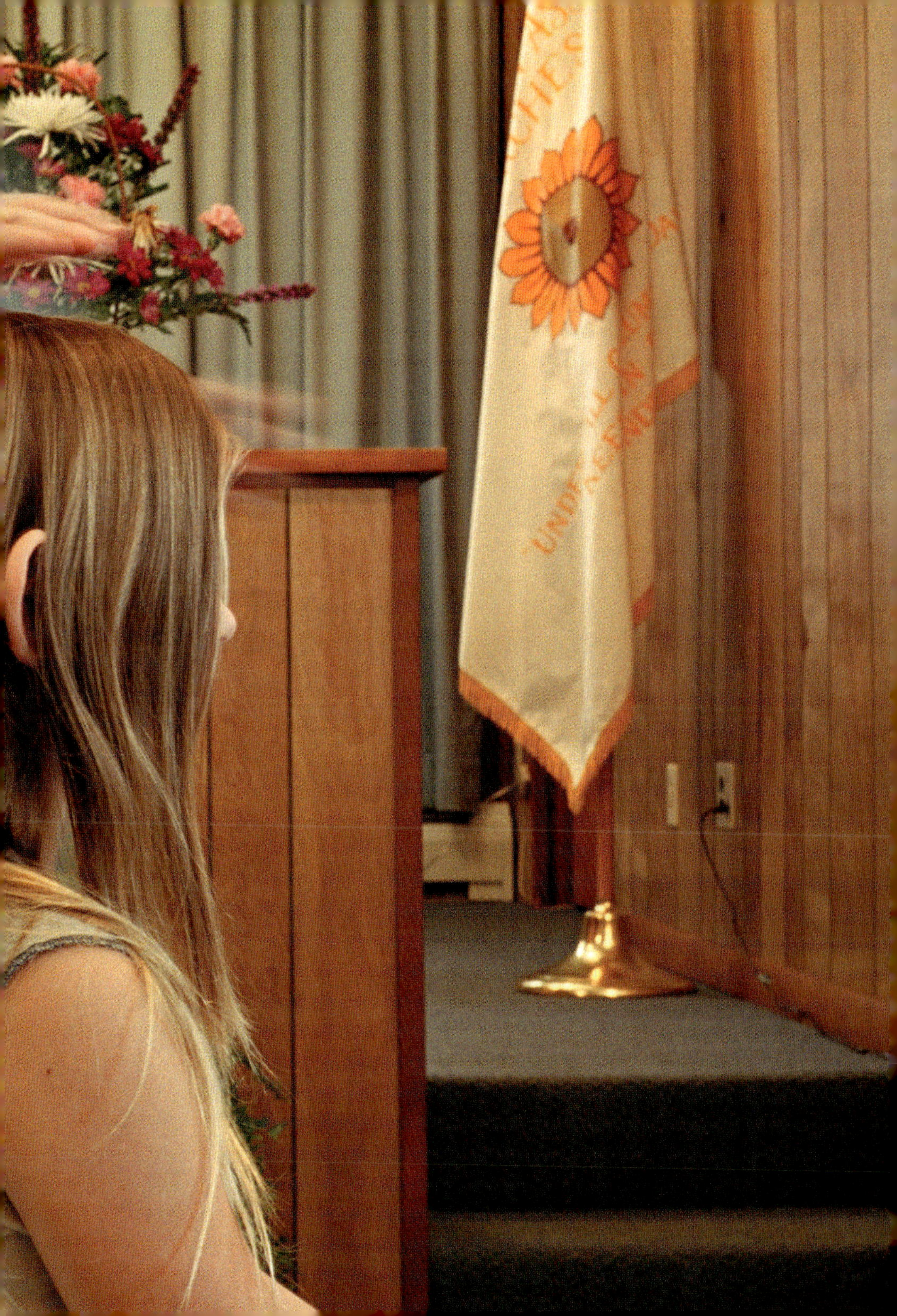

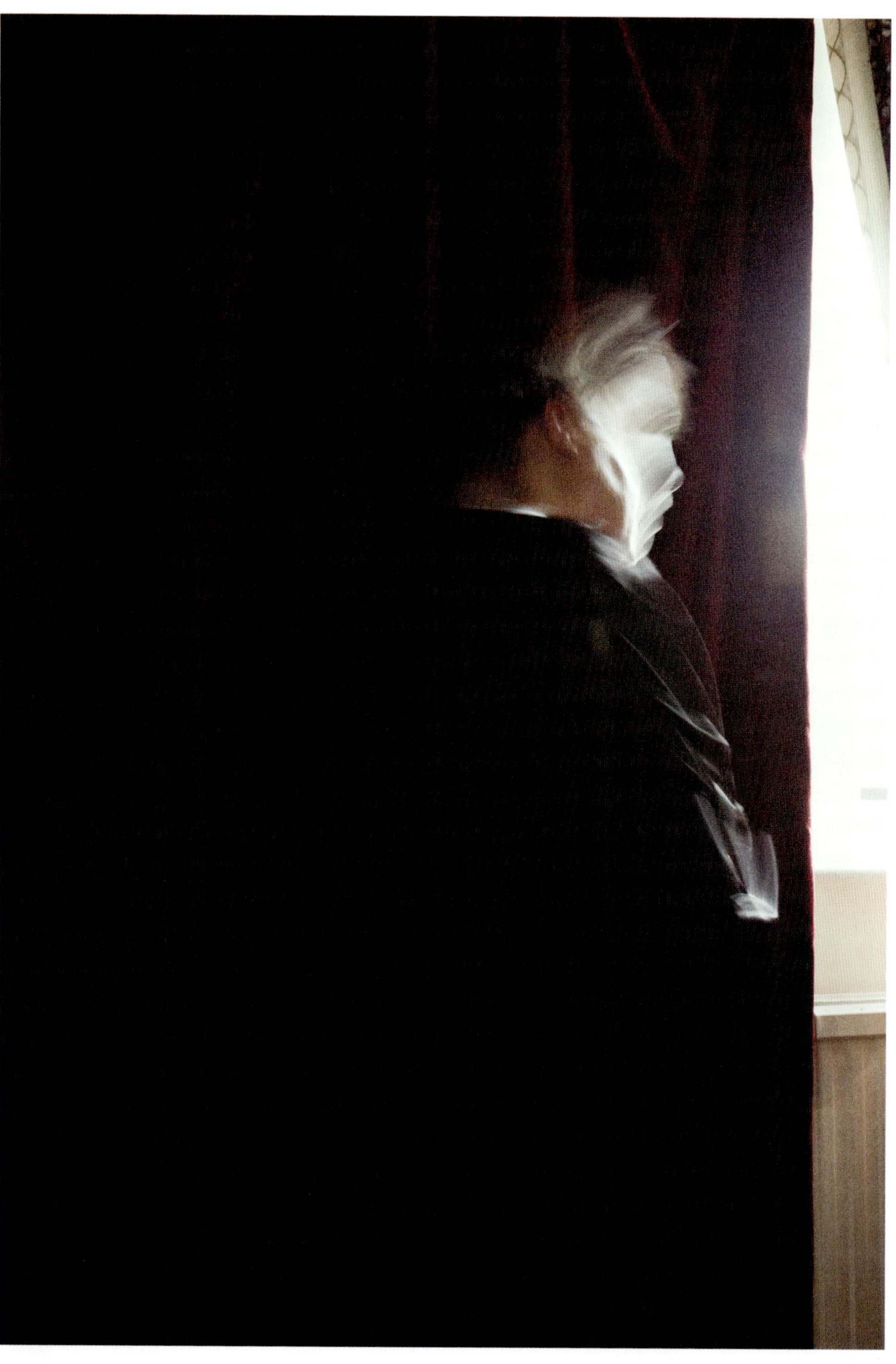

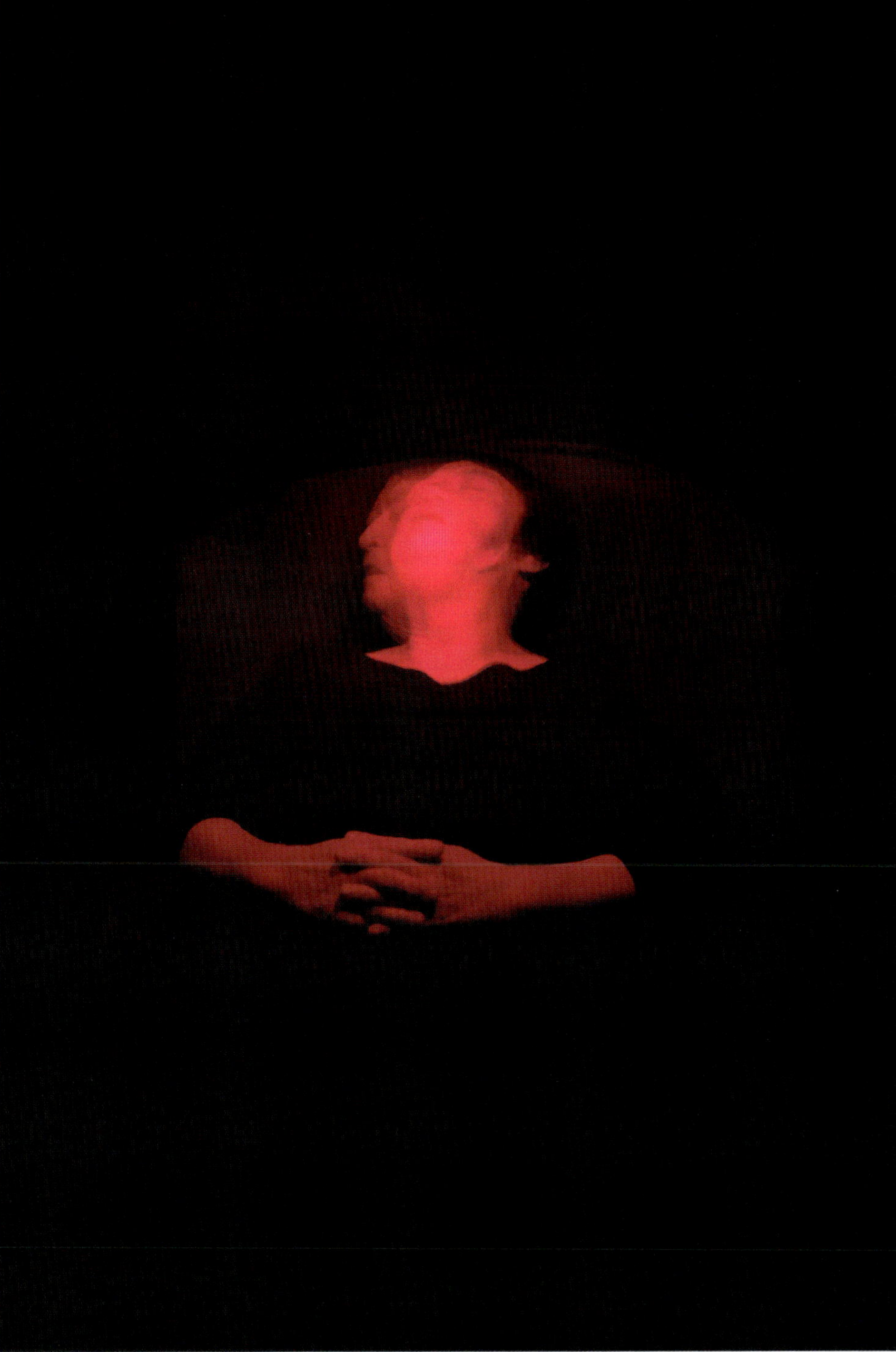

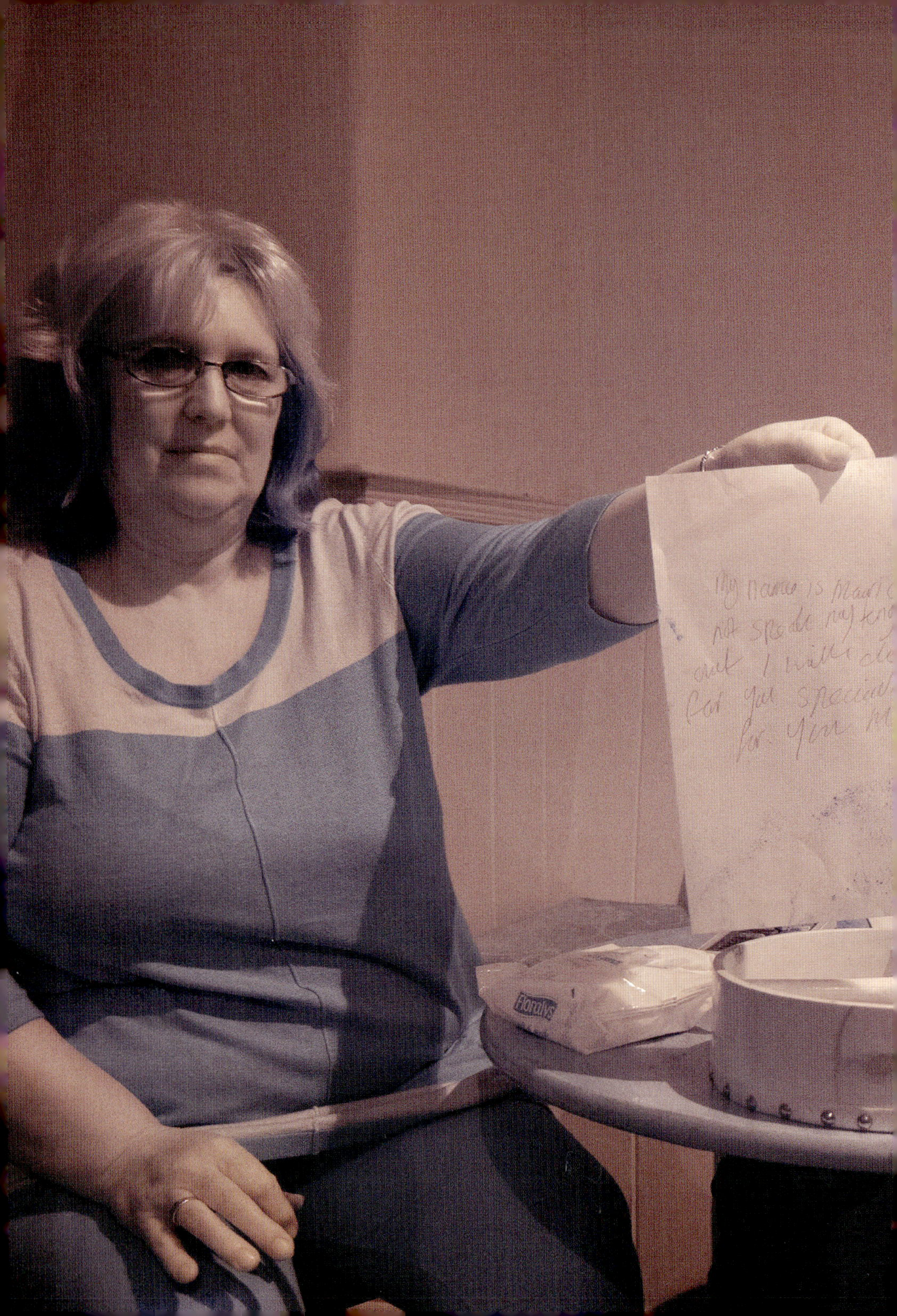

My name is
Floralys

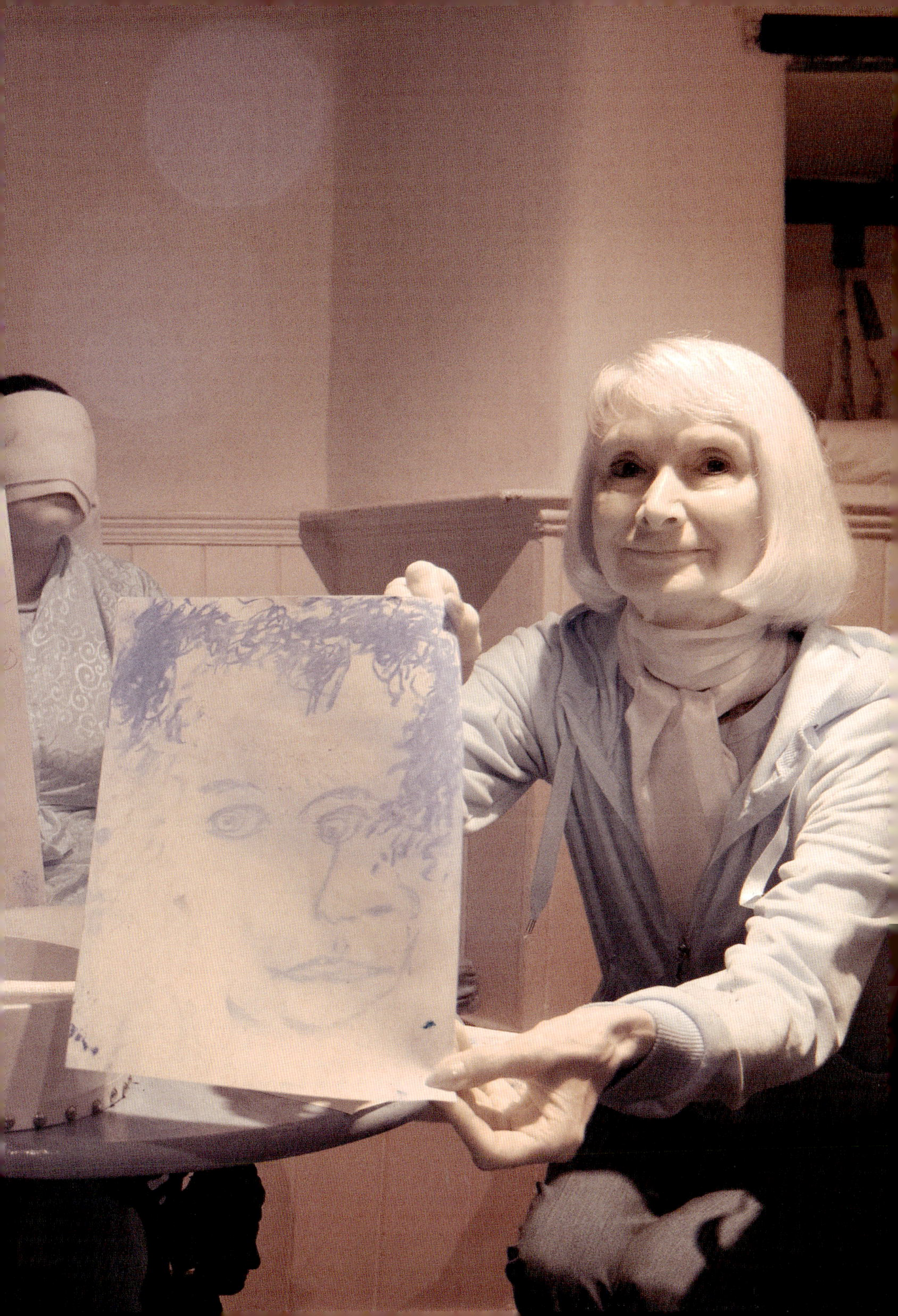

ON THE NON-DENIAL DENIAL OF DEATH

JOHN TROYER

FOR A LONG TIME, THE STORY GOES, WE TWENTY-FIRST CENTURY humans supported a post-Victorian, death-denying culture, and we continue to be dominated by it even today. Thus the image of the late twentieth century/early twenty-first century death-denying prude is emblazoned on our restrained and mute denials of death. So this epic story goes and is repeated on a daily basis.

Readers familiar with late twentieth century writing on human sexuality will quickly note that I am introducing this essay by freely adopting and adapting Michel Foucault's introduction to his 1976 book *The History of Sexuality, Volume 1: An Introduction.*[1] Foucault's central argument was that contrary to popular belief, the Victorians (across the English-speaking "first world") did not repress human sexuality, rather they embraced it at every turn. Books on sex, classroom lessons on sex, and male doctors' preoccupation with sex (especially women's sexuality), were a constant staple in Victorian discourse. Yet twentieth-century understandings of a more modern, politically "liberated" sexuality came to rely on the nineteenth century's "repressed" sexuality.

In a most peculiar switch, the exact opposite cultural and historical juxtaposition has supposedly now occurred with death. Whereas the Victorians were much more aware and fluent in discussions regarding death, we twenty-first century, English-speaking, first-world inhabitants have become horribly repressed when it comes to dying. Somehow, during the nineteenth century, the Victorians produced a liberated death discourse that became lost during the twentieth century.

But was it lost? And what, exactly, is a liberated notion of death? I raise these questions and do so provocatively for the following reasons. First and foremost, we see and hear discussions of death *every day*. It would be rare indeed for any person reading this book (which might be an audience already prone to seeing death in daily life, so point taken) to not hear or see or even partake in a discussion regarding death. These everyday discussions involving death lead to me to my second point, that while it is true we discuss death (or hear discussions of dying) on a daily basis, what we do not always discuss is our own deaths. But is this death repression? Or could it be that given changes to how life is lived in the twenty-first-century first world, we do not live in a "death-denying culture" but actually a cultural moment in which people are simply never asked to discuss their own deaths. There is a significant difference between death denial, i.e., individuals actively avoiding anything to do with the end of life, and a more common situation where very few people are ever asked to contemplate their own demise.[2]

I have two questions to ask then: (1) what do you want done with your dead body after you die and (2) do your next of kin, i.e., the legally recognized individuals responsible for your dead body, know what you want done with your dead body?[3] I have routinely started asking these questions whenever and wherever possible, not to make audiences uncomfortable (which rarely happens) but to provoke a series of thoughts about death, dying, and the dead body. The single most-common response I receive to these questions is this: "No one has ever asked me that before."

[1] *Michel Foucault,* The History of Sexuality, Volume 1: An Introduction, *trans. Robert Hurley (New York: Vintage Books, 1978).*

[2] *For more on the denial of death and death repression thesis see Ernest Becker,* The Denial of Death *(New York: Free Press, 1973).*

[3] *See olhn Troyer,* Technologies of the Human Corpse *(Durham: University of North Carolina Press, 2013), for a further development of these questions.*

Followed by a close, "I have never thought of these things before." None of this suggests death denial. It really suggests a twenty-first century first-world social milieu in which death questions regarding the self rarely come up.

To further demonstrate the paradoxical social prevalence of the death-denial thesis, Internet-based searches reveal some suggestive numbers. These numbers are hardly scientific proof (my data-driven empirical death friends will cringe right now), and I would never claim that running Google or Amazon searches produces infallible evidence. Yet the general, overall findings do suggest a couple of things. If death denial is so rampant, then it (i.e., death denial) is counterintuitively discussed almost every day in millions of different ways on the Internet, in books, and in workshops. Stated another way, a good number of people certainly seem interested in talking at great lengths and quite often about how much death is repressed.

The videos, for example, range from reflections on the denial of death thesis to popular songs about dying. A whole set of videos also involves medical doctors learning how to speak with patients about death and dying. Many of the text-based examples link to popular press and academic articles on death, as well as blog posts and personal accounts about dying. Death and dying, it becomes clear, is anything but repressed on the Internet.

Google:
Death denial culture: 12,300,000 hits
Death denial America: 14,400,000 hits
Denial of death: 46,900,000 hits
Discussing death: 61,400,000 hits
Discussing death workshop: 30,900,000 hits

Amazon:
Discussing death: 1,635 results
Death denial: 6,173 results

YouTube:
Death denial: 124,000 videos
Discussing death: 201,000 videos
Talking about death: 2,270,000 videos

Even when the discussions focus more on "talking about death," or "talking about dying," the launching point for these same discussions is usually about the current culture of postmortem denial and repression. What all these numbers suggest to me is that many people seem extremely dedicated to discussing the denial of death as opposed to just death. Perhaps just talking about death is too boring compared to talking about death denial and how a certain book (usually written by the person speaking) can change that situation.

Funeral Director's Son

One of the fundamental reasons that I became interested in how the very idea of death denial is positioned in contemporary culture is through my own lifelong relationship with human mortality. My father, Ron Troyer, was a funeral director in America for over thirty years before retiring. He worked in both the funeral industry and funeral education, at both the Cincinnati College of Mortuary Science and the Program of Mortuary Science at the University of Minnesota.[4] Despite my father's profession, and even though I grew up around death, it was not until my teenage years that I realized how unique my own childhood had been. The key difference during my youth was not the persistence of funerals or relatively common conversations about dead bodies (both things certainly occurred over the years) but the frequent and ongoing discussions about how and why people died. Death was literally a daily discussion topic that began during my childhood and that I continue

[4] Cincinnati College of Mortuary Science (http://www.ccms.edu) and the University of Minnesota Program of Mortuary Science (http://www.mortuaryscience.umn.edu). At no point during my life did my father and I ever discuss my eventually working in the Centre for Death and Society at the University of Bath (http://www.bath.ac.uk/cdas), one of the world's only research centers dedicated to the interdisciplinary study of death, but this is how death works sometimes.

discussing today. Every day. These early childhood discussions also meant thinking about what death, dying, and the dead body meant for everyday life, even though I did not fully comprehend this fact until my late teens and early twenties. Growing up the way that I did also demonstrated that far from being denied, death was everywhere, every day for most people—with the following caveat. While it is true that dying and the funerals that result from an individual's death occur every day, a living person's encounter with that death is usually limited to the moment that he/she attends the funeral. Death, in this context, is still not denied—it just isn't visible in the way that a funeral director's son or daughter sees the end of life. Is it possible, I have begun asking, to not only encourage individuals to contemplate death on a more daily basis (similar to how I grew up) but to also begin answering questions about their own funerals? The answer to both queries is of course "yes," but a singular universal method does not work. I want to now discuss two specific examples of different ways that individuals can (and often do) make death both more visible and prepared for in the future: memorial tattoos and funeral planning worksheets.

Memorial Tattoos: Making Death More Visible

One of the contemporary memorialization practices which I find compelling and that explicitly involves death and visibility is memorial tattooing.[5] Memorial tattoos are tattoos that individuals have done after a person (or often a pet) dies. The tattoos represent the memory of the deceased but can also, sometimes, contain a very small portion of the dead person's cremated remains. These memorial pieces are often quite visible (even if the tattoo itself is not automatically recognizable as a memorial), but the tattoos can also be hidden underneath clothing. The visibility of the memorial tattoo is often practically related to

[5] *Discussions of contemporary memorialization practices can easily involve numerous examples: social networking sites (e.g., Facebook, Instagram, etc.), roadside memorials, memorial T-shirts, memorial bumper stickers, etc. I focused on memorial tattoos in part because these memorials are both so portable and permanent (as opposed to many others), and because for a long time these tattoos slipped under the radar. If you know a person with tattoos, ask him or her if any are memorials. Ask a complete stranger, for that matter. It opens up fascinating conversations about human mortality.*

where exactly the design is placed on the body and the local climate, i.e., how much clothing a person needs to stay warm. More than anything, these tattoos represent an individual remembering a dead person and choosing to do so by having ink permanently etched into their skin. While tattooing might not seem the obvious practice to makes death more visible, memorial tattoos function as increasingly *difficult-to-ignore* visual and historiographical opportunities to discuss a person's death. No discussion is necessarily forced (which is a good thing), but the opportunity to discuss how the tattoo represents a death or the end of a life is both opened up and even encouraged by the memorial tattoo itself.

The exact numbers of individuals with memorial or memorial-like tattoos remains difficult to quantify. In speaking with working tattoo artists, it becomes apparent that almost all of them have anecdotes about memorial designs for customers of all ages, genders, social classes, and ethnic backgrounds. And given the extremely personal nature of memorial tattoos, the designs themselves come in a diverse aesthetic range. A tattoo might have RIP and a name, or maybe just a date. Some parents have the footprint or handprint of a deceased newborn or child tattooed into their skin. Still other people choose a portrait tattoo taken from a photograph of the now-deceased individual. A memorial tattoo is also just as likely to be an abstract design or symbol. All of the designs, regardless of type, pointedly embrace the deceased individual attached to the tattoo in order to remember the death, and do so for a significant period of time.

Most memorial tattoos will presumably remain visible on a person's body (unless covered over by a new tattoo or removed by a laser) until the bearer of the tattoo also dies. That commitment to physically carrying the memory of the deceased person in the skin illustrates how these memorials remain portable and resist being temporary. It is this portability, the ability to bring the memorial wherever an individual goes, that I think makes death more tangible. The memorial tattoo is a constant reminder to remember mortality and fundamentally represents a choice about bringing memories and conversations about death back into daily life. A memorial tattoo is not about never letting go; it is an embrace of death.

Funeral Planning: Answering Questions about Death

Given that the two questions which I asked at the beginning of this essay ("what do you want done with your dead body" and "have you told your next-of-kin") require explicitly engaging with death, I want to circle back and delve into answering them. Again, it seems more likely that instead of denying death many individuals are simply never asked to think about their own mortality. A very simple way to go about working through (and answering) these death, dying, and end-of-life questions is with a planning sheet. While I am not necessarily a huge advocate of worksheets for all occasions (smartphone planning apps already run amok), this specific funeral-planning document opens up questions that help answer some important issues.

The Centre for Death and Society at the University of Bath (where I hold an academic post) put this particular funeral planning form together, and it is often used in diverse settings, e.g., with professional groups, such as funeral directors, or university students studying the sociology of death.[6] The point of the planning sheet is to engage the future certainty of death, and, I will add, demonstrate that death is hardly repressed once people start discussing what they want done after they die. I have slightly adapted the planning document, but the core questions remain the same. Some quick examples:

[6] The CDAS funeral planning document is not a legally binding form so if you want or need documents that legally guarantee your postmortem wishes then you should have pre-arranged funeral plans and advanced medical directives drawn up by the appropriate authorities.

Do you want to be embalmed?

Do you want to be cremated?

Do you want to be organ, bone, and tissue donor?

What kind of casket or burial shroud do you want?

What music do you want played or *not* played?

Which funeral director should handle your funeral? If any?

Do you want a secular, religious, or secular-religious funeral?[7]

If you're not religious but identify with a certain religious group, do you want a hybrid funeral service?

Do you want financial donations made in your name to certain organizations?

What clothes do you want to be wearing? Do you care?

The full funeral planning document contains many more questions and it can function as a catalyst for discussions with next of kin that are best had before a person is incapacitated or dies. As the son of a funeral director who heard story after story about families who never discussed funerals until they suddenly had to, I strongly suggest that you start thinking about and discussing these end-of-life questions now.

The funeral planning form also brings me back to my larger point on death denial. What many twenty-first century, first-world humans lack is a location to conveniently answer and then document anything to do with funerals. It is this particular "access to death" gap (for lack of a better term) that fosters much of the death denial argument. The questions contained in the Centre for Death and Society's funeral planning form, and the space provided for writing down answers, will most certainly help limit the possibility of death remaining in this seemingly forever-repressed state. Again, do not wait to answer these

[7] Many funeral directors have stories about families planning strictly secular funeral services, but then still requesting that the Lord's Prayer be said or that certain hymns be sung. Just in case.

questions but keep in mind that your answers can change, and probably will over time. What will not change is the certainty of death.

A final point to conclude on is this: What would death liberation (in contrast to denial) resemble? How would it work? Liberating one's self with death (not *from* death) means comprehending both the inevitability of human mortality as well as knowing what you want done with your dead body. It is one thing to say, "I know that I am going to die." It is quite another to say, "I know that I am going to die and I want the following things done with my body after my death." In the end, I am not really sure that we twenty-first century, first-world humans want total death liberation. Just as Michel Foucault warned readers against believing that sexual "liberation" is in the balance when discussing the modern politics of sexuality, I too remain skeptical about the political motivations that support the constant identification of death denial and repression.[8] What we twenty-first century, post-Victorian humans need, it seems to me, are constant opportunities for individuals to discuss not only their own personal deaths but to also think about and identify a broader understanding of how death is entirely visible in everyday life. Just take a minute. And look.

[8] *Foucault, 159.*

FUNERAL PLANNING

Indicate your dead body and funeral wishes by completing the following sentence. Include a very brief explanation for your choices.

- ☐ I would like my body to be (laid out and kept at home/taken to a funeral home's chapel for a visitation or wake/other)

____

____

- ☐ I would like my body to be (embalmed/not embalmed)

____

____

- ☐ I would like my body to be dressed in (everyday clothes/special clothes/costume)

____

____

- ☐ I would like my body to be viewed by (my next-of-kin only/extended family/friends/work colleagues/anybody who wants to)

____

____

- ☐ I would like my body to be transported to the church/chapel/cemetery in a (hearse/my own vehicle/other)

____

____

- ☐ The funeral director, cemetery, or crematorium I prefer is

____

____

- ☐ The price range I would like spent on my funeral is

____

____

☐ I would like the final disposition of my body to be (burial, cremation, scattering of remains, etc.)

☐ If I am buried, I would like a gravestone or a marker to read

---

☐ If I am cremated, I want my ashes

☐ I (would/would not) like flowers sent by (close family/friends/anyone)

☐ I (would/would not) like monetary donations made to

☐ I would like a funeral or memorial service to be led by (religious minister – state which religion/secular and/or humanist celebrant/civil celebrant/other)

☐ During the funeral service I would like the following music (none/hymns/classical music chosen by funeral director/special piece of music chosen my me)

☐ I would prefer to leave all the choices of arrangements for my funeral to

---

☐ I (aim to, have already) planned my funeral

☐ I want to be an Organ, Bone, and Tissue Donor after I die and why? (yes/no)

☐ What I would most like my family and friends to understand about my life, what was important to me, and what I learned from life are described below. The last thing I would like to say is

HELL ÉPOQUE

Death-themed Cabarets & Other Macabre Entertainments of Nineteenth-Century Paris

VADIM KOSMOS

THE FRENCH, THE FRENCH; JUST WHAT IS IT WITH THE FRENCH AND their lust for the lurid? From the tortured torch songs of Piaf and Brel to the diabolical deeds of that fictional fiend Fantômas; our Gallic friends seem to revel in their romance with everything that is ghastly and gloomy.

Ever since I can recall I have been obsessed with the French and their popular culture—not obsessed enough to learn their language to any degree of fluidity beyond a meager *"Quand est le dentifrice?"*—but it's fair to say seriously fixated. And for that same duration inquiries have been made toward the possible motivations for this obsession, and the glib reply I usually supplied was a simple *"French Girls."*

And yet, upon mounting my research for this piece, I was given pause to ponder; was there indeed a deeper motivation for my Francophilia? A Proustian recollection rooted in my childhood that rendered this result inevitable?

TO BE OR NOT TO BE
AVIS
CABARET DU NÉANT - Paris-Montmartre — n° 1. Salle d'Intoxication

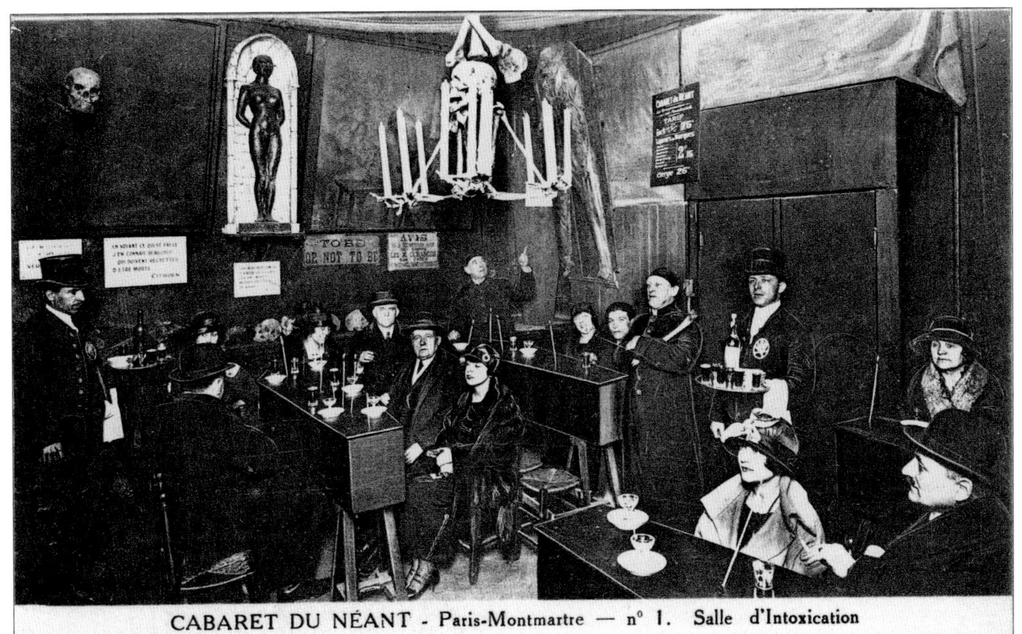

Postcard from Cabaret du Néant. *Courtesy of the author.*

Southport—So Much to Answer for (and yet So Little to Recommend It).

And thus we begin this tale, as all good stories about France do, in Southport, England (the northwest of England to be precise), that listless, lackluster seaside resort to where I was so cruely confined for so many of my miserable formative years. A town so torpid that a visiting (and I can only presume lost) Nathaniel Hawthorne had this to say about it in 1856: "an interminable breadth of sands, stretching out to the horizon—brown or yellow sands ... dull and dreary little watering-place."

But if Hawthorne saw nothing in Southport but bleak desolation, another foreign-born guest derived quite a different and entirely more positive impression of the town. In May 1846 (ten years before that great American novelist's ill-

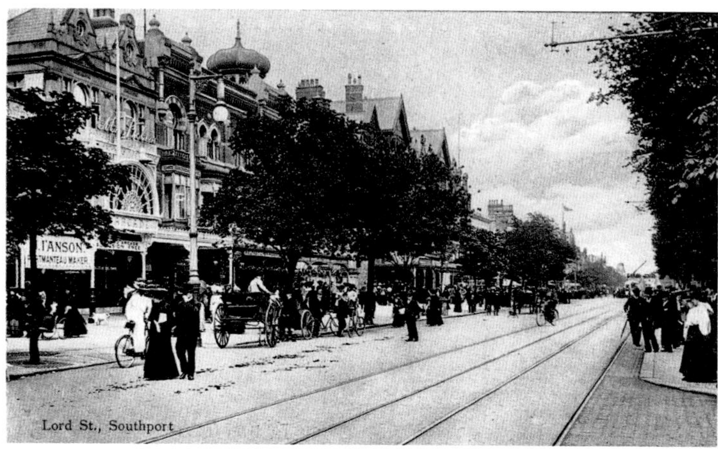

Postcard of Southport. Courtesy of the author.

located vacation) an exiled French nobleman, Louis-Napoléon Bonaparte, nephew of the more famous and fêted military and political leader, obtained lodgings off Lord Street, where he resided until his triumphant return to his homeland two years later. Stretching for exactly one mile down the length of the Southport's town center, Lord Street is a wide and tree-lined shopping street flanked with grand buildings, gardens, fountains, canopied walkways and arcades and—at one time—an opera house.

It was this image of Southport that Bonaparte took with him back to his homeland. Upon ascending his self-appointed throne, the now-Emperor Napoléon III of the Second Empire initiated a series of reforms designed to create a more ordered and modern France and begat a wave of ameliorations that would firmly establish Paris as the world cultural capital of the nineteenth century. One of Napoléon III's first initiatives, in 1853, was to instruct his *préfet de la Seine*, Baron Georges Eugène Haussmann, to level sixty percent of Paris' putrid, pretzelled, Medieval lanes and replace them with eighty miles of wide and tree-lined shopping streets flanked with grand buildings, gardens, fountains, canopied walkways and arcades—and, of course, *an opera house.* According to Vanessa R. Schwartz's splendid tome *Spectacular Realities* (1998), the establishing of a sanitary city center created the conditions for a new form of mass entertainment in Paris. The division between low street entertainments and the high arts dissolved towards "Boulevard Culture"— a culture of *flâneurs* and *badauds,* where middlebrow amusements arose that relied upon a high turnover of paying spectators.

Paris had long ago developed an appetite for dark divertissements. During the one-year period known as "The Reign of Terror" from 1793–1794, between sixteen thousand and forty thousand unlucky souls had been put to the guillotine. "The Terror" drew daily family audiences numbering in the thousands, with vendors touting programs listing each day's schedule of decapitation. As Boulevard Culture began to flourish in the second half of the nineteenth century, the city's new entertainments reflected this.

Phantasmagoria and Les Diableries

First established in the mid-seventeenth century, magic lanterns resembled an early version of Don Draper's favored tearful nostalgia delivery device—the slide projector. Berlin-based Paul Philidor (or *Paul de Philipsthal*—his true origins and name remain unclear) began his own lantern performances in 1789, initially inspired by the use of ghostly magic lantern projections in the charlatan séances of German fraud Joann Georg Schröpfer. Moving to Paris in 1793, Philidor's diabolic portraits of revolutionary heroes Marat, Danton and Robespierre failed to amuse local authorities, precipitating his swift relocation to London.

Within Philidor's Paris audience had sat a certain Belgian by the name of Étienne-Gaspard Robert—later anglicizing himself as "Robertson," he would develop Philidor's concept

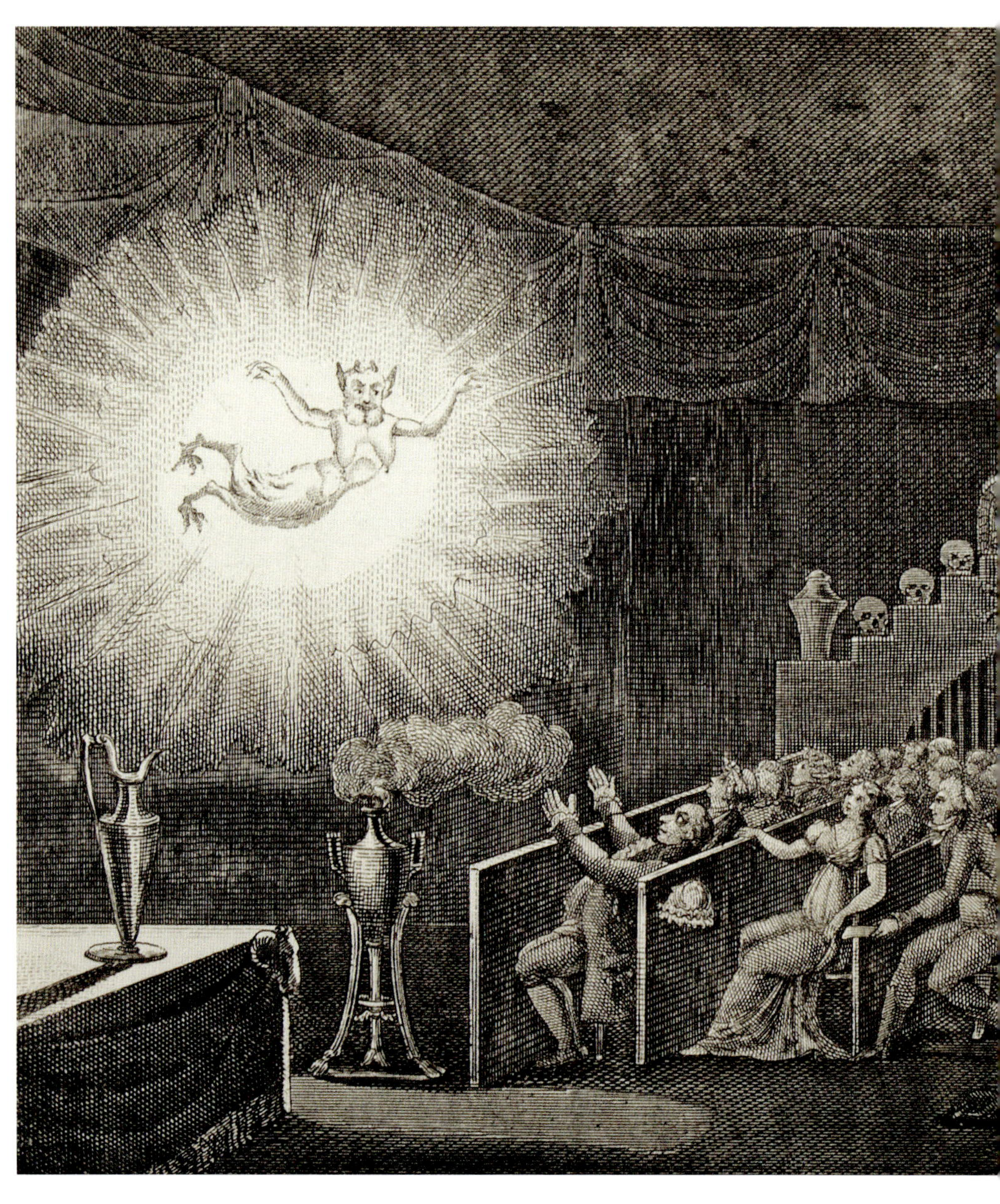

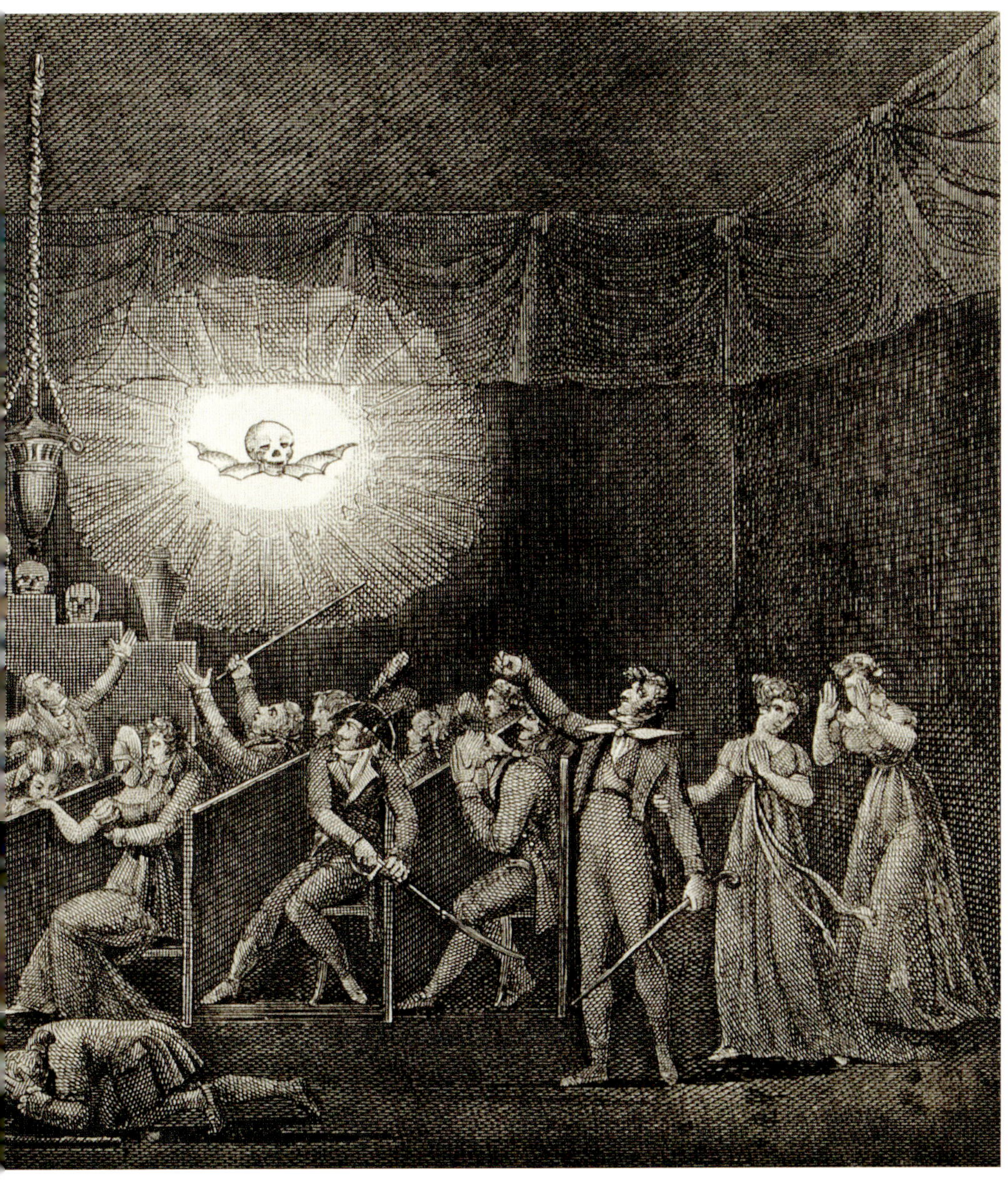

Image previous page: Phantasmagoria de Robertson dans la Cour des Capuchines en 1797, Frontspiece to Robertson, E. G. Mémoires: récréatifs, scientifiques et anecdotiques. Paris: Chez l'auteur et à la Librairie de Wurtz, 1831. Photograph of image by Nicole Neenan, courtesy of The New York Public Library.

further. Robertson's "Fantasmagorie" (Phantasmagoria, from the Old French "Fantasme"—"ghost"—and the Greek "agora," or "gathering") show opened at Paris' Pavillon de l'Echiquier in 1798, where he too drew the wrath of local authorities when accused of claiming the power to resurrect enemy-of-the-revolution Louis XVI's headless spirit. After fleeing briefly to Bordeaux, Robertson retooled his show, taking the Phantasmagoria to new heights of horror with an elaborately choreographed new production and his newly developed mobile, wheeled lantern, the *'Fantascope.'*

Robertson established his new spooky spectacular at the crumbling Gothic ruins of the Convent des Capuchines near the Place Vendôme in January 1799. After approaching the convent's auditorium via dark cloisters and sepulchres piled high with broken gravestones and skeletal friars, Robertson would first explain in "scientific" terms the "galvanic fluid" principles of contacting the dead and conjuring their manifestations into the physical world. Then, obscured behind a gauze scrim and with the aid of his six assistants, Robertson's audience were subjected to a fright fest such as they had never seen before. Multiple lanterns, fitted with a prototype zoom lens, would rush and retreat at the screen—giving the illusion of impending spectral collision. As mock-thunder boomed and lightning flashed, Robertson would incant ghoulish visions from within a burning brazier, filling the room with sulphurous smoke and thus providing yet another canvas for these infernal illusions. The audience—augmented with planted "stooge" actors—were treated to eldritch voices thrown via ventriloquism, the eerie tones of the Benjamin Franklin-invented instrument the "Glass Armonica" while hand-held lanterns projected bats bombarding the bouffants of the many madames and mademoiselles there present.

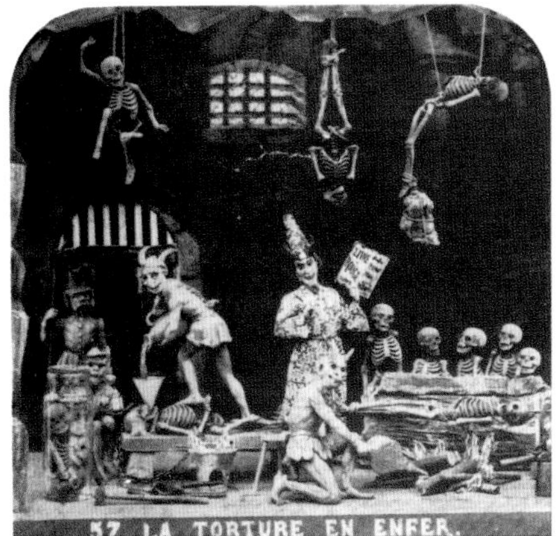

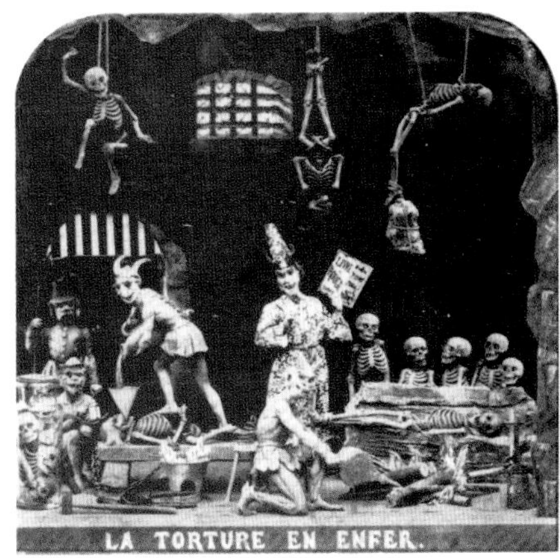

Diablerie stereo card. Courtesy of the author.

The rise to power of Napoléon III coincided with a more portable infernal entertainment than the Phantasmagoria, one that any Parisian could enjoy in the comfort of their *l'appartement*. Tissue-backed photographic transparencies, viewed via a handheld device; the Stereoscope was the nineteenth century's precursor to that baby boomer novelty the View-Master. However, in place of Yogi Bear or Pebbles and Bamm-Bamm resplendent in all their 3D glory, we might instead have expected to see a stirring photographic transparency of the Egyptian Pyramids in all their magnificence, a fine selection of the famed cheeses of Amsterdam or—increasingly as the century wore on—hardcore pornography.

Brits Sir Charles Wheatstone and David Brewster had invented and developed the handheld device itself, but it was Queen Victoria's enthusiasm for Parisian optician Jules Duboscq's stereoscopic daguerreotype display at London's Great Exhibition of 1851 that caused the Stereoscope craze to spread like syphilis throughout Europe and the United States. By 1858, the London Stereoscopic Company boasted of having over a hundred thousand images for sale, and in 1901, New York's

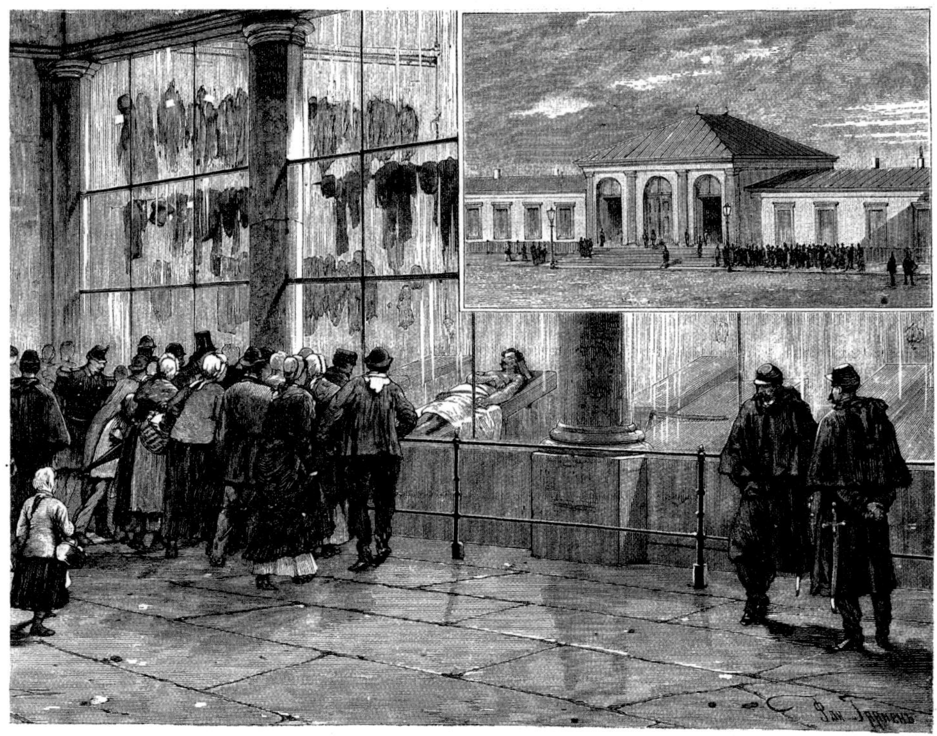

The Paris Morgue. Courtesy of the author.

Underwood & Underwood claimed to manufacture 23,000 stereocards a day. The stereoscopic series "Les Diableries" were a series of highly detailed, sculpted-plaster-and-clay tabletop tableaux depicting the denizens of the underworld engaged in various visions of hell. When beams of backlight penetrated the pierced transparency, dabs of colored gelatin gave the illusion of demonic eyes glowing ember red.

Napoléon III's rule had not sat well with all of his subjects. Much of the center of Paris' modern center had been bequeathed to Louis' allies and supporters, there was ever-widening economic inequality and the nouveau riche created by Napoleon fell into decadent excess. Each stereoscopic scenario made mockery of the emperor's rule with the skeletal forms of Louis' bony cronies bowing in cringing chorus while Napoléon III's cloven-hoofed caliph held court. The first set of numbered cards (72 in total) was released in 1860, surreptitiously and understandably anonymously, as swift imprisonment awaited any who dare to mock Napoléon III's authoritarian reign, though recent research has revealed that sculptor Louis "Alfred" Habert with photographer and publisher Francois Benjamin Lamiche originated and were responsible for the bulk of the slides.

The Morgue and Catacombs

If you happened to stroll through central Paris one bright afternoon in the late nineteenth century you may well have observed a curious sight; a steady stream of customers queuing before a nondescript administrative building in the shadow of Notre Dame Cathedral. But these spectators were not indulging in the newly created concept of "window-shopping," nor were they idly viewing an example of the "Panorama" phenomena that had gripped the city.

No, they were staring at human corpses.

The term "morgue" derives from the archaic French verb *morguer*—"to stare, to have a fixed or questioning gaze"—and originally referred to a prison-holding cell where newly arrived convicts were observed and inspected. By the eighteenth century the morgue at Paris' Grand Châtelet prison changed its purpose permanently to a public viewing room where the unclaimed dead were displayed for identification through a grilled skylight. The first officially named and purposefully built "La Morgue" was established in 1804, initially at the Marché-Neuf on the Île de la Cité, and then at the nearby Quai de l'Archevêché when Baron Haussmann's reorganization of the city center forced the morgue's relocation in 1864.

Drawing curious crowds from the outset, both morgues allowed for public inspection of anonymous cadavers claimed from the neighboring Seine, and known by the slang term "Macchabées" (the Latin phrase *Machabaeorum chorea*, "Dance of the Martyred Maccabees," possibly providing the origin for the word "macabre"). The damp deceased were displayed naked behind high windows on tilted marble slabs in two rows of six, their genitals obscured for the sake of propriety—their remaining clothes hung above to abet identification. Large curtains would regularly obscure the spectators' view while the decaying array was revised like a museum exhibit or a Macy's window display.

The morgue's popularity led to its listing in almost every guidebook and being featured on Thomas Cook's package tour of the city. At its peak the morgue could command an audience of up to ten thousand visitors a day, powered by a prurient popular press concocting sensationalist narratives around suicide, murder and the mysterious deaths of women and young children (the latter thankfully displayed clothed and propped upright in chairs).

"Les Catacombes de Paris," perhaps sensing this appetite for morbid tourism, swung open its sepulchre door in 1874 to any citizen with the price of admission. Initially established as a resolution to the bulging, oozing *Cimetière des Innocents*—the largest, oldest and overwhelmingly the most malodorous cemetery in old Paris, almost from its inception the catacombs received visits from curious dignitaries.

From 1786, in a process lasting fifteen months, the exhumed and rendered bones of *des Innocents'* deceased were transported by night in priestly procession to the aptly-named *Place D'Enfer* (Later punningly renamed after Franco-Prussian War hero Pierre Denfert-Rochereau), and dropped down chutes and

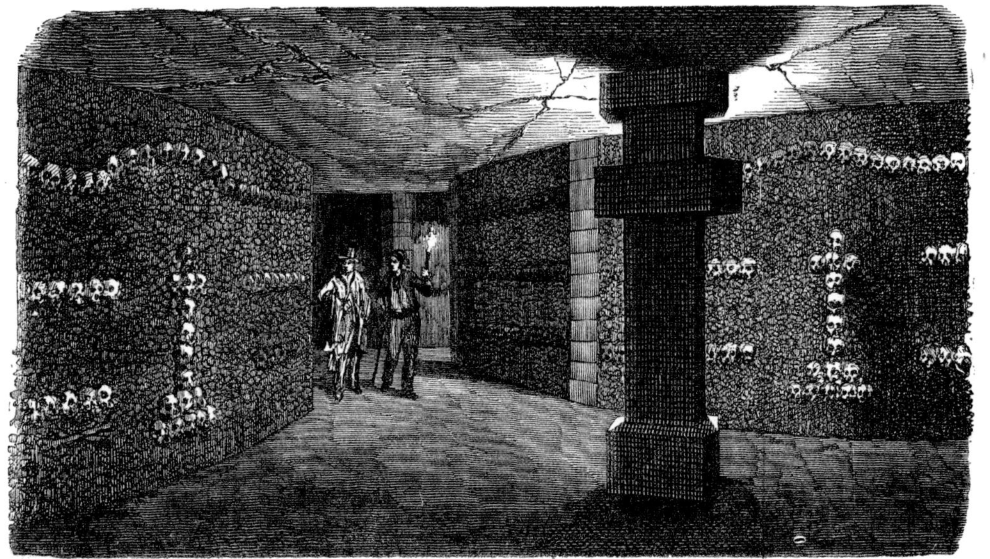

stored away by workers below. The contents of Paris' remaining cemeteries followed until eventually the remains of an estimated six million people were contained within the ossuary.

The Paris Catacombs. Courtesy of the author.

Magic & Méliès

Midnight: you brood in your room, alone. You silently tiptoe to your window to peer into the dark to see only your double glaring back; standing as equidistant to the window as yourself. It is merely a mirage, your illuminated reflection—but is also the basis for the illusion known as "Pepper's Ghost."

London had long held a conversation with Paris over the subject of stage magic. In the earlier part of the nineteenth century, both Philidor and Robertson had introduced their Phantasmagoria shows to the London stage—the former with the young Madame Tussaud and her waxworks in tow. Then, in the 1840s, Jean Eugène Robert-Houdin had created in Paris a new, sophisticated form of stage prestidigitation—far from the primitive fairground conjurers that had preceded him—and this new form of legerdemain found its natural successor in the form of England's John Nevil Maskelyne and George Alfred Cooke. Maskelyne and Cooke were initially inspired toward a conjuring career after viewing a séance performed by spurious Spiritualists the Davenport Brothers in the 1860s. Maskelyne's insight into the Brothers' deceit drove the duo to create a show exposing the Davenport's duplicity. In 1873, Maskelyne and Cooke began a thirty-year tenancy at the Egyptian Hall on Piccadilly (a former exhibition hall built in the mock-Pharaonic style that proved so popular following Napoleon's conquest of Egypt in the late eighteenth century), transforming it into "England's Home of Mystery" and creating many of the illusions common to most modern magician's repertoire, most notably "the levitation."

The London of 1884 witnessed a new arrival from Paris; Georges Méliès, a 23 year-old youth sent at his parents' bidding to work at a Piccadilly gent's outfitters—to improve his anglophone skills and possibly add an additional branch to his father's successful boot-making empire. Méliès became obsessed with the nearby Maskelyne's show and discovered a pursuit more diverting than shoe soles and saddle stitching.

A short walk away from Piccadilly, at the north end of Regent's Street, the Royal Polytechnic was established in 1838 as much as a permanent "World's Fair"-type science exhibit as a seat of learning. Displays of all the latest inventions and scientific innovations were exhibited at the hall; the Royal seal of approval was received in 1840 after Queen Victoria's consort Prince Albert's delighted descent within the working diving bell display.

1848 saw the addition of a theater to the exhibition hall—perfect for magic lantern projections and microscopic slide images enlarged to fill the 425-square foot screen. That same year, chemist John Henry Pepper delivered his first lecture to the Polytechnic. A highly skilled orator and showman, by 1854 "Professor Pepper" was director of the Polytechnic, introducing a succession of crowd-pleasing diversions. Ten years later saw the introduction of Liverpudlian engineer Henry Dircks' *"Dircksian Phantasmagoria,"* a device for projecting ghost illusions onto a pane of onstage glass, invisible to the theater audience. Pepper modified the device to render it simpler and more cost effective, and though he tried in vain to share the credit, the device nonetheless became known as Pepper's Ghost.

Returning to Paris in 1885, Méliès sold his share of his father's business and in 1888 bought the now-derelict Théâtre Robert-Houdin and attempted to replicate, with fewer resources, the narrative illusion shows of Maskelyne's theater. In 1895, Méliès was one of only thirty-three people to witness the premiere of *La Sortie des usines Lumière à Lyon* ("Workers Leaving the Lumière Factory in Lyon"), the Lumière Brothers' first film performance and the event that ushered in the era of the motion picture. Méliès realised in an instant that this new technology would provide a fine addition to his theater show.

Historically, the earliest films were simple examples of "cinéma vérité"—naturalistic scenes of everyday life—but due to a chance camera malfunction while shooting a street scene sequence, Méliès discovered to his delight that movies could also be magic tricks, first putting this new technique into practice in *Escamotage d'une dame au théâtre Robert Houdin* ("The Vanishing Lady"). With his devilish goatee, Méliès delighted in presenting himself in the Mephistophelean role in the many short films he produced on an infernal theme; conjuring up the first-ever satanic imagery on celluloid with his 1896 short, *Le Manoir du Diable* ("The Haunted Castle")—frequently cited as the first ever vampire/horror film.

Art and Montmarte

Let us pause a moment to reflect again on my tortured youth.

Each dreary school-day morning as I stumbled bleary eyed from my pit of slumber, I would draw aside my bedroom curtains and gaze across the bay towards Southport's seaside neighbor and rival: Blackpool. Dominating the skyline, clearly visible through the grey haze of a Northern English morning was Blackpool Tower, a half-scale replica of Gustave Eiffel's vastly more celebrated 1,050 foot tall tower built for Paris' Exposition Universelle of 1889. Held in celebration of the hundredth anniversary of the storming of the Bastille, the Exposition Universelle of 1889 was the third such Parisian World's Fair since Napoleon III's 1855 response to London's Great Exhibition of 1851. A global sensation, the Exposition attracted thirty-two million visitors—over five times as many attendees as the London event.

And with these tourists came tourist money, eager to be spent on the outrageous diversions and in pursuit of the scandalous *demimondaine* lifestyle on which Paris had now built a somewhat notorious reputation. No area of Paris was more notorious than Montmartre. One of the first establishments in Montmartre to exploit the huge influx of disposable tourist income was the more-than-a-little-bit-famous Moulin Rouge cabaret, opened in the autumn of 1889. Located on the Moulin Rouge's *Jardin de Paris* back patio was one of the Exposition Universelle's less well-remembered attractions—an enormous stucco elephant, modeled after Napoleon Bonaparte's ill-fated, 78-foot plaster Place de la Bastille monument erected in 1813. A spiral staircase contained within this particular Parisian pachyderm's leg led to an opium den where any gentlemen with a franc free were entertained by undulating belly dancers.

Though by far the most famous, the Moulin Rouge was by no means the first or only cabaret in Montmartre. "Les

Hydropathes" was a rather rambunctious literary and drinking club (so named for their aversion to water passing their lips), founded by poet and novelist Émile Goudeau in 1878 in Paris' Latin Quarter. In 1881, outgrowing their *Rive Gauche* location, Goudeau led these literary libertines in a mock-solemn torchlit procession across the Seine to friend and artist Rodolphe Salis' newly acquired tavern, Le Chat Noir, in Montmartre. Switching locations a number of times, Le Chat Noir became famed for its shadow theater and baroque interior.

Writers, artists and composers were eager to engage in cabaret's new style of anarchic entertainment. F*in de siècle* Montmatre's art scene was significant for the prevalence of Symbolists within its ranks; Verlaine and Mallarmé were regulars at Le Chat Noir, Debussy performed there, and Satie was the house pianist. Like its late eighteenth-century forebear Romanticism (and its literary offshoot, the gothic novel)—a movement inspired by dramatic passions, occult practices, nightmares, dreams and the unconscious—Symbolism arose in reaction to Enlightenment ideals and the rationality of the Industrial Revolution. But while Romanticism held in awe the natural world—from the tundra-like wastes of Shelley's *Frankenstein* to Caspar David Friedrich's blasted landscapes—in contrast the Symbolists worshipped artifice and decadence. A revived interest in Roman Catholicism's more cultish, unorthodox aspects was also experienced amongst French intellectuals of this period. An occult underground had prospered in Paris since at least the Black Masses held in the court of Louis XIV; Cardinal Richelieu was also said to have privately engaged in such practices. But it was within the Symbolist movement that the popularizing of occult ritual really took root.

Decadent author J. K. Huysmans' 1891 roman-à-clef *Là-Bas* describes his own investigations into Paris' esoteric underworld.

Included among the pseudonymous proxies within *Là-Bas* were thinly veiled versions of the feuding defrocked priest Joseph-Antoine Boullan and Rosicrucian mystic Stanislas de Guiata. The following year de Guita's Rosicrucian companion Joséphin Péladan—an associate of Gustav Moreau, Stravinsky, Claude Debussy, Fèlicien Rops, Georges Rouault and Erik Satie—established the *Salon de la Rose + Croix,* a series of six hugely popular annual art and music salons hosted to promote the works of Symbolist painters, writers and composers. Charles Baudelaire's hugely popular translations of the fevered nightmare and deductive crime writings of Edgar Allan Poe, an outsider writer in his homeland, also inspired a whole generation of Symbolist poets; translations by Stéphane Mallarmé and Paul Valéry would follow.

Death is a Cabaret, Old Chum

In 1885 Georges Méliès debuted as professional magician on stage at the Cabinet Fantastique—part of the Musée Grevin waxworks. The Grevin was curated as a form of 3D living newspaper, with regularly updated displays of the most sensationalist current events of the day—murders, kidnappings, suicides—presented in waxen dioramas. Some of the earliest experiments in pre-Lumière Brothers' cinema and earliest X-ray demonstrations also occurred there.

It was while performing at Musée Grevin that Méliès would meet another young magician, a man who would create illusions for and be featured in Méliès' short movies—a man known only by the name "Dorville." The only surviving image I can locate of Dorville derives from the theater poster collection of the late magic enthusiast and authority Christian Fechner, a film producer and the former teen-pop Svengali behind beat group *Antoine et les Problems.* The color lithograph reveals a lean, dapper gent—dark, glossy haired and wax moustachioed in black evening attire, the magician's uniform created by Robert-Houdin to blend in with the attire of his evening-dressed audience.

Cabarets had spread like a fungal infection all over Montmartre since the success of Le Chat Noir. Dorville would distill the dark spirit of his age in the creation of three cabarets—Néant, L'Enfer and Ciel—but Dorville's cabarets would have a singular twist—magic.

Dorville's first cabaret opened its doors in Brussels in 1892, but would soon move to the Boulevard Rochechouart in Paris, changing its name from *Cabaret du Mort* ("Cabaret of Death") to *Cabaret du Néant* ("Cabaret of Nothingness") following the death of a resident of the quartier.

On the exterior wall of 34 Boulevard de Clichy, Néant's new home, yellow lamps cast sallow, pallid light upon the cabaret's patrons, greeted by a doorman with the top-hatted, black silhouette of a pallbearer, as were the waiters within.

Those who dared to delve through the dark drapes into the *Salle d'Intoxication* ("Room of Intoxication") were confronted by the sight of coffins laid out as table-tops, a skeletal ceiling fitting known as "Robert Macaire's chandelier" (the legendary criminal bogeyman, immortalized in Daumier's satirical engravings) and walls decorated with skulls, images of grim mortality and trick paintings that transformed into scenes of horror. Drink orders were translated into concoctions named for vile pestilence: "one microbe of Asiatic cholera from the last corpse," "one leg of a lively cancer," and "one sample of our consumption germ." The returning waiter would encourage imbibing with the incantation "Drink, Macchabées! Drink these noxious potions, which contain the vilest and deadliest poisons!" Presently, a guide in hooded vestments escorted

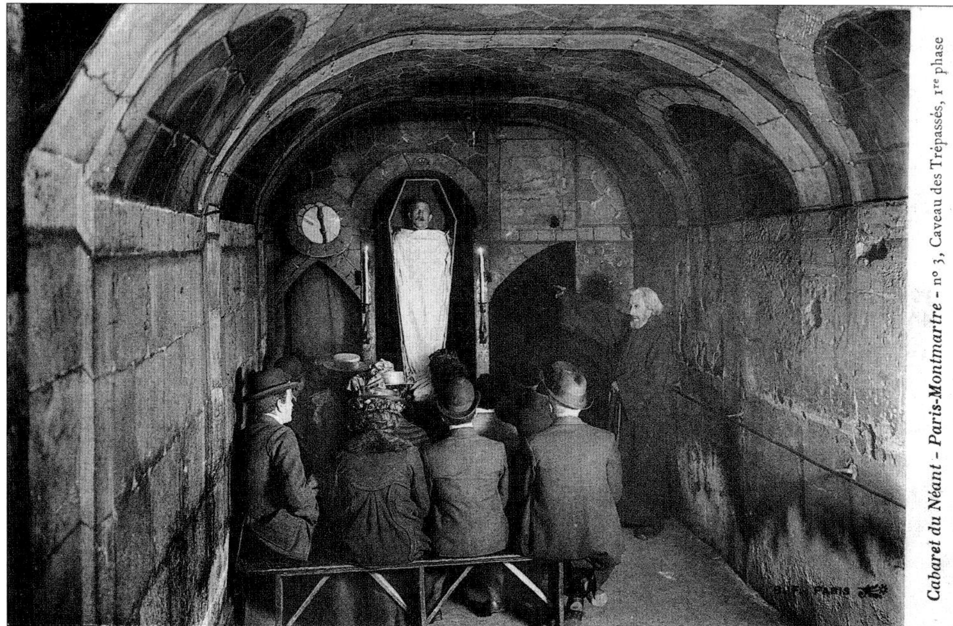

the gathered occupants to a second chamber where his ghoulish presentation would begin. As a harmonium dirged and bell tolled, an audience volunteer, placed within a coffin at the narrow room's far end, was seen to dissolve, his flesh corrupting into osseous form and then later restored to his previous tonicity—all possible due to a concealed Pepper's Ghost illusion.

A swift trip across to 53 Boulevard de Clichy led to *Cabaret du Ciel* ("Cabaret of Heaven") and *Cabaret de L'Enfer* ("Cabaret of Hell") the neighboring nightspots established by Dorville in 1896. Customers entered L'Enfer via the yawning demon's maw that dominated the building's façade. Inside, stucco stalactites and carved renderings of the dancing damned dangled from the low ceiling. Fiery lantern projections gleamed and sulphurous smoke billowed as waiters dressed as horned imps served drinks with customary gusto: "Three seething bumpers of molten sins,

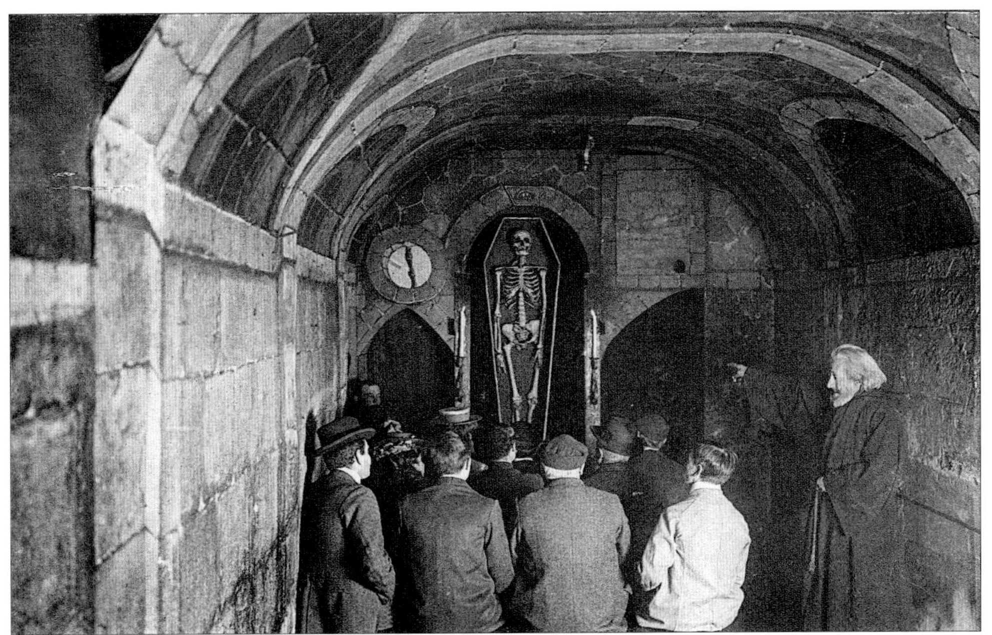

Postcards from Cabaret du Néant. *Both courtesy of the author.*

with a dash of brimstone intensifier!" As a small orchestra of devils played extracts from Faust, the host, decked out in full Mephistophelean goatee and garb, appeared and proceeded to mock the gathered crowd and taunt uncooperative members of the public placed in a facsimile cauldron. Ushered into an adjoining antechamber; the paying guests were treated to a contortion show.

In contrast, the conjoined Ciel offered more saintly fare, but with a typical Montmartre mocking twist, where patrons were invited to sit within a heavenly banquet hall and sip their liquor from a golden chalice. Saint Peter (complete with supersized celestial key), lantern-projected through fleecy clouds, gave blessings to the assembled audience while his disciple Onésime sprinkled sinners with holy water via toilet brush and chamber pot. The congregation was then encouraged to bow down in idolatrous fashion before a large golden pig cast in effigy; while

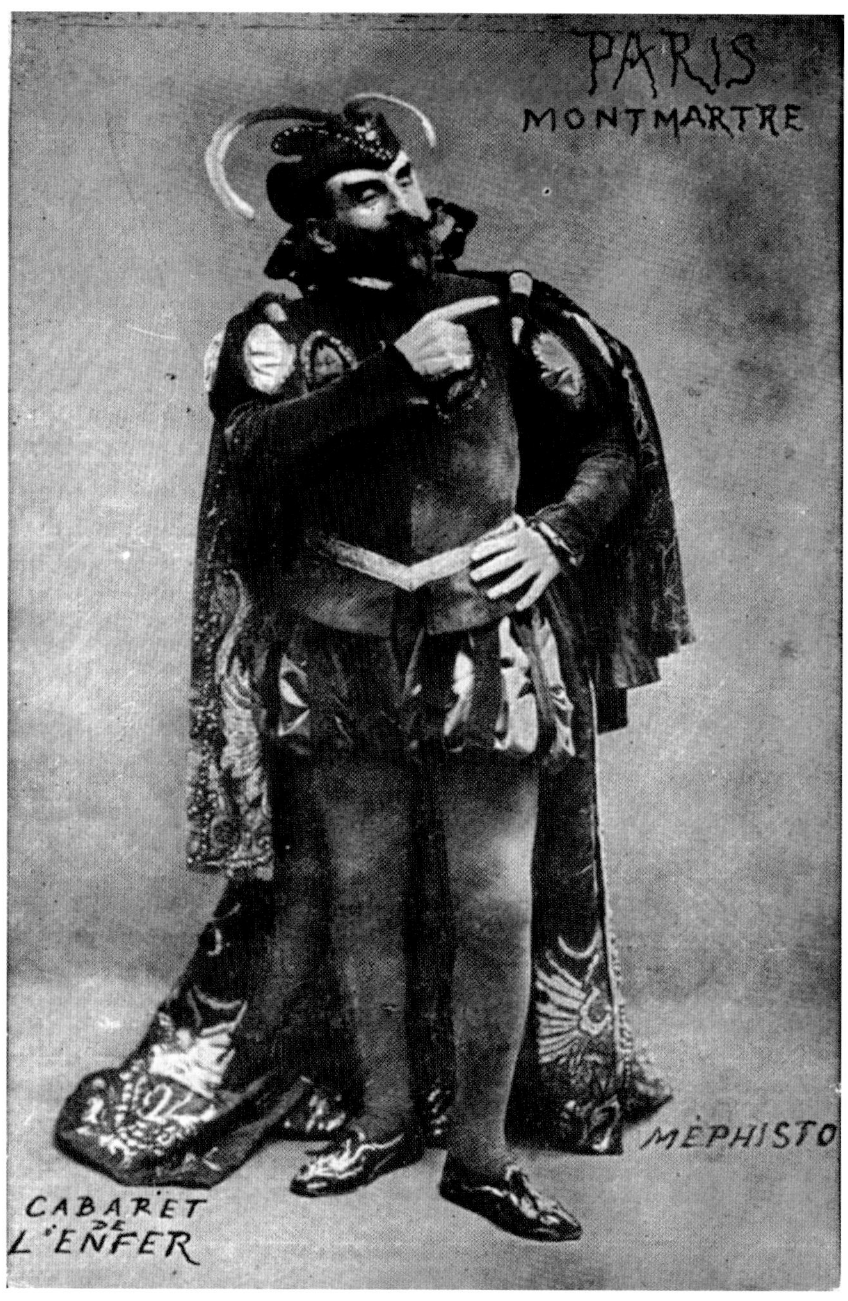
PARIS
MONTMARTRE
MÉPHISTO
CABARET
DE
L'ENFER

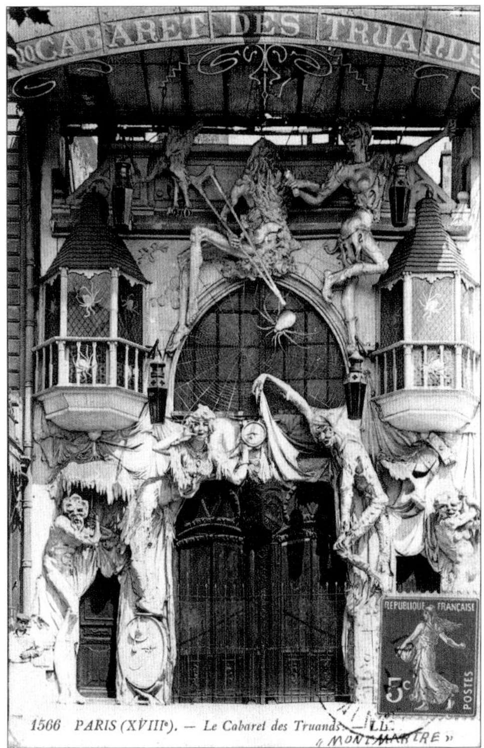

admittance to the Angel room provided a grand finale where scantily clad female cherubim frolicked and teased their spectators.

The baroque aesthetic and tone of Dorville's cabarets inspired at least two Montmartre imitators in *Cabaret des Truands* ("Cabaret of Hoodlums") and *Cabaret des Métèques* ("Cabaret of 'Wogs'"), dens of iniquity both by all accounts. The troika of taverns' notoriety seeped beyond Montmartre's environs as their Stygian exploits were regularly recounted within the pages of the British and American press.

Flushed with success and international attention, Dorville had grand plans for franchising his phantasmal formula, long before the days of the Hard Rock Café or Planet Hollywood.

Image above: Postcard from Cabaret des Truands. *Image left: Postcard from* Cabaret de L'Enfer. *Both courtesy of the author.*

In 1896, a *Cabaret du Néant* concession opened at New York's Casino Chambers on Broadway and 39th Street, and a *Cabaret de la Mort* existed in the early 1900s at the San Francisco Chutes Amusement Park, before transferring to the Bay Area's Idora Park in 1906.

Like Hard Rock Café or Planet Hollywood, Dorville's cabarets fell victim to their own success and changing tastes. After awhile, only the most guileless of tourist would be seen mocking the dead there. L'Enfer and Ciel were no more by 1955 and Néant—relocated one final time to no. 64—was gone by the early 70s; their original locations put to more mundane purpose: Néant is now a pharmacy, L'Enfer and Ciel a supermarket. The only surviving evidence of their existence are some stray beer mats and menus, a series of souvenir post cards depicting various staged scenes from within the cabaret's interiors or images immortalized via the street photography of Eugène Atget and Robert Doisneau.

Despite their fall into oblivion, the cabarets' legacy and influence lingered with London's La Macabre and Heaven & Hell, contributing to SoHo's 1950s coffee house craze and continuing today in Disney's Haunted Mansion and Phantom Manor rides, NYC's Jekyll & Hyde horror-themed restaurants and its Edinburgh offshoot Frankenstein, and a Steampunk bar dubbed Cabaret du Néant in Paris' Ménilmontant district.

Fin

So, in closing, I return to my childhood recollections and ponder my fascination *avec tout le choses françaises*. Hi-res winter skies cast sharp shadows upon my hometown—the castellated hotels and retirement homes that stand in opposition along those silent, slumbering streets, like pieces in some long abandoned titanic chess game. And I recall the many times, each wretched school-day morning, I viewed La Tour Eiffel upon awakening, and remember my many blackboard-bound journeys along the Avenue des Champs-Élysées, and it would seem my fate was so very securely sealed.

[SELECTED BIBLIOGRAPHY]

During, Simon. Modern *Enchantments: The Cultural Power of Secular Magic.* Cambridge, Mass: Harvard University Press, 2004.

Evans, Henry Ridgely, and Adrian Plate. *The Old and the New Magic.* Chicago: Open Court Publishing Co, 1906.

Heard, Mervyn. *Phantasmagoria: The Secret Life of the Magic Lantern : a Full-Blooded Account of an Extraordinary Theatrical Ghost-Raising Entertainment of the Early Nineteenth-Century and the True Exploits of Its Mysterious Inventor, Paul De Philipsthal, in Britain and Abroad.* Hastings: Projection Box, 2006.

Hopkins, Albert A. *Magic; Stage Illusions and Scientific Diversions, Including Trick Photography.* New York: B. Blom, 1967.

Kaba, Mitch. "Les Diableries: 3D Visions of Hell from the 19th Century," Cine-Graphics: 3D & Motion Picture Media, 2011.

Koudounaris, Paul. *The Empire of Death: A Cultural History of Ossuaries and Charnel Houses.* New York, New York: Thames & Hudson, 2011.

Morrow, W. C., and Edouard Cucuel. *Bohemian Paris of to-Day.* London: Chatto & Windus, 1899.

Schwartz, Vanessa R. *Spectacular Realities: Early Mass Culture in Fin-De-Siècle Paris*. Berkeley [u.a.]: Univ. of California Press, 1998.

Schreck, Nikolas. *The Satanic Screen: An Illustrated Guide to the Devil in Cinema*. [London]: Creation, 2001.

Steinmeyer, Jim. *Hiding the Elephant: How Magicians Invented the Impossible and Learned to Disappear.* New York: Carroll & Graf Publishers, 2003.

Williams, Heather. *Mallarmé's Ideas in Language.* Oxford: P. Lang, 2004.

CONTRIBUTOR BIOGRAPHIES

CHIARA AMBROSIO is a filmmaker working with animation, experimental film, documentary and sound to explore the ways in which we perceive, remember, articulate and preserve personal and collective histories and place through the filter of memory and the imagination. Her most recent works include " A Walk Through Woods," a film-cycle developed and filmed on location in North Cornwall, and "La Frequenza Fantasma (The Ghost Frequency)", a feature-length documentary film-poem developed as part of a Fellowship in the Visual Anthropology department of Goldsmith University and filmed in a village in the South of Italy. Her first animation was produced and scored by British composer Michael Nyman, and her subsequent work has included collaborations with performance artists, musicians and writers, and has been shown in a number of venues including national and international film festivals, galleries and site-specific events. Chiara is also the founder and curator of The Light & Shadow Salon, a monthly film salon at The Horse Hospital in Bloomsbury. More information can be found at: www.acuriousroom.com.

STEPHEN T. ASMA is Professor of Philosophy at Columbia College Chicago, where he is a Fellow of the "Research Group in Mind, Science and Culture." Asma is the author of seven books, including *On Monsters: an Unnatural History of Our Worst Fears* (Oxford), and *Stuffed Animals and Pickled Heads: The Culture and Evolution of Natural History Museums* (Oxford). Professor Asma has written articles for the *New York Times*, the *Sunday Times*, the *Chronicle of Higher Education*, the *Chicago Tribune*, *Aeon Magazine*, *Skeptic*, and many others. In 2003, he was Visiting Professor at the Buddhist Institute in Phnom Penh, Kingdom of Cambodia, and in 2007 he lived and studied in Shanghai, China. In 2013 Asma won a Fulbright Award to teach in Beijing.

ZOE BELOFF is an artist and professor at Queens College CUNY. She works with a wide range of media including film, projection performance, installation and drawing. Each project aims to connect the present to past so that it might illuminate the future in new ways. Her projects have presented internationally at venues that include the Whitney Museum of American Art, Site Santa Fe, and the Pompidou Center in Paris. She has been awarded fellowships from Guggenheim Foundation, The Foundation for Contemporary Arts, The Radcliffe Institute at Harvard and the New York Foundation for the Arts. Her publications include T*he Coney Island Amateur Psychoanalytic Society* and its Circle and *The Somnambulists: A Compendium of Source Material.*

ELIZABETH L. BRADLEY is a Brooklyn-based historian whose interests include the human archaeology of New York City as well as the intersections of literature, science, and American popular culture. Her books include *Knickerbocker: The Myth Behind New York* (Rutgers University Press, 2009) and *New York* (forthcoming from Reaktion Books). Dr. Bradley is also the editor of the Penguin Classics edition of Washington Irving's *A History of New York*. She has contributed articles on New York's singular features to numerous anthologies, as well as to publications such as *Edible Brooklyn*, *Bookforum*, and the *New York Times*. She is currently at work on a history of the eugenics movement in New York.

SIMON CHAPLIN is a London-based curator-turned librarian with an interest in the history of anatomy and medical museums. Since 2010 he's been head of the Wellcome Library, the free library for the incurably curious. Before joining the library he worked at the Royal College of Surgeons of England where he was responsible for the Hunterian Museum, based on the anatomy and pathology collections of the eighteenth-century surgeon John Hunter, and at the Science Museum in London.

MARK DERY is a cultural critic. He has been a professor of journalism at NYU, a Chancellor's Distinguished Fellow at UC Irvine, a Hertog author in Columbia University's Hertog Fellowship program, and a Visiting Scholar at the American Academy in Rome. His books include *The Pyrotechnic Insanitarium: American Culture on the Brink* and *Escape Velocity: Cyberculture at the End of the Century*. His latest book is the essay collection *I Must Not Think Bad Thoughts: Drive-by Essays on American Dread, American Dreams*. Dery is at work on a biography of the author, illustrator, and legendary eccentric Edward Gorey for Little, Brown.

COLIN DICKEY is the author of *Afterlives of the Saints: Stories from the Ends of Faith,* and *Cranioklepty: Grave Robbing and the Search for Genius.* He is also the co-editor (with Nicole Antebi and Robby Herbst) of *Failure! Experiments in Social and Aesthetic Practices,* and is a regular contributor to *Lapham's Quarterly* and the *LA Review of Books.* He is the former managing director of the Morbid Anatomy Museum.

CAITLIN DOUGHTY is a mortician and writer living in Los Angeles. She is the host of the "Ask a Mortician" web series and the founder of The Order of the Good Death, a group of artists, academics, and funeral professionals dedicated to changing how we look at death. Caitlin's academic passion is the late Middle Ages, having majored in Medieval History at the University of Chicago before entering the death industry.

JOANNA EBENSTEIN is a New York based artist, curator and independent scholar. She is the creative director of the Morbid Anatomy Museum in Brooklyn, and founder of the Morbid Anatomy Blog and Library. She is co-author (and featured photographer) of *Walter Potter's Curious World of Taxidermy, with Dr. Pat Morris* and acted as curatorial consultant on the Wellcome Collection's "Exquisite Bodies" exhibition (2009). Her photography and writing have been exhibited and published internationally, and she lectures regularly around the world.

RICHARD FAULK is the author of the seminal grossological text *Gross America: Your Coast-to-Coast Guide to All Things Gross* and the upcoming companion volume, *An Awful Almanac.* His writing on natural prodigies, medical oddities, music, and popular culture has appeared on *CNN.com*, *The Huffington Post*, and *The Faster Times*, and in *Penthouse, Metro Silicon Valley*, and *Content* magazine. His latest book His latest book is *The Next Big Thing: A History of the Boom-or-Bust Moments That Shaped the Modern World.*

KATE FORDE is Senior Curator of Temporary Exhibitions at Wellcome Collection, London. She has worked on exhibitions examining the mysteries of sleep, the relationship between war and medicine, the history of anatomical waxworks, and the iconography of death. She is particularly interested in the display of fine art within scientific institutions and is currently developing an exhibition about the history of sexology.

MEL GORDON is professor of Theatre Arts at University of California, Berkeley. He is a director and the author of fourteen books on theatre history, acting, and popular culture. His most recent book is *Stanislavsky in America* (London: Routledge, 2010), which *Choice Magazine* awarded its "Outstanding Academic Title of 2010."

RICHARD HARRIS grew up in New York and graduated from Queens College with a degree in Economics and a strong background in art history. He started his career path at an art reproductions business selling copies of old master paintings to businesses. His introduction to antique prints began as he worked for two dealers who bought and sold botanical prints and prints with birds and animals. He has since accumulated over 1500 objects exploring the related themes of death and mortality.

AMY HERZOG is Coordinator of the Film Studies Program at The CUNY Graduate Center, and Associate Professor of Media Studies at Queens College, CUNY. She is the author of *Dreams of Difference, Songs of the Same: The Musical Moment in Film* (Minnesota, 2010). Her current research involves the evolution of peep show arcades in Times Square in the 1960s and 70s.

AMBER MAYKUT is Senior Staff Writer and Editor for the children's educational websites BrainPOP and BrainPOP Jr., creating comics, jokes, science experiments, arts and crafts activities, and assorted content. She was an assistant teacher of the Anthropomorphic Mouse Taxidermy class at Observatory, was featured on the Science Channel's hit TV series *Oddities*, and is a taxidermy collector, hobbyist, and dealer in Brooklyn, New York.

VADIM KOSMOS is a DJ, writer, musician and authority on post-war French popular culture. He is also the manager of the "Last Tuesday Society" curiosity shop and Wunderkammer in deepest, darkest Hackney, London.

PAUL KOUDOUNARIS has a PhD in Art History and specializes in macabre imagery and the cultural reception of death. He is the author of a the historical and photographic study of ossuaries, *The Empire of Death* (Thames and Hudson: 2011), and *Heavenly Bodies* (Thames and Hudson: 2013), a history of jeweled skeletons from the Roman Catacombs and Memento Mori (Thames and Hudson: 2015), a global exploration of sacred sites where the dead are preserved.

ROSS MACFARLANE is Research Engagement Officer in the Wellcome Library, where he is heavily involved in promoting the Library's collections. He has researched, lectured and written on such topics as the history of early recorded sound, freak shows and notions of urban folklore in Edwardian London. He has led guided walks around London on the occult past of Bloomsbury and on the intersection of medicine, science and trade in Greenwich and Deptford. As an archivist, he has worked at a number of London institutions including King's College, Tate Britain, the Royal Society and the Reform Club. Whilst doing so he has handled a mermaid, discovered a lost alchemical manuscript written by Isaac Newton and found out almost too much about Henry Wellcome.

DÁNIEL MARGÓCSY is assistant professor of early modern European history at Hunter College CUNY. He was the 2012-3 Birkelund fellow at the Cullman Center for Scholars and

Writers, the New York Public Library. A historian of science by training, he has published articles on the development of taxonomy, the visual culture of early modern anatomy, and the aesthetics of curiosities. He is co-editor of States of Secrecy, a special issue of the *British Journal for the History of Science* and author of *Commercial Visions: Science, Trade and Visual Culture in the Dutch Golden Age* (University of Chicago Press, 2014).

EVAN MICHELSON is an antiques dealer, lecturer, writer, musician and co-owner of Obscura Antiques and Oddities in New York City. She is also one of the stars of the international hit TV series *Oddities* on the Science Channel. She has been collecting, researching, buying and selling natural history specimens, medical and scientific antiques, objects of mourning, taxidermy, wax ladies and random inexplicable objects for more than two decades. She has spoken on the history of Gothic culture and fashion at FIT and delivered regular lectures at Brooklyn's *Observatory* and the *Coney Island Museum* on a wide array of topics including *The Saddest Object in the World*, the *Culture of Curiosity* and the history of sacred relics. She currently holds the post of Scholar in Residence at Morbid Anatomy Library, and is writing a book on the human corpse as cultural artifact.

DR. PAT MORRIS was Senior Lecturer in Zoology at Royal Holloway, University of London, and retired in 2002. He is well known for his studies on mammal ecology (hedgehogs, water voles, bats, red squirrels) and major research and conservation projects on dormice. He is a past Chairman of the Mammal Society (and holder of its Silver Medal). He was also a nominated, then an elected member of the Council of the National Trust and Chairman of its Nature Conservation

Advisory Panel for 11 years. He is a former Vice President of the London Wildlife Trust and a member of several other Natural History and conservation organizations. He has published over 50 scientific papers, mostly about mammals and also written books on bats, dormice and the natural history of lakes. He acted as consultant to several major publishers as well as the BBC. In his spare time he has pursued a longstanding interest in the history of taxidermy and has published many papers and books on this topic. He is one of the Government's taxidermy inspectors for the purpose of assessing age and authenticity of antique taxidermy in connection with CITES controls, and was appointed as the first Honorary Life member of the Guild of Taxidermists. He is also co-author of the book *Walter Potter and his Curious World of Taxidermy.*

SALVADOR OLGUÍN was born in Monterrey, Mexico. He currently lives in Brooklyn, New York. He finished a Masters degree in Humanities and Social Thought at NYU, where he studied the connection between writing, photography and death. His work includes critical studies on posthumanism and cultural representations of death. Work by Olguín focusing on the role of postmortem photography in contemporary Mexican culture has recently been published in journals and book chapters in New York and Spain. He was the curator of *La Loteria Mexicana*, a 2011 international art exhibit that took place at Observatory, an art and events space in Brooklyn. *La Carabela Portuguesa*, Salvador Olguín's first poetry book, received the Carmen Alardin Poetry Award granted by Mexico's National Council for Culture and the Arts in 2010.

DAVID PESCOVITZ is managing partner and co-editor of Boing Boing and head of the creative studio at Medium, a platform for sharing stories and ideas. He also has written for *Wired, Scientific American, New Scientist, the New York Times,* and many other publications. An earlier version of this essay appeared as a response to the EDGE.org Annual Question of 2007, "What Are you Optimistic About?," and in a book of the same name.

CARL SCHOONOVER is a neuroscientist at Columbia University where he studies instinctual fear behaviors. He is the author of *Portraits of the Mind.*

DANIEL K. SMITH has been involved with books as a collector, binder and now the proprietor of Strike Three Press, for over 30 years. The press was founded with the simple desire to keep the experience of books alive. Strike Three Press won an Award of Excellence from Communication Arts Illustration Annual 53 for their book *Black White and Blues.* Their books are in the permanent collections of Haverford College, Schromberg Center of The New York Public Library, The John and Mable Ringling Museum of Art, UC Santa Cruz McHenry Library, Butler Library at Columbia University and Denver University. By day he is a husband, father of two, grandfather of one and an Art Director at the *Wall Street Journal.*

SHANNON TAGGART is a photographer and independent researcher based in Brooklyn, NY. Her photographs have been exhibited and featured internationally including the publications *Newsweek, New York Times Magazine* and *TIME.* She curates a lecture series about the science and aesthetics of the miraculous. Currently, she is working on a book about Spiritualism and physical mediumship.

RONNI THOMAS is a filmmaker born and raised in Brooklyn, NY. His short films have received critical acclaim worldwide, most notably in the UK and his home town of New York City. He co-produced *Hey is Dee Dee Home* with Lech Kowalski, an art-house documentary about Dee Dee Ramone. In 2006, his short, *Mime and Punishment,* won Best Digital Short at the Raindance Film Festival in London, and his film *The Old Song and Dance* won Best Music Video at NYC's Royal Flush Film Festival. His film *Radio Girl,* which features the music of longtime collaborator Stephen Coates of The Real Tuesday Weld, received Best Short honors at Boston's Underground Film Festival in 2010. In 2011 he created *The Midnight Archive,* a web docuseries that has over 20 episodes, and has been critically acclaimed and honored worldwide. The series takes a cutting edge and passionate look at morbidity, the strange, unusual, and truly unique. In addition to filmmaking, Ronni is a frequent lecturer for Morbid Anatomy on his various perverse interests.

DR. JOHN TROYER is the Deputy Director of the Centre for Death and Society at the University of Bath. His inter-disciplinary research focuses on contemporary memorialization practices, concepts of spatial historiography, and the dead body's relationship with technology. Dr. Troyer is also a theatre director and installation artist with extensive experience in site-specific performance across the United States and Europe. He is a co-founder of the Death Reference Desk website (http://www.deathreferencedesk.org) and a frequent commentator for the BBC. His forthcoming book, *Technologies of the Human Corpse* (published by the University of North Carolina Press), will appear in 2013. His father, Ron Troyer, is a funeral director.

ACKNOWLEDGEMENTS

For five years, the Morbid Anatomy Library in Gowanus, Brooklyn, has hosted dozens of scholars, artists, writers and artisans of the macabre and the spectacular, and we would like to thank all of our presenters who have made Morbid Anatomy what it is today.

This book began its life as a Kickstarter project, could not have been made without the generous support and vision of our Kickstarter backers, who made this project a reality.

Very special thanks are also due to Tracy Hurley Martin as well as Thomas Campbell Jackson, Andrew Davidson, and Jennifer Butkevich for their generous support.

In addition, we are grateful to the institutions, libraries, museums, artists and private collectors who provided images and other resources for this book, specifically: The Wellcome Collection, The Wellcome Library and Wellcome Images; the New York Academy of Medicine; The Gordon Museum, King's College, London; The Mütter Museum of the College of Physicians of Philadelphia; The American Museum of Natural History Library Special Collections; The National Library of Medicine; The Coney Island Museum;

The George Eastman International Museum of Photography and Film; The Hunterian Museum at the Royal College of Surgeons; The Family Coolen Collection; Palazzo Poggi; The Musée Orfila; The Countway Library of Medicine; The Thanatos Archive/Thanatos.net; The Library of Congress; Museo Nacional de la Muerte; The John Hay Library at Brown University; The Boston Athenaeum; University College, London; and the Palermo Catacombs.

Joanna and Colin would also like to thank the following for their invaluable support: Tonya Hurley, Laetitia Barbier, Erica Saunders, Cristina Preda, Mark Dion, Davin Kuntze, Dan Smith, Esther McGowan, Emmet Liston, Mark Pilkington, Stefanie Rookis, Michael Sappol, Sasha Chavchavadze and Tamara Pittman of Proteus Gowanus, Sina Najafi, Ronni Thomas, Charlie Mounter, Eric Huang, Danielle Sommer, MikeJohns, Gemma Angel, Mark Dery, Michelle Legro, Susan Jeiven, Zoe Beloff, Paul Koudounaris, Stephen T. Asma, Viktor Wynd and The Last Tuesday Society, Aaron Beebe, Richard Barnett, Heather Skinner, Jocelyn Marzec, Venita Bryant, Arlene Shaner, William Edwards, Anna Dhoty, Evi Numen, Barbara Mathé, Thomas Baione, Dick Zigun, Katie Karkheck, Sam Alberti, Sarah Pearson, Jack and Beverly Wilgus, Nicole Neenan, Jenn Chittick, Susan Coolen, Patrice Le Floch-Prigent, Alfonso Rodríguez Baeza, Jack Mord, Jeffrey Kraus, Errol Fuller, Pat Morris, Dario Piombino-Mascali, Subhadra Das, Corey Schjoth, Mervyn Heard, Laris Kreslins, Marisa Ortega-Sánchez, Crestina Forcina, Fulvio Simoni, John Whitenight, Fred LaValley, and Meaghan O'Connell.

Special thanks also to JR Pepper and GF Newland for image corrections and Cristina Preda and Amy Slonaker for text edits.

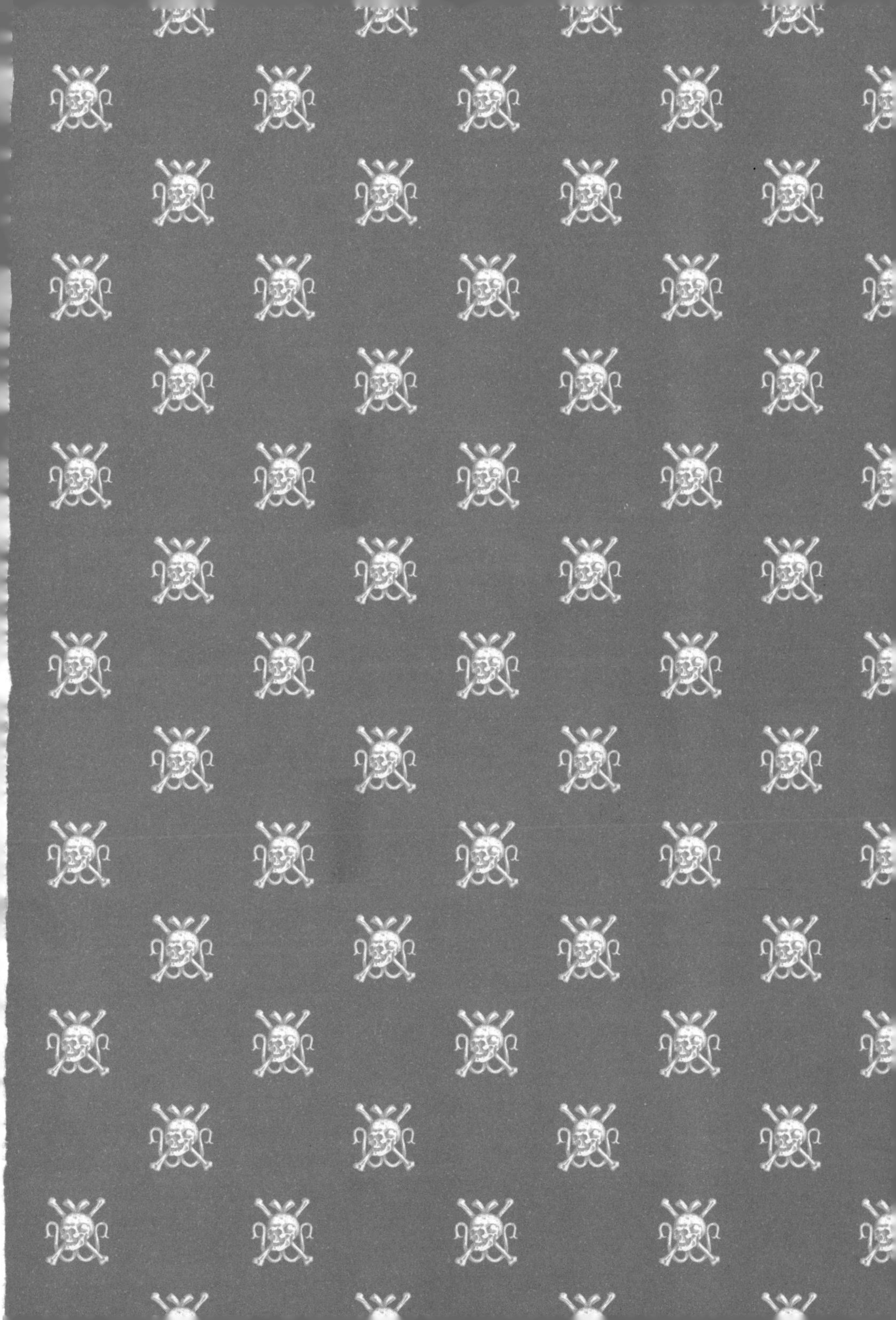